Advanced Life Support

6th Edition January 2011

Reprinted in March 2011 (with corrections)
Reprinted in August 2011 (with corrections)
Reprinted in January 2012 (with corrections)
Reprinted in July 2012 (with corrections)

ISBN – 978-1-903812-22-8

Advanced Life Support
6th Edition January 2011

Editors

Jerry Nolan
Jasmeet Soar
Andrew Lockey
Gavin Perkins
David Pitcher

Carl Gwinnutt
David Gabbott
Mike Scott
Sarah Mitchell

Contributors

Gamal Abbas
Annette Alfonzo
Alessandro Barelli
Joost Bierens
Leo Bossaert
Hermann Brugger
Mat Cordingly
Robin Davies
Charles Deakin
Sarah Dickie
Joel Dunning
Hans Domanovits
James Fullerton
David Gabbott

Marios Georgiou
Carl Gwinnutt
Anthony Handley
Bob Harris
Sara Harris
Jenny Lam
Freddy Lippert
Andrew Lockey
David Lockey
Carsten Lott
Oliver Meyer
Sarah Mitchell
Koen Monsieurs
Jerry Nolan

Peter Paal
John Pawlec
Gavin Perkins
David Pitcher
Rani Robson
Helen Routledge
Maureen Ryan
Claudio Sandroni
Mike Scott
Gary Smith
Jasmeet Soar
Karl-Christian Thies
David Zideman
Elizabeth Norris

Acknowledgements

We thank Mike Scott for his dual talents as photographer and ALS instructor – he has shot and digitally prepared all the photographs in this manual. We also thank the staff of the Guildford Clinic for the use of their facilities, Oliver Meyer for digital preparation of the all the 12-lead ECGs and rhythm strips, Correen Cleggett for help with the final preparation for printing, and the models for their help with the photographs.

Environmental friendly paper has been used. 15% recycled, elemental chlorine free fibre sourced from well managed forests.

Published by Resuscitation Council (UK)
5th Floor, Tavistock House North, Tavistock Square, London WC1H 9HR
Tel: 020 7388 4678   Fax: 020 7383 0773   E-mail: enquiries@resus.org.uk   Website: http://www.resus.org.uk

Printed by: TT Litho Printers Limited
Corporation Street, Rochester, Kent. ME1 1NN
Tel: 01634 845397   Fax: 01634 846807   Email: admin@ttlitho.co.uk   Website: http://www.ttlitho.co.uk

Contents

Glossary

Throughout this publication:
- The masculine pronouns he, him and his are used generically.
- The terms cardiopulmonary arrest, cardiorespiratory arrest and cardiac arrest have been used interchangeably.
- Adrenaline is the preferred term for adrenaline/epinephrine.
- The terms DNAR and DNACPR are both in common use and are interchangeable

A	Amperes
AC	alternating current
ACEI	angiotensin converting enzyme inhibitor
ACS	acute coronary syndrome
AED	automated external defibrillator
AF	atrial fibrillation
ALS	advanced life support
AMI	acute myocardial infarction
AV	atrioventricular as in atrioventricular node
AVNRT	AV nodal re-entry tachyarrhythmia
AVRT	AV re-entry tachyarrhythmia
BLS	basic life support- no equipment is used except protective devices
BP	blood pressure
CABG	coronary artery bypass grafting
CCU	coronary care unit
CK	creatine kinase
CHB	complete heart block
CPR	cardiopulmonary resuscitation - refers to chest compressions and ventilations
CVP	central venous pressure
DC	direct current
DNAR	do not attempt resuscitation
DNACPR	do not attempt cardiopulmonary resuscitation
ECG	electrocardiogram
ED	emergency department
EMS	emergency medical services, e.g. ambulance service
ETCO$_2$	end tidal carbon dioxide
h	hour
HDU	high dependency unit
ICD	implantable cardioverter-defibrillator
ICU	intensive care unit
IM	intramuscular
IO	intraosseous
IV	intravenous
JVP	jugular venous pressure
LBBB	left bundle branch block
LMA	laryngeal mask airway
LT	laryngeal tube
LV	left ventricular
MET	medical emergency team
MILS	manual in-line stabilisation
NSTEMI	non-ST-elevation myocardial infarction
PCI	percutaneous coronary intervention
PEA	pulseless electrical activity
PLMA	ProSeal laryngeal mask airway
ROSC	return of spontaneous circulation
RV	right ventricular
s	second
SA	sino-atrial as in sino-atrial node
SBP	systolic blood pressure
STEMI	ST-elevation myocardial infarction
SVT	supraventricular tachycardia
TDP	torsade de pointes
VF	ventricular fibrillation
VT	ventricular tachycardia
VF/VT	VF/pulseless VT
WPW	Wolff-Parkinson-White syndrome

Advanced Life Support in Perspective

CHAPTER 1

The problem

Ischaemic heart disease is the leading cause of death in the world. In Europe, cardiovascular disease accounts for around 40% of all deaths under the age of 75 years. Sudden cardiac arrest is responsible for more than 60% of adult deaths from coronary heart disease. Summary data from 37 communities in Europe indicate that the annual incidence of emergency medical system (EMS)-treated out-of-hospital cardiopulmonary arrests (OHCAs) for all rhythms is 38 per 100,000 population. Based on these data, the annual incidence of EMS-treated ventricular fibrillation (VF) arrest is 17 per 100,000 and survival to hospital discharge is 10.7% for cardiac arrest from all rhythms and 21.2% for VF cardiac arrest. Recent data from 10 North American sites are remarkably consistent with these figures: median rate of survival to hospital discharge was 8.4% after EMS-treated cardiac arrest from any rhythm and 22.0% after VF. There is some evidence that long-term survival rates after cardiac arrest are increasing. On initial heart rhythm analysis, about 28 - 35% of OHCA victims have VF, a percentage that has declined over the last 20 years. It is likely that many more victims have VF or rapid ventricular tachycardia (VT) at the time of collapse but, by the time the first electrocardiogram (ECG) is recorded by EMS personnel, the rhythm has deteriorated to asystole. When the rhythm is recorded soon after collapse, the proportion of patients in VF is about 60%.

One third of all people developing a myocardial infarction die before reaching hospital; most of them die within an hour of the onset of acute symptoms. In most of these deaths the presenting rhythm is VF or pulseless ventricular tachycardia (VF/VT). The only effective treatment for these arrhythmias is attempted defibrillation and, in the absence of bystander CPR, with each minute's delay the chances of a successful outcome decrease by about 10 - 12%. Once the patient is admitted to hospital the incidence of VF after myocardial infarction is approximately 5%.

The incidence of in-hospital cardiac arrest is difficult to assess because it is influenced heavily by factors such as the criteria for hospital admission and implementation of a do-not-attempt-resuscitation (DNAR) policy. The reported incidence of in-hospital cardiac arrest is in the range of 1 - 5 per 1000 admissions. Preliminary data from the UK National Cardiac Arrest Audit (NCAA) indicate that survival to hospital discharge after in-hospital cardiac arrest is 13.5% (all rhythms). The initial rhythm is VF or pulseless VT in 18% of cases and, of these, 44% survive to leave hospital; after PEA or asystole, 7% survive to hospital discharge. These preliminary NCAA data are based on 3,184 adults (aged ≥ 16 y) in 61 hospitals participating in NCAA (increasing numbers of hospitals during Oct 2009 to Oct 2010) with known presenting/first documented rhythm and complete data for return of spontaneous circulation (ROSC) and survival to hospital discharge. All these individuals received chest compressions and/or defibrillation from the resuscitation team in response to a 2222 call. Many in-hospital cardiac arrests did not fulfil these criteria and were not included. Many patients sustaining an in-hospital cardiac arrest have significant comorbidity, which influences the initial rhythm and, in these cases, strategies to prevent cardiac arrest are particularly important.

The Chain of Survival

The interventions that contribute to a successful outcome after a cardiac arrest can be conceptualised as a chain - the Chain of Survival (Figure 1.1). The chain is only as strong as its weakest link; all four links of the Chain of Survival must be strong. They are:

- Early recognition and call for help

- Early cardiopulmonary resuscitation (CPR)

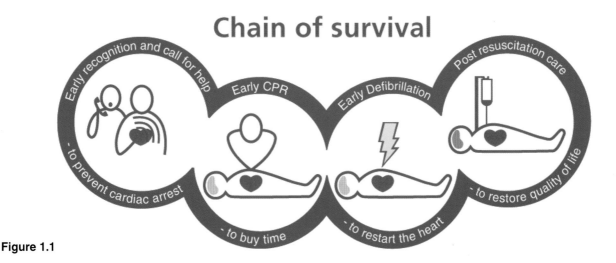

Figure 1.1

- Early defibrillation

- Post-resuscitation care.

Early recognition and call for help

Out of hospital, early recognition of the importance of chest pain will enable the victim or a bystander to call the EMS so that the victim can receive treatment that may prevent cardiac arrest. After out-of-hospital cardiac arrest, immediate access to the EMS is vital. In most countries access to the EMS is achieved by means of a single telephone number (e.g. 999, 112).

In-hospital, early recognition of the critically ill patient who is at risk of cardiac arrest and a call for the resuscitation team or medical emergency team (MET) will enable treatment to prevent cardiac arrest (Chapter 3). A universal number for calling the resuscitation team or MET should be adopted in all hospitals - in the UK this number is 2222. If cardiac arrest occurs, do not delay defibrillation until arrival of the resuscitation team - clinical staff should be trained to use a defibrillator.

Early CPR

Chest compressions and ventilation of the victim's lungs will slow down the rate of deterioration of the brain and heart. After out-of-hospital cardiac arrest, bystander CPR extends the period for successful resuscitation and at least doubles the chance of survival after VF cardiac arrest. Performing chest-compression-only CPR is better than giving no CPR at all. Despite the well-accepted importance of CPR, in most European countries bystander CPR is carried out in only a minority of cases (approximately 30%). After in-hospital cardiac arrest, chest compressions and ventilation must be undertaken immediately, but should not delay attempts to defibrillate those patients in VF/VT. Interruptions to chest compressions must be minimised and should occur only very briefly during defibrillation attempts and rhythm checks.

Early defibrillation

After out-of-hospital cardiac arrest, the goal is to deliver a shock (if indicated) within 5 min of the EMS receiving the call. In many areas, achievement of this goal will require the introduction of Public Access Defibrillation (PAD) programs using automated external defibrillators (AEDs). In hospitals, sufficient healthcare personnel should be trained and authorised to use a defibrillator to enable the first responder to a cardiac arrest to attempt defibrillation when indicated, without delay, in virtually every case.

Post-resuscitation care

Return of a spontaneous circulation (ROSC) is an important phase in the continuum of resuscitation; however, the ultimate goal is to return the patient to a state of normal cerebral function, a stable cardiac rhythm, and normal haemodynamic function, so that they can leave hospital in reasonable health at minimum risk of a further cardiac arrest. The quality of treatment in the post-resuscitation period influences the patient's ultimate outcome. The post-resuscitation phase starts at the location where ROSC is achieved. The ALS provider must be capable of providing high quality post-resuscitation care until the patient is transferred to an appropriate high-care area.

Science and guidelines

The 2010 International Consensus on Cardiopulmonary Resuscitation and Emergency Cardiovascular Care Science with Treatment Recommendations was the culmination of a prolonged period of collaboration between resuscitation experts from around the world. It followed a similar format to the 2005 International Consensus on CPR Science. The European Resuscitation Council (ERC) Guidelines for Resuscitation 2010 are derived from the 2010 consensus document and the contents of this ALS provider manual are consistent with these guidelines. Most resuscitation organisations in Europe have ratified and adopted the ERC guidelines.

ALS algorithm

The ALS algorithm (Figure 1.2) is the centre point of the ALS course and is applicable to most cardiopulmonary resuscitation situations. Some modifications may be required when managing cardiac arrest in special circumstances (Chapter 12).

The ALS course

The ALS course provides a standardised approach to cardiopulmonary resuscitation in adults. The course is targeted at doctors, nurses, and other healthcare professionals who are expected to provide ALS in and out of hospital. The multidisciplinary nature of the course encourages efficient teamwork. By training together, all ALS providers are given the opportunity to gain experience as both resuscitation team members and team leaders. The course comprises workshops, skill stations, cardiac arrest simulation (CAS) training, and lectures. Candidates' knowledge is assessed by means of a multiple choice question paper. Practical skills in airway management and the initial approach to a collapsed patient (including defibrillation where appropriate) are assessed continuously. There is also assessment of a simulated cardiac arrest (CASTest). Candidates reaching the required standard receive an ALS provider certificate. Resuscitation knowledge and skills deteriorate with time and therefore recertification is required for those who have not recently undertaken the course. Recertification provides the opportunity to refresh resuscitation skills and to be updated on resuscitation guidelines, and can be undertaken by attending a provider course or an accredited recertification course. All ALS providers have a responsibility to maintain their skills in resuscitation and to keep up to date with changes in guidelines and practice, and the requirement for recertification should be seen as an absolute minimum frequency of refreshing skills and knowledge.

Adult Advanced Life Support

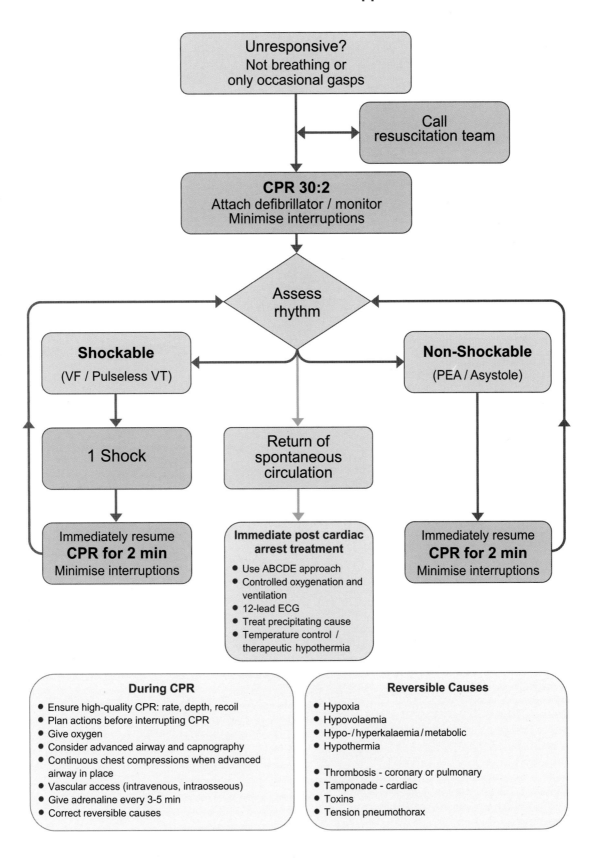

Figure 1.2 Adult Advanced Life Support

Further reading

Atwood C, Eisenberg MS, Herlitz J, Rea TD. Incidence of EMS-treated out-of-hospital cardiac arrest in Europe. Resuscitation 2005;67:75-80.

Berdowski J, Berg RA, Tijssen JG, Koster RW. Global incidences of out-of-hospital cardiac arrest and survival rates: systematic review of 67 prospective studies. Resuscitation 2010;81:1479-87.

Deakin CD, Nolan JP, Soar J, et al. European Resuscitation Council Guidelines for Resuscitation 2010. Section 4. Adult Advanced Life Support. Resuscitation 2010;81:1305-52.

Hollenberg J, Herlitz J, Lindqvist J, et al. Improved survival after out-of-hospital cardiac arrest is associated with an increase in proportion of emergency crew—witnessed cases and bystander cardiopulmonary resuscitation. Circulation 2008;118:389-96.

Iwami T, Nichol G, Hiraide A, et al. Continuous improvements in "chain of survival" increased survival after out-of-hospital cardiac arrests: a large-scale population-based study. Circulation 2009;119:728-34.

Meaney PA, Nadkarni VM, Kern KB, Indik JH, Halperin HR, Berg RA. Rhythms and outcomes of adult in-hospital cardiac arrest. Crit Care Med 2010;38:101-8.

Murray CJ, Lopez AD. Mortality by cause for eight regions of the world: Global Burden of Disease Study. Lancet 1997;349:1269-76.

Nichol G, Thomas E, Callaway CW, et al. Regional variation in out-of-hospital cardiac arrest incidence and outcome. JAMA 2008;300:1423-31.

Nolan JP, Hazinski MF, Billi JE, et al. 2010 International Consensus on Cardiopulmonary Resuscitation and Emergency Cardiovascular Care Science with Treatment Recommendations. Part 1: Executive Summary. Resuscitation 2010;81:e1-e25.

Nolan J, Soar J, Eikeland H. The chain of survival. Resuscitation 2006;71:270-1.

Nolan JP, Soar J, Zideman DA, et al. European Resuscitation Council Guidelines for Resuscitation 2010. Section 1. Executive Summary. Resuscitation 2010;81:1219-76.

Sandroni C, Nolan J, Cavallaro F, Antonelli M. In-hospital cardiac arrest: incidence, prognosis and possible measures to improve survival. Intensive Care Med 2007;33:237-45.

Sans S, Kesteloot H, Kromhout D. The burden of cardiovascular diseases mortality in Europe. Task Force of the European Society of Cardiology on Cardiovascular Mortality and Morbidity Statistics in Europe. Eur Heart J 1997;18:1231-48.

Weisfeldt ML, Sitlani CM, Ornato JP, et al. Survival after application of automatic external defibrillators before arrival of the emergency medical system: evaluation in the resuscitation outcomes consortium population of 21 million. J Am Coll Cardiol 2010;55:1713-20.

Zheng ZJ, Croft JB, Giles WH, Mensah GA. Sudden cardiac death in the United States, 1989 to 1998. Circulation 2001;104:2158-63.

Human Factors and Quality in Resuscitation

Human factors

The skills of chest compressions, defibrillation, intravenous cannulation and rhythm recognition are considered typically to be the most important factors in managing a cardiac arrest. These are all technical skills that are learnt from books, lectures, courses and peers. Although they are important for the successful resuscitation of a patient, there is another group of skills that is becoming increasingly recognised in medicine - human factors or non-technical skills. Non-technical skills can be defined as the cognitive, social and personal resource skills that complement technical skills and contribute to safe and efficient task performance. More simply, they are the things that affect our personal performance.

Deficiencies in the requisite non-technical skills are a common cause of adverse incidents. The introduction and practice of non-technical skills has been one of the key factors in increasing aviation safety - pilots undergo regular, rigorous assessment of their non-technical skills in order to maintain their licence. Until recently little attention had been paid to the importance of non-technical skills in medicine. The pioneers of this aspect of training in medicine were anaesthetists. Analysis of adverse incidents in anaesthesia showed that in up to 80%, failures in non-technical skills such as communication, checking drug doses, planning and team organisation were responsible, rather than equipment failure or lack of knowledge. As a result the Anaesthetic Crisis Resource Management course was developed in America, followed by the Anaesthetists Non-Technical Skills (ANTS) system, pioneered by a team of anaesthetists and psychologists in Scotland (www.abdn.ac.uk/iprc/ants). The principles used to promote good non-technical skills in the ALS course are based on the principles of ANTS:

- Situational awareness

- Decision making

- Team working, including team leadership

- Task management

Situational awareness

This can be described as an individual's awareness of the environment at the moment of an event and the analysis of this to understand how an individual's actions may impact on future events. This becomes particularly important when many events are happening simultaneously, e.g. at a cardiac arrest. High information input with poor situational awareness may lead to poor decision making and serious consequences. At a cardiac arrest, all those participating will have varying degrees of situational awareness. In a well functioning team, all members will have a common understanding of current events, or shared situational awareness. It is important that only the relevant information is shared otherwise there is too much distraction or noise. At a cardiac arrest, important situational awareness factors include:

- consideration of the location of the arrest, which can give clues to the cause;

- obtaining information from staff about the events leading up to the arrest;

- confirmation of the diagnosis;

- determining who is present - including names, roles, and who is leading;

- noting the actions already initiated e.g. chest compressions;

- checking that a monitor has been attached and interpreting what it shows;

- communicating with the team, gathering information;

- implementing any immediate action necessary;

- consideration of the likely impact of interventions;

- determining the immediate needs.

Decision making

This is defined as the cognitive process of choosing a specific course of action from several alternatives. At a cardiac arrest, the many decisions to be made usually fall to the team leader. The leader will assimilate information from the team members and from personal observation and will use this to determine appropriate interventions. Typical decisions made at a cardiac arrest include:

- diagnosis of the cardiac arrest rhythm;

- choice of shock energy to be used for defibrillation;

- likely reversible causes of the cardiac arrest;

- how long to continue resuscitation.

Once a decision has been made, clear unambiguous communication with the team members is essential to ensure that it is implemented.

Team working, including team leadership

This is one of the most important non-technical skills that contribute to successful management of critical situations. A team is a group of individuals working together with a common goal or purpose. In a team, the members usually have complementary skills and, through coordination of effort, work synergistically. Teams work best when everyone knows each other's name, when they are doing something they perceive to be important, and when their role is within their experience and competence. Optimal team function mandates a team leader. There are several characteristics of a good resuscitation team member:

- Competence – has the skills required at a cardiac arrest and performs them to the best of their ability.

- Commitment – strives to achieve the best outcome for the patient.

- Communicates – openly, indicating their findings and actions taken, and be prepared to raise concerns about clinical or safety issues, but also by listening to briefings and instructions from the team leader.

- Supportive – allows others to achieve their best.

- Accountable – for their own and the team's actions.

- Prepared to admit when help is needed.

- Creative – suggests different ways of interpreting the situation.

- Participates in providing feedback.

Team leadership

A team leader provides guidance, direction and instruction to the team members to enable successful completion of their stated objective. They lead by example and integrity. Team leaders need experience not simply seniority. Team leadership can be considered a process; thereby it can become available to everyone with training and not restricted to those with leadership traits. There are several attributes recognisable in good team leaders:

- Knows everyone in the team by name and knows their capability.

- Accepts the leadership role.

- Is able to delegate tasks appropriately.

- Is knowledgeable and has sufficient credibility to influence the team through role modelling and professionalism.

- Stays calm and keeps everyone else focused and controls distractions.

- Is a good communicator – not just good at giving instructions, but also a good listener and decisive in action. Is empathic towards the whole team.

- Is assertive and authoritative when appropriate.

- Shows tolerance towards hesitancy or nervousness in the emergency setting.

- Has good situational awareness; has the ability to constantly monitor the situation, with an up to date overview, listening and deciding on a course of action.

During a cardiac arrest, the role of team leader is not always immediately obvious. The leader should state early on that they are assuming the role of team leader. Specifically, at a cardiac arrest the leader should:

- Follow current resuscitation guidelines or explain a reason for any significant deviation from standard protocols.

- If they are unsure, he or she should consult with the team or call for senior advice and assistance if appropriate.

- Play to the strengths of team members and allow them some autonomy if their skills are adequate.

- Allocate roles and tasks throughout the resuscitation and be specific. This avoids several people or nobody attempting the task!

- Use the two-minute periods of chest compressions to plan tasks and safety aspects of the resuscitation attempt with the team.

- At the end of the resuscitation attempt, thank the team and ensure that staff and relatives are being supported. Complete all documentation and ensure an adequate handover.

Task management

During the resuscitation of a patient, either in a peri-arrest or full cardiac arrest situation, there are numerous tasks to be carried out by the team members, either sequentially or simultaneously. The coordination and control, or management, of these tasks is the responsibility of the team leader (Figure 2.1). They include:

- Planning, where appropriate and briefing the team, prior to the arrival of the patient.

- Being inclusive of team members.

- Being prepared for both the expected and the unexpected.

- Identification of resources required - ensure that equipment is checked and specifics organised and delegated.

- Prioritising actions of the team.

- Watching out for fatigue, stress and distress amongst the team.

- Managing conflict.

- Communicating with relatives.

- Communicating with experts for safe handover both by telephone and in person.

- Debriefing the team.

- Reporting untoward incidents, particularly equipment or system failures (see below).

- Participation in audit.

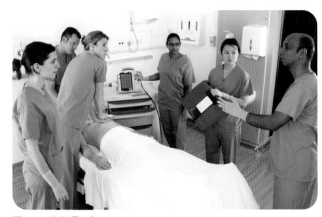

Figure 2.1 Task management

The importance of communication when managing a sick patient

Communication problems are a factor in up to 80% of adverse incidents or near miss reports in hospitals. This failure of communication is also evident when a medical emergency occurs on a ward and a doctor or nurse summons senior help. The call for help is often suboptimal, with failure by the caller to communicate the seriousness of the situation and to convey information in a way that informs the recipient of the urgency of the situation. The poor-quality information heightens the anxiety of the person responding to the call, who is then uncertain of the nature of the problem

they are about to face. A well-structured process that is simple, reliable and dependable, will enable the caller to convey the important facts and urgency, and will help the recipient to plan ahead. It was for similar reasons that the ABCDE approach was developed as an aide memoire of the key technical skills required to manage a cardiac arrest.

The use of the SBAR (Situation, Background, Assessment, Recommendation) or RSVP (Reason, Story, Vital signs, Plan) tool enables effective, timely communication between individuals from different clinical backgrounds and hierarchies (Table 2.1).

Resuscitation teams

The resuscitation team may take the form of a traditional cardiac arrest team, which is called only when cardiac arrest is recognised. Alternatively, hospitals may have strategies to recognise patients at risk of cardiac arrest and to summon a team (e.g. medical emergency team) before cardiac arrest occurs (Chapter 3). The term resuscitation team reflects the range of response teams. As the team may change daily or more frequently, as shift pattern working is introduced, members may not know each other or the skill mix of the team members. The team should therefore meet at the beginning of their period on duty to:

- Introduce themselves; communication is much easier and more effective if people can be referred to by their name.

- Identify everyone's skills and experience.

- Allocate the team leader. Skill and experience takes precedence over seniority.

- Allocate responsibilities; if key skills are lacking, e.g. nobody skilled in tracheal intubation, work out how this deficit can be managed.

- Review any patients who have been identified as 'at risk' during the previous duty period.

Finally, every effort should be made to enable the team members to meet to debrief (Figure 2.2), e.g. difficulties or concerns about their performance, problems or concerns with equipment and submit incident reports. It may also be possible to carry out a formal handover to the incoming team.

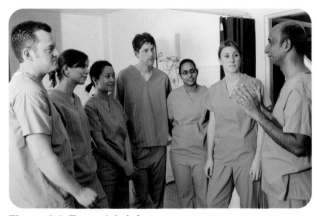

Figure 2.2 Team debrief

SBAR	RSVP	Content	Example
SITUATION	**R**EASON	<ul><li>Introduce yourself and check you are speaking to the correct person</li><li>Identify the patient you are calling about (who and where)</li><li>Say what you think the current problem is, or appears to be</li><li>State what you need advice about</li><li>Useful phrases:<ul><li>- The problem appears to be cardiac/respiratory/neurological/sepsis</li><li>- I'm not sure what the problem is but the patient is deteriorating</li><li>- The patient is unstable, getting worse and I need help</li></ul></li></ul>	<ul><li>Hi, I'm Dr Smith the medical F2</li><li>I am calling about Mr Brown on acute medical admissions who I think has a severe pneumonia and is septic</li><li>He has an oxygen saturation of 90% despite high-flow oxygen and I am very worried about him</li></ul>
BACKGROUND	**S**TORY	<ul><li>Background information about the patient</li><li>Reason for admission</li><li>Relevant past medical history</li></ul>	<ul><li>He is 55 and previously fit and well</li><li>He has had fever and a cough for 2 days</li><li>He arrived 15 minutes ago by ambulance</li></ul>
ASSESSMENT	**V**ITAL SIGNS	<ul><li>Include specific observations and vital sign values based on ABCDE approach</li><li>Airway</li><li>Breathing</li><li>Circulation</li><li>Disability</li><li>Exposure</li><li>The early warning score is…</li></ul>	<ul><li>He looks very unwell and is tiring</li><li>Airway - he can say a few words</li><li>Breathing - his respiratory rate is 24, he has bronchial breathing on the left side. His oxygen saturation is 90% on high - flow oxygen. I am getting a blood gas and chest X-ray</li><li>Circulation - his pulse is 110, his blood pressure is 110/60</li><li>Disability - he is drowsy but can talk a few words</li><li>Exposure - he has no rashes</li></ul>
RECOMMENDATION	**P**LAN	<ul><li>State explicitly what you want the person you are calling to do</li><li>What by when?</li><li>Useful phrases:<ul><li>- I am going to start the following treatment; is there anything else you can suggest?</li><li>- I am going to do the following investigations; is there anything else you can suggest?</li><li>- If they do not improve; when would you like to be called?</li><li>- I don't think I can do any more; I would like you to see the patient urgently</li></ul></li></ul>	<ul><li>I am getting antibiotics ready and he is on IV fluids</li><li>I need help - please can you come and see him straight away</li></ul>

Table 2.1 SBAR and RSVP communication tools

High quality care

The Institute of Medicine defines that quality care is safe, effective, patient-centred, timely, efficient and equitable. Hospitals, resuscitation teams and ALS providers should ensure they deliver these aspects of quality to improve the care of the deteriorating patient and patients in cardiac arrest. Two aspects of this are safety incident reporting (also called adverse or critical incident reporting) and collecting good quality data.

Safety incident reporting

In England and Wales, hospitals can report patient safety incidents to the National Patient Safety Agency (NPSA) National Reporting and Learning System (NRLS) (http://www.nrls.npsa.nhs.uk/report-a-patient-safety-incident/). A patient safety incident is defined as 'any unintended or unexpected incident that could have harmed or did lead to harm for one or more patients being cared for by the National Health Service (NHS)'. Previous reviews of this database have identified patient safety incidents associated with airway devices in critical care units and led to recommendations to improve safety. A review of NPSA safety incidents relating to cardiac arrest and patient deterioration by the Resuscitation Council (UK) shows that the commonest reported incidents are associated with equipment problems, communication, delays in the resuscitation team attending, and failure to escalate treatment.

Audit and outcome after cardiac arrest

Measurement of processes and outcomes provides information about whether interventions and changes made to resuscitation guidelines improve patient care. Published survival rates from in-hospital cardiac arrest vary substantially and range from 13 - 59% at 24 h and 3 - 27% to discharge, with a median survival to discharge of about 15%. There are probably two main reasons for such variation: firstly, there are many confounders that influence outcome following cardiac arrest. These include:

- differences in the type of EMS system (e.g. availability of defibrillators, differences in response intervals);

- differences in the incidence of bystander CPR;

- different patient populations (e.g. a study may be confined to in-hospital cardiac arrests or may include pre-hospital arrests);

- the prevalence of co-morbid conditions;

- the frequency of implementing do-not-attempt-resuscitation (DNAR) policies;

- the primary arrest rhythm;

- the definition of cardiac arrest (e.g. inclusion of primary respiratory arrests);

- availability of cardiac arrest and medical emergency teams.

Secondly, there is lack of uniformity in reporting both the process and results of resuscitation attempts; for example, the definition of survival is reported variously as return of spontaneous circulation, or survival at 5 min, 1 h, 24 h, or to discharge from hospital. The lack of uniformity in cardiac arrest reporting makes it difficult to evaluate the impact on survival of individual factors, such as new drugs or techniques.

New interventions that improve survival rate only slightly are important because of the many victims of cardiac arrest each year. Local hospitals or healthcare systems are unlikely to have sufficient patients to identify these effects or eliminate confounders. One way around this dilemma is by adopting uniform definitions and collecting standardised data on both the process and outcome of resuscitation on many patients in multiple centres. Changes in the resuscitation process can then be introduced and evaluated using a reliable measure of outcome. This methodology enables drugs and techniques developed in experimental studies to be evaluated reliably in the clinical setting.

In the UK, the National Cardiac Arrest Audit (NCAA) is an ongoing, national, comparative outcome audit of in-hospital cardiac arrests. It is a joint initiative between the Resuscitation Council (UK) and the Intensive Care National Audit & Research Centre (ICNARC) and is open to all acute hospitals in the UK and Ireland. The audit monitors and reports on the incidence of, and outcome from, in-hospital cardiac arrest in order to inform practice and policy. It aims to identify and foster improvements in the prevention, care delivery and outcomes from cardiac arrest. The initial scope of data collection is patients who meet all of the following criteria:

- Adults or children over 28 days of age

- Receive chest compressions and/or defibrillation

- Attended by the hospital-based resuscitation team (or equivalent) in response to a 2222 call.

Data are collected according to standardised definitions and entered onto the NCAA secure web-based system. Once data are validated, hospitals are provided with activity reports and comparative reports, allowing a comparison of to be made not only within, but also between, hospitals locally, nationally and internationally. Furthermore it also enables the effects of introducing changes to guidelines, new drugs, new techniques etc to be monitored that would not be possible on a hospital-by-hospital basis.

Key learning points

- Human factors are important during resuscitation.

- Use SBAR or RSVP for effective communication.

- Report safety incidents and collect cardiac arrest data to help improve patient care.

Further reading

Featherstone P, Chalmers T, Smith GB. RSVP: a system for communication of deterioration in hospital patients. Br J Nurs 2008;17:860-64.

Flin R, O'Connor P, Crichton M. Safety at the Sharp End: a Guide to Non-Technical Skills. Aldershot: Ashgate, 2008.

Flin R, Patey R, Glavin R, Maran N. Anaesthetists' non-technical skills. Br J Anaesth 2010;105:38-44.

Acknowledgment

The Resuscitation Council (UK) would like to express its thanks to Professor Rhona Flin, University of Aberdeen, for permission to use the Anaesthetists Non-Technical Skills (ANTS) system.

Recognition of the Deteriorating Patient and Prevention of Cardiorespiratory Arrest

CHAPTER 3

Learning outcomes

To understand:

▶ **The importance of early recognition of the deteriorating patient**

▶ **The causes of cardiorespiratory arrest in adults**

▶ **How to identify and treat patients at risk of cardiorespiratory arrest using the Airway, Breathing, Circulation, Disability, Exposure (ABCDE) approach**

Introduction

Early recognition of the deteriorating patient and prevention of cardiac arrest is the first link in the chain of survival. Once cardiac arrest occurs, fewer than 20% of patients having an in-hospital cardiac arrest will survive to go home. Prevention of in-hospital cardiac arrest requires staff education, monitoring of patients, recognition of patient deterioration, a system to call for help, and an effective response.

Survivors from in-hospital cardiac arrest usually have a witnessed and monitored ventricular fibrillation (VF) arrest, primary myocardial ischaemia as the cause, and receive immediate and successful defibrillation.

Most cardiorespiratory arrests in hospital are not sudden or unpredictable events: in approximately 80% of cases there is deterioration in clinical signs during the few hours before cardiac arrest. These patients often have slow and progressive physiological deterioration, particularly hypoxia and hypotension (i.e. Airway, Breathing, Circulation problems) that is unnoticed by staff, or is recognised but treated poorly. The cardiac arrest rhythm in this group is usually non-shockable (PEA or asystole) and the survival rate to hospital discharge is very low.

Early recognition and effective treatment of the deteriorating patient might prevent cardiac arrest, death or an unanticipated intensive care unit (ICU) admission. Closer attention to patients who have a 'false' cardiac arrest (i.e. a 'cardiac arrest team' call when the patient has not had a cardiac arrest) may also improve outcome, because up to one third of these patients die during their in-hospital stay. Early recognition will also help to identify individuals for whom cardiorespiratory resuscitation is not appropriate or who do not wish to be resuscitated.

Prevention of in-hospital cardiac arrest: the Chain of Prevention

The Chain of Prevention can assist hospitals in structuring care processes to prevent and detect patient deterioration and cardiac arrest. The five rings of the chain represent: staff education; the monitoring of patients; the recognition of patient deterioration; a system to call for help; and an effective response (Figure 3.1):

● **Education**: how to observe patients; interpretation of observed signs; the recognition of signs of deterioration; and the use of the ABCDE approach and simple skills to stabilise the patient pending the arrival of more experienced help.

● **Monitoring**: patient assessment and the measurement and recording of vital signs, which may include the use of electronic monitoring devices.

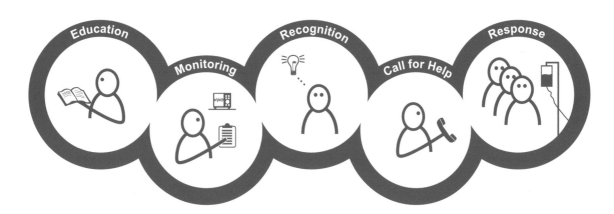

Figure 3.1 Chain of Prevention

Score	3	2	1	0	1	2	3
Pulse (min⁻¹)		≤ 40	41 - 50	51 - 90	91 - 110	111 - 130	≥ 131
Respiratory rate (min⁻¹)	≤ 8		9 - 11	12 - 20		21 - 24	≥ 25
Temperature (°C)	≤ 35.0		35.1 - 36.0	36.1 - 38.0	38.1 - 39.0	≥ 39.1	
Systolic BP (mmHg)	≤ 90	91 - 100	101 - 110	111 - 249	≥ 250		
Oxygen saturation (%)	≤ 91	92 - 93	94 - 95	≥ 96			
Inspired oxygen				Air			Any oxygen therapy
AVPU				Alert (A)			Voice (V) Pain (P) Unresponsive (U)

TABLE 3.1 Example of early warning scoring (EWS) system*

* From Prytherch et al. ViEWS - Towards a national early warning score for detecting adult in-patient deterioration. Resuscitation. 2010;81(8):932-7

- **Recognition** encompasses the tools available to identify patients in need of additional monitoring or intervention, including suitably designed vital signs charts and sets of predetermined 'calling criteria' to 'flag' the need to escalate monitoring or to call for more expert help.

- **Call for help** protocols for summoning a response to a deteriorating patient should be universally known and understood, unambiguous and mandated. Doctors and nurses often find it difficult to ask for help or escalate treatment as they feel their clinical judgement may be criticised. Hospitals should ensure all staff are empowered to call for help. A structured communication tool such as SBAR (Situation, Background, Assessment, Recommendation) or RSVP (Reason, Story, Vital signs, Plan) should be used to call for help.

- **Response** to a deteriorating patient must be assured, of specified speed and by staff with appropriate acute or critical care skills, and experience.

Recognising the deteriorating patient

In general, the clinical signs of critical illness are similar whatever the underlying process because they reflect failing respiratory, cardiovascular, and neurological systems i.e. ABCDE problems (see below). Abnormal physiology is common on general wards, yet the measurement and recording of important physiological observations of acutely ill patients occurs less frequently than is desirable. The assessment of very simple vital signs, such as respiratory rate, may help to predict cardiorespiratory arrest. To help early detection of critical illness, many hospitals use early warning scores (EWS) or calling criteria. Early warning scoring systems allocate points to measurements of routine vital signs on the basis of their derangement from an arbitrarily agreed 'normal' range. The weighted score of one or more vital sign

observations, or the total EWS, indicates the level of intervention required, e.g. increased frequency of vital signs monitoring, or calling ward doctors or resuscitation teams to the patient. An example of an EWS system is shown in Table 3.1.

Early warning scores are dynamic and change over time and the frequency of observations should be increased to track improvement or deterioration in a patient's condition. If it is clear a patient is deteriorating help should be called for early rather than waiting for the patient to reach a specific score.

The patient's EWS is calculated based on Table 3.1. An increased score indicates an increased risk of deterioration and death. There should be a graded response to scores according to local hospital protocols (Table 3.2).

Alternatively, systems incorporating calling criteria are based on routine observations, which activate a response when one or more variables reach an extremely abnormal value. It is not clear which of these two systems is better. Some hospitals combine elements of both systems.

Even when doctors are alerted to a patient's abnormal physiology, there is often delay in attending to the patient or referring to higher levels of care.

Response to critical illness

The traditional response to cardiac arrest is reactive: the name 'cardiac arrest team' implies that it will be called only after cardiac arrest has occurred. In some hospitals the cardiac arrest team has been replaced by other resuscitation teams (e.g. rapid response team, critical care outreach team, medical emergency team). These teams can be activated according to the patient's EWS (see above) or according to specific calling criteria. For example, the medical emergency team (MET) responds

EWS	Minimal observation frequency	Escalation	
		Recorder's action	Doctor's action
3 - 5	4 hourly	Inform nurse in charge	
6	4 hourly	Inform doctor	Doctor to see within 1 h
7 - 8	1 hourly	Inform doctor Consider continuous monitoring	Doctor to see within 30 min and discuss with senior doctor and/or outreach team
≥9	30 min	Inform doctor Start continuous monitoring	Doctor to see within 15 min and discuss with senior doctor and ICU team

TABLE 3.2 Example escalation protocol based on early warning score (EWS)

not only to patients in cardiac arrest, but also to those with acute physiological deterioration. The MET usually comprises medical and nursing staff from intensive care and general medicine and responds to specific calling criteria (Table 3.3). Any member of the healthcare team can initiate a MET call. Early involvement of the MET may reduce cardiac arrests, deaths and unanticipated ICU admissions, and may facilitate decisions about limitation of treatment (e.g. do-not-attempt-resuscitation [DNAR] decisions). Medical emergency team interventions often involve simple tasks such as starting oxygen therapy and intravenous fluids. The benefits of the MET system remain to be proved.

MET calling criteria	
Airway	Threatened
Breathing	All respiratory arrests Respiratory rate < 5 min⁻¹ Respiratory rate > 36 min⁻¹
Circulation	All cardiac arrests Pulse rate < 40 min⁻¹ Pulse rate > 140 min⁻¹ Systolic BP < 90 mmHg
Neurology	Sudden decrease in level of consciousness Decrease in GCS of > 2 points Repeated or prolonged seizures
Other	Any patient causing concern who does not fit the above criteria

TABLE 3.3 Medical emergency team (MET) calling criteria

In the UK, a system of pre-emptive ward care known as critical care outreach, has developed. Outreach services

exist in many forms ranging from a single nurse to a 24-hour, seven days per week multiprofessional team. An outreach team or system may reduce ward deaths, postoperative adverse events, ICU admissions and readmissions, and increase survival.

All critically ill patients should be admitted to an area that can provide the greatest supervision and the highest level of organ support and nursing care. This is usually in a critical care area, e.g. ICU, high dependency unit (HDU), or resuscitation room. These areas should be staffed by doctors and nurses experienced in advanced resuscitation and critical care skills.

Hospital staffing tends to be at its lowest during the night and at weekends. This influences patient monitoring, treatment and outcomes. Admission to general wards in the evening, or to hospital at weekends, is associated with increased mortality. Studies have shown that in-hospital cardiac arrests occurring in the late afternoon, at night or at weekends are more often non-witnessed and have a lower survival rate. Patients discharged at night from ICUs to general wards have an increased risk of ICU readmission and in-hospital death compared with those discharged during the day and those discharged to HDUs.

Causes of deterioration and cardiorespiratory arrest

Deterioration and cardiorespiratory arrest can be caused by primary airway and/or breathing and/or cardiovascular problems.

Airway obstruction

For a detailed review of airway management see Chapter 7.

Causes

Airway obstruction can be complete or partial. Complete airway obstruction rapidly causes cardiac arrest. Partial obstruction often precedes complete obstruction. Partial airway obstruction can cause cerebral or pulmonary oedema, exhaustion, secondary apnoea, and hypoxic brain injury, and eventually cardiac arrest.

Causes of airway obstruction

- Central nervous system depression
- Blood
- Vomitus
- Foreign body (e.g. tooth, food)
- Direct trauma to face or throat
- Epiglottitis
- Pharyngeal swelling (e.g. infection, oedema)
- Laryngospasm
- Bronchospasm – causes narrowing of the small airways in the lung
- Bronchial secretions
- Blocked tracheostomy

Central nervous system depression may cause loss of airway patency and protective reflexes. Causes include head injury and intracerebral disease, hypercarbia, the depressant effect of metabolic disorders (e.g. diabetes mellitus), and drugs, including alcohol, opioids and general anaesthetic agents. Laryngospasm can occur with upper airway stimulation in a semi-conscious patient whose airway reflexes remain intact.

In some people, the upper airway can become obstructed when they sleep (obstructive sleep apnoea). This is more common in obese patients and obstruction can be worsened in the presence of other factors (e.g. sedative drugs).

Recognition

Assess the patency of the airway in anyone at risk of obstruction. A conscious patient will complain of difficulty in breathing, may be choking, and will be distressed. With partial airway obstruction, efforts at breathing will be noisy. Complete airway obstruction is silent and there is no air movement at the patient's mouth. Any respiratory movements are usually strenuous. The accessory muscles of respiration will be involved, causing a 'see-saw' or 'rocking-horse' pattern of chest and abdominal movement: the chest is drawn in and the abdomen expands on inspiration, and the opposite occurs on expiration.

Treatment

The priority is to ensure that the airway remains patent. Treat any problem that places the airway at risk; for example, suck blood and gastric contents from the airway and, unless contraindicated, turn the patient on their side. Give oxygen as soon as possible to achieve an arterial blood oxygen saturation by pulse oximetry (SpO_2) in the range of 94 - 98%. Assume actual or impending airway obstruction in anyone with a depressed level of

consciousness, regardless of cause. Take steps to safeguard the airway and prevent further complications such as aspiration of gastric contents. This may involve nursing the patient on their side or with a head-up tilt. Simple airway opening manoeuvres (head tilt/chin lift or jaw thrust), insertion of an oropharyngeal or nasal airway, elective tracheal intubation or tracheostomy may be required. Consider insertion of a nasogastric tube to empty the stomach.

Breathing problems

Causes

Breathing inadequacy may be acute or chronic. It may be continuous or intermittent, and severe enough to cause apnoea (respiratory arrest), which will rapidly cause cardiac arrest. Respiratory arrest often occurs because of a combination of factors; for example, in a patient with chronic respiratory inadequacy, a chest infection, muscle weakness, or fractured ribs can lead to exhaustion, further depressing respiratory function. If breathing is insufficient to oxygenate the blood adequately (hypoxaemia), a cardiac arrest will occur eventually.

Respiratory drive

Central nervous system depression may decrease or abolish respiratory drive. The causes are the same as those for airway obstruction from central nervous system depression.

Respiratory effort

The main respiratory muscles are the diaphragm and intercostal muscles. The latter are innervated at the level of their respective ribs and may be paralysed by a spinal cord lesion above this level. The innervation of the diaphragm is at the level of the third, fourth and fifth segment of the spinal cord. Spontaneous breathing cannot occur with severe cervical cord damage above this level.

Inadequate respiratory effort, caused by muscle weakness or nerve damage, occurs with many diseases (e.g. myasthenia gravis, Guillain-Barré syndrome, and multiple sclerosis). Chronic malnourishment and severe long-term illness may also contribute to generalised weakness.

Breathing can also be impaired with restrictive chest wall abnormalities such as kyphoscoliosis. Pain from fractured ribs or sternum will prevent deep breaths and coughing.

Lung disorders

Lung function is impaired by a pneumothorax or haemothorax. A tension pneumothorax causes a rapid failure of gas exchange, a reduction of venous return to the heart, and a fall in cardiac output. Severe lung disease will impair gas exchange. Causes include infection, aspiration, exacerbation of chronic obstructive pulmonary disease (COPD), asthma, pulmonary embolus, lung contusion, acute respiratory distress syndrome (ARDS) and pulmonary oedema.

Recognition

A conscious patient will complain of shortness of breath and be distressed. The history and examination will usually indicate the underlying cause. Hypoxaemia and hypercarbia can cause irritability, confusion, lethargy and a decrease in the level of consciousness. Cyanosis may be visible but is a late sign. A fast respiratory rate (>25 min⁻¹) is a useful, simple indicator of breathing problems. Pulse oximetry is an easy, non-invasive measure of the adequacy of oxygenation (see Chapter 15). However, it is not a reliable indicator of ventilation and an arterial blood gas sample is necessary to obtain values for arterial carbon dioxide tension ($PaCO_2$) and pH. A rising $PaCO_2$ and a decrease in pH are often late signs in a patient with severe respiratory problems.

Treatment

Give oxygen to all acutely ill hypoxaemic patients and treat the underlying cause. Give oxygen at 15 l min⁻¹ using a high-concentration reservoir mask. Once the patient is stable, change the oxygen mask and aim for a SpO_2 in the range of 94 - 98%. For example, suspect a tension pneumothorax from a history of chest trauma and confirm by clinical signs and symptoms. If diagnosed, decompress it immediately by inserting a large-bore (14 G) cannula into the second intercostal space, in the mid-clavicular line (needle thoracocentesis).

Patients who are having difficulty breathing or are becoming tired will need respiratory support. Non-invasive ventilation using a face mask or a helmet can be useful and prevent the need for tracheal intubation and ventilation. For patients who cannot breathe adequately, sedation, tracheal intubation and controlled ventilation is needed.

Circulation problems

Causes

Circulation problems may be caused by primary heart disease or by heart abnormalities secondary to other problems. Most often, circulation problems in acutely ill patients are due to hypovolaemia. The heart may stop suddenly or may produce an inadequate cardiac output for a period of time before stopping.

Primary heart problems

The commonest cause of sudden cardiac arrest is an arrhythmia caused by either ischaemia or myocardial infarction. Cardiac arrest can also be caused by an arrhythmia due to other forms of heart disease, by heart block, electrocution and some drugs.

Sudden cardiac arrest may also occur with cardiac failure, cardiac tamponade, cardiac rupture, myocarditis and hypertrophic cardiomyopathy.

Causes of ventricular fibrillation

- Acute coronary syndromes (Chapter 4)
- Hypertensive heart disease
- Valve disease
- Drugs (e.g. antiarrhythmic drugs, tricyclic antidepressants, digoxin)
- Inherited cardiac diseases (e.g. long QT syndromes)
- Acidosis
- Abnormal electrolyte concentration (e.g. potassium, magnesium, calcium)
- Hypothermia
- Electrocution

Secondary heart problems

The heart is affected by changes elsewhere in the body. For example, cardiac arrest will occur rapidly following asphyxia from airway obstruction or apnoea, tension pneumothorax, or acute severe blood loss. Severe hypoxia and anaemia, hypothermia, oligaemia and severe septic shock will also impair cardiac function and this may lead to cardiac arrest.

Recognition

The signs and symptoms of cardiac disease include chest pain, shortness of breath, syncope, tachycardia, bradycardia, tachypnoea, hypotension, poor peripheral perfusion (prolonged capillary refill time), altered mental state, and oliguria.

Most sudden cardiac deaths (SCDs) occur in people with pre-existing cardiac disease, which may have been unrecognised previously. Although the risk is greater for patients with known severe cardiac disease, most SCDs occur in people with unrecognised disease. Asymptomatic or silent cardiac disease may include hypertensive heart disease, aortic valve disease, cardiomyopathy, myocarditis, and coronary disease.

Recognition of risk of sudden cardiac death out of hospital

Coronary artery disease is the commonest cause of SCD. Non-ischaemic cardiomyopathy and valvular disease account for some other SCD events. A small percentage of SCDs are caused by inherited abnormalities (e.g. long and short QT syndromes, Brugada syndrome, hypertrophic cardiomyopathy, arrhythmogenic right ventricular cardiomyopathy), and by congenital heart disease.

In patients with a known diagnosis of cardiac disease, syncope (with or without prodrome - particularly recent or recurrent) is as an independent risk factor for increased risk of death. Apparently healthy children and young adults who have SCD may also have symptoms and signs (e.g. syncope/pre-syncope, chest pain, palpitation, heart murmur) that should alert healthcare professionals to seek expert help to prevent cardiac arrest. Features that indicate a high probability of arrhythmic syncope include:

- syncope in the supine position;

- syncope occurring during or after exercise (although syncope after exercise is often vasovagal);

- syncope with no or only brief prodromal symptoms;

- repeated episodes of unexplained syncope;

- syncope in individuals with a family history of sudden death or inherited cardiac condition.

Assessment in a clinic specialising in the care of those at risk for SCD is recommended in family members of young victims of SCD or those with a known cardiac disorder resulting in an increased risk of SCD. Specific and detailed guidance for the care of individuals with transient loss of consciousness is available (http://guidance.nice.org.uk/CG109).

Treatment

Treat the underlying cause of circulatory failure. In many sick patients, this means giving intravenous fluids to treat hypovolaemia. Assess patients with chest pain for an acute coronary syndrome (ACS). A comprehensive description of the management of ACS is given in Chapter 4.

Most patients with cardiac ischaemic pain will be more comfortable sitting up. In some instances lying flat may provoke or worsen the pain. Consider using an anti-emetic, especially if nausea is present.

Survivors of an episode of VF are likely to have a further episode unless preventative treatment is given. These patients may need percutaneous coronary intervention, coronary artery bypass grafting, or an implantable defibrillator.

Treating the underlying cause should prevent many secondary cardiac arrests; for example, early goal-directed therapy to optimise vital organ perfusion decreases the risk of death in severe sepsis. Cardiovascular support includes correction of underlying electrolyte or acid-base disturbances, and treatment to achieve a desirable cardiac rate, rhythm and output. Advanced cardiovascular monitoring and echocardiography may be indicated. Appropriate manipulation of cardiac filling may require fluid therapy and vasoactive drugs. Inotropic drugs and vasoconstrictors may be indicated to support cardiac output and blood pressure. In some situations, mechanical circulatory support (e.g. intra-aortic balloon pump) or consideration of heart transplantation will be necessary.

The ABCDE approach

Underlying principles

The approach to all deteriorating or critically ill patients is the same. The underlying principles are:

1. Use the **A**irway, **B**reathing, **C**irculation, **D**isability, **E**xposure approach to assess and treat the patient.

2. Do a complete initial assessment and re-assess regularly.

3. Treat life-threatening problems before moving to the next part of assessment.

4. Assess the effects of treatment.

5. Recognise when you will need extra help. Call for appropriate help early.

6. Use all members of the team. This enables interventions, e.g. assessment, attaching monitors, intravenous access, to be undertaken simultaneously.

7. Communicate effectively - use the SBAR or RSVP approach (see Chapter 2).

8. The aim of the initial treatment is to keep the patient alive, and achieve some clinical improvement. This will buy time for further treatment and making a diagnosis.

9. Remember - it can take a few minutes for treatments to work.

First steps

1. Ensure personal safety. Wear apron and gloves as appropriate.

2. First look at the patient in general to see if the patient appears unwell.

3. If the patient is awake, ask "How are you?". If the patient appears unconscious or has collapsed, shake him and ask "Are you alright?" If he responds normally he has a patent airway, is breathing and has brain perfusion. If he speaks only in short sentences, he may have breathing problems. Failure of the patient to respond is a clear marker of critical illness.

4. This first rapid 'Look, Listen and Feel" of the patient should take about 30 s and will often indicate a patient is critically ill and there is a need for urgent help. Ask a colleague to ensure appropriate help is coming.

5. If the patient is unconscious, unresponsive, and is not breathing normally (occasional gasps are not normal) start CPR according to the guidance in Chapter 5. If you are confident and trained to do so, feel for a pulse to determine if the patient has a respiratory arrest. If there are any doubts about the presence of a pulse start CPR.

6. Monitor the vital signs early. Attach a pulse oximeter, ECG monitor and a non-invasive blood pressure monitor to **all** critically ill patients, as soon as possible.

7. Insert an intravenous cannula as soon as possible. Take bloods for investigation when inserting the intravenous cannula.

Airway (A)

Airway obstruction is an emergency. Get expert help immediately. Untreated, airway obstruction causes hypoxia and risks damage to the brain, kidneys and heart, cardiac arrest, and death.

1. Look for the signs of airway obstruction:

- Airway obstruction causes paradoxical chest and abdominal movements ('see-saw' respirations) and the use of the accessory muscles of respiration. Central cyanosis is a late sign of airway obstruction. In complete airway obstruction, there are no breath sounds at the mouth or nose. In partial obstruction, air entry is diminished and often noisy.

- In the critically ill patient, depressed consciousness often leads to airway obstruction.

2. Treat airway obstruction as a medical emergency:

- Obtain expert help immediately. Untreated, airway obstruction causes hypoxaemia (low PaO_2) with the risk of hypoxic injury to the brain, kidneys and heart, cardiac arrest, and even death.

- In most cases, only simple methods of airway clearance are required (e.g. airway opening manoeuvres, airways suction, insertion of an oropharyngeal or nasopharyngeal airway). Tracheal intubation may be required when these fail.

3. Give oxygen at high concentration:

- Provide high-concentration oxygen using a mask with an oxygen reservoir. Ensure that the oxygen flow is sufficient (usually 15 l min⁻¹) to prevent collapse of the reservoir during inspiration. If the patient's trachea is intubated, give high concentration oxygen with a self-inflating bag.

- In acute respiratory failure, aim to maintain an oxygen saturation of 94 - 98%. In patients at risk of hypercapnic respiratory failure (see below) aim for an oxygen saturation of 88 - 92%.

Breathing (B)

During the immediate assessment of breathing, it is vital to diagnose and treat immediately life-threatening conditions, e.g. acute severe asthma, pulmonary oedema, tension pneumothorax, and massive haemothorax.

1. Look, listen and feel for the general signs of respiratory distress: sweating, central cyanosis, use of the accessory muscles of respiration, and abdominal breathing.

2. Count the respiratory rate. The normal rate is 12 - 20 breaths min⁻¹. A high (≥ 25 min⁻¹), or increasing, respiratory rate is a marker of illness and a warning that the patient may deteriorate suddenly.

3. Assess the depth of each breath, the pattern (rhythm) of respiration and whether chest expansion is equal on both sides.

4. Note any chest deformity (this may increase the risk of deterioration in the ability to breathe normally); look for a raised jugular venous pulse (JVP) (e.g. in acute severe asthma or a tension pneumothorax); note the presence and patency of any chest drains; remember that abdominal distension may limit diaphragmatic movement, thereby worsening respiratory distress.

5. Record the inspired oxygen concentration (%) and the SpO_2 reading of the pulse oximeter. The pulse oximeter does not detect hypercapnia. If the patient is receiving supplemental oxygen, the SpO_2 may be normal in the presence of a very high $PaCO_2$.

6. Listen to the patient's breath sounds a short distance from his face: rattling airway noises indicate the presence of airway secretions, usually caused by the inability of the patient to cough sufficiently or to take a deep breath. Stridor or wheeze suggests partial, but significant, airway obstruction.

7. Percuss the chest: hyper-resonance may suggest a pneumothorax; dullness usually indicates consolidation or pleural fluid.

8. Auscultate the chest: bronchial breathing indicates lung consolidation with patent airways; absent or reduced sounds suggest a pneumothorax or pleural fluid or lung consolidation caused by complete bronchial obstruction.

9. Check the position of the trachea in the suprasternal notch: deviation to one side indicates mediastinal shift (e.g. pneumothorax, lung fibrosis or pleural fluid).

10. Feel the chest wall to detect surgical emphysema or crepitus (suggesting a pneumothorax until proven otherwise).

11. The specific treatment of respiratory disorders depends upon the cause. Nevertheless, all critically

ill patients should be given oxygen. In a subgroup of patients with chronic obstructive pulmonary disease (COPD), high concentrations of oxygen may depress breathing (i.e. they are at risk of hypercapnic respiratory failure - often referred to as type 2 respiratory failure). Nevertheless, these patients will also sustain end-organ damage or cardiac arrest if their blood oxygen tensions are allowed to decrease. In this group, aim for a lower than normal PaO_2 and oxygen saturation. Give oxygen via a Venturi 28% mask (4 l min^{-1}) or a 24% Venturi mask (4 l min^{-1}) initially and reassess. Aim for target SpO_2 range of 88 - 92% in most COPD patients, but evaluate the target for each patient based on the patient's arterial blood gas measurements during previous exacerbations (if available). Some patients with chronic lung disease carry an oxygen alert card (that documents their target saturation) and their own appropriate Venturi mask.

12. If the patient's depth or rate of breathing is judged to be inadequate, or absent, use bag-mask or pocket mask ventilation to improve oxygenation and ventilation, whilst calling immediately for expert help. In cooperative patients who do not have airway obstruction consider the use of non-invasive ventilation (NIV). In patients with an acute exacerbation of COPD, the use of NIV is often helpful and prevents the need for tracheal intubation and invasive ventilation.

Circulation (C)

In almost all medical and surgical emergencies, consider hypovolaemia to be the primary cause of shock, until proven otherwise. Unless there are obvious signs of a cardiac cause, give intravenous fluid to any patient with cool peripheries and a fast heart rate. In surgical patients, rapidly exclude haemorrhage (overt or hidden). Remember that breathing problems, such as a tension pneumothorax, can also compromise a patient's circulatory state. This should have been treated earlier on in the assessment.

1. Look at the colour of the hands and digits: are they blue, pink, pale or mottled?

2. Assess the limb temperature by feeling the patient's hands: are they cool or warm?

3. Measure the capillary refill time (CRT). Apply cutaneous pressure for 5 s on a fingertip held at heart level (or just above) with enough pressure to cause blanching. Time how long it takes for the skin to return to the colour of the surrounding skin after releasing the pressure. The normal value for CRT is usually < 2 s. A prolonged CRT suggests poor peripheral perfusion. Other factors (e.g. cold surroundings, poor lighting, old age) can prolong CRT.

4. Assess the state of the veins: they may be under-filled or collapsed when hypovolaemia is present.

5. Count the patient's pulse rate (or preferably heart rate by listening to the heart with a stethoscope).

6. Palpate peripheral and central pulses, assessing for presence, rate, quality, regularity and equality. Barely palpable central pulses suggest a poor cardiac output, whilst a bounding pulse may indicate sepsis.

7. Measure the patient's blood pressure. Even in shock, the blood pressure may be normal, because compensatory mechanisms increase peripheral resistance in response to reduced cardiac output. A low diastolic blood pressure suggests arterial vasodilation (as in anaphylaxis or sepsis). A narrowed pulse pressure (difference between systolic and diastolic pressures; normally 35 - 45 mmHg) suggests arterial vasoconstriction (cardiogenic shock or hypovolaemia) and may occur with rapid tachyarrhythmia.

8. Auscultate the heart. Is there a murmur or pericardial rub? Are the heart sounds difficult to hear? Does the audible heart rate correspond to the pulse rate?

9. Look for other signs of a poor cardiac output, such as reduced conscious level and, if the patient has a urinary catheter, oliguria (urine volume < 0.5 ml kg^{-1} h^{-1}).

10. Look thoroughly for external haemorrhage from wounds or drains or evidence of concealed haemorrhage (e.g. thoracic, intra-peritoneal, retroperitoneal or into gut). Intra-thoracic, intra-abdominal or pelvic blood loss may be significant, even if drains are empty.

11. The specific treatment of cardiovascular collapse depends on the cause, but should be directed at fluid replacement, haemorrhage control and restoration of tissue perfusion. Seek the signs of conditions that are immediately life threatening, e.g. cardiac tamponade, massive or continuing haemorrhage, septicaemic shock, and treat them urgently.

12. Insert one or more large (14 or 16 G) intravenous cannulae. Use short, wide-bore cannulae, because they enable the highest flow.

13. Take blood from the cannula for routine haematological, biochemical, coagulation and microbiological investigations, and cross-matching, before infusing intravenous fluid.

14. Give a rapid fluid challenge (over 5 - 10 min) of 500 ml of warmed crystalloid solution (e.g. Hartmann's solution or 0.9% sodium chloride) if the patient is normotensive. Give one litre, if the patient is hypotensive. Use smaller volumes (e.g. 250 ml) for patients with known cardiac failure or trauma and use closer monitoring (listen to the chest for crackles after each bolus, consider a CVP line).

15. Reassess the heart rate and BP regularly (every 5 min), aiming for the patient's normal BP or, if this is unknown, a target > 100 mmHg systolic.

16. If the patient does not improve, repeat the fluid challenge.

17. If symptoms and signs of cardiac failure (dyspnoea, increased heart rate, raised JVP, a third heart sound and pulmonary crackles on auscultation) occur, decrease the fluid infusion rate or stop the fluids altogether. Seek alternative means of improving tissue perfusion (e.g. inotropes or vasopressors).

18. If the patient has primary chest pain and a suspected ACS, record a 12-lead ECG early, and treat initially with aspirin, nitroglycerine, oxygen, and morphine.

19. Immediate general treatment for ACS includes:

- Aspirin 300 mg, orally, crushed or chewed, as soon as possible.

- Nitroglycerine, as sublingual glyceryl trinitrate (tablet or spray).

- Oxygen, aiming at a SpO_2 of 94 - 98%; do not give supplementary oxygen if the patient's SpO_2 is within this range when breathing air alone.

- Morphine (or diamorphine) titrated intravenously to avoid sedation and respiratory depression.

Disability (D)

Common causes of unconsciousness include profound hypoxia, hypercapnia, cerebral hypoperfusion, or the recent administration of sedatives or analgesic drugs.

1. Review and treat the ABCs: exclude or treat hypoxia and hypotension.

2. Check the patient's drug chart for reversible drug-induced causes of depressed consciousness. Give an antagonist where appropriate (e.g. naloxone for opioid toxicity).

3. Examine the pupils (size, equality and reaction to light).

4. Make a rapid initial assessment of the patient's conscious level using the AVPU method: **A**lert, responds to **V**ocal stimuli, responds to **P**ainful stimuli or **U**nresponsive to all stimuli. Alternatively, use the Glasgow Coma Scale score.

5. Measure the blood glucose to exclude hypoglycaemia using a rapid finger-prick bedside testing method. If the blood sugar is below 4.0 mmol l⁻¹, give an initial dose of 50 ml of 10% glucose solution intravenously. If necessary, give further doses of intravenous 10% glucose every minute until the patient has fully regained consciousness, or a total of 250 ml of 10%

glucose has been given. Repeat blood glucose measurements to monitor the effects of treatment. If there is no improvement consider further doses of 10% glucose.

6. Nurse unconscious patients in the lateral position if their airway is not protected.

Exposure (E)

To examine the patient properly full exposure of the body may be necessary. Respect the patient's dignity and minimise heat loss.

Additional information

1. Take a full clinical history from the patient, any relatives or friends, and other staff.

2. Review the patient's notes and charts:

- Study both absolute and trended values of vital signs.

- Check that important routine medications are prescribed and being given.

3. Review the results of laboratory or radiological investigations.

4. Consider which level of care is required by the patient (e.g. ward, HDU, ICU).

5. Make complete entries in the patient's notes of your findings, assessment and treatment. Where necessary, hand over the patient to your colleagues.

6. Record the patient's response to therapy.

7. Consider definitive treatment of the patient's underlying condition.

Key learning points

- Most patients who have an in-hospital cardiac arrest have warning signs and symptoms before the arrest.

- Early recognition and treatment of the deteriorating patient will prevent some cardiorespiratory arrests.

- Use strategies such as early warning scoring (EWS) systems to identify patients at risk of cardiorespiratory arrest.

- Airway, breathing and circulation problems can cause cardiorespiratory arrest.

- Use the ABCDE approach to assess and treat critically ill patients.

Further reading

Armitage M, Eddleston J, Stokes T. Recognising and responding to acute illness in adults in hospital: summary of NICE guidance. BMJ 2007;335:258-9.

Deakin CD, Nolan JP, Soar J, et al. European Resuscitation Council Guidelines for Resuscitation 2010. Section 4. Adult Advanced Life Support. Resuscitation 2010;81:1305-52.

Deakin CD, Morrison LJ, Morley PT, et al. 2010 International Consensus on Cardiopulmonary Resuscitation and Emergency Cardiovascular Care Science with Treatment Recommendations. Part 8: Advanced Life Support. Resuscitation 2010;81:e93-e169.

DeVita MA, Bellomo R, Hillman K, et al. Findings of the first consensus conference on medical emergency teams. Crit Care Med. 2006;34:2463-2478.

DeVita MA, Smith GB, Adam SK, et al. "Identifying the hospitalised patient in crisis"— a consensus conference on the afferent limb of rapid response systems. Resuscitation 2010;81:375-82.

Featherstone P, Chalmers T, Smith GB. RSVP: a system for communication of deterioration in hospital patients. Br J Nurs 2008;17:860-4.

Luettel D, Beaumont K, Healey F. Recognising and responding appropriately to early signs of deterioration in hospitalised patients. London: National Patient Safety Agency; 2007.

Marshall S, Harrison J, Flanagan B. The teaching of a structured tool improves the clarity and content of interprofessional clinical communication. Qual Saf Health Care 2009;18:137-40.

Meaney PA, Nadkarni VM, Kern KB, Indik JH, Halperin HR, Berg RA. Rhythms and outcomes of adult in-hospital cardiac arrest. Crit Care Med 2010;38:101-8.

National Confidential Enquiry into Patient Outcome and Death. An Acute Problem? London: National Confidential Enquiry into Patient Outcome and Death; 2005.

NICE clinical guideline 50 Acutely ill patients in hospital: recognition of and response to acute illness in adults in hospital. London: National Institute for Health and Clinical Excellence; 2007.

O'Driscoll BR, Howard LS, Davison AG. BTS guideline for emergency oxygen use in adult patients. Thorax 2008;63 Suppl 6:vi1-68.

Smith GB. In-hospital cardiac arrest: Is it time for an in-hospital 'chain of prevention'? Resuscitation 2010;81:1209-11.

Soar J, Mancini ME, Bhanji F, et al. 2010 International Consensus on Cardiopulmonary Resuscitation and Emergency Cardiovascular Care Science with Treatment Recommendations. Part 12: Education, Implementation, and Teams. Resuscitation 2010;81:e283-e325.

Acute Coronary Syndromes

Introduction

Whilst rapid resuscitation offers the best chance of recovery from cardiac arrest, it is clearly better to prevent cardiac arrest whenever possible. Many cardiac arrests are caused by underlying coronary artery disease and occur in the context of an acute coronary syndrome (ACS). It is therefore important that the ALS provider understands how to recognise an ACS, how to assess a patient with an ACS, and what treatments may reduce the risk of cardiac arrest and death.

Definitions and pathogenesis

The acute coronary syndromes (ACS) comprise:

- Unstable angina

- Non-ST-segment-elevation myocardial infarction

- ST-segment-elevation myocardial infarction

These clinical syndromes form parts of a spectrum of the same disease process. In the vast majority of cases this process is initiated by the fissuring of an atheromatous plaque in a coronary artery causing:

- haemorrhage into the plaque causing it to swell and restrict the lumen of the artery;

- contraction of smooth muscle within the artery wall, causing further constriction of the lumen;

- thrombus formation on the surface of the plaque, which may cause partial or complete obstruction of the lumen of the artery, or distal embolism.

The extent to which these events reduce the flow of blood to the myocardium largely determines the nature of the clinical ACS that ensues.

Angina (stable and unstable)

Angina is pain or discomfort caused by myocardial ischaemia and is felt usually in or across the centre of the chest as tightness or an indigestion-like ache. As with acute myocardial infarction (AMI), the pain/discomfort often radiates into the throat, into one or both arms, and into the back or into the epigastrium. Some patients experience angina predominantly in one or more of these areas rather than in the chest. Many patients perceive it as discomfort rather than pain. As with AMI, angina is sometimes accompanied by belching and this may be misinterpreted as evidence of indigestion as the cause of the discomfort. Pain of this nature, which is provoked only by exercise and which settles promptly when exercise ceases, is referred to as stable angina and is not an ACS.

In contrast, **unstable angina** is defined by one or more of:

1. Angina on exertion, occurring over a few days with increasing frequency, provoked by progressively less exertion. This is referred to as 'crescendo angina'.

2. Episodes of angina occurring recurrently and unpredictably, without specific provocation by exercise. These episodes may be relatively short-lived (e.g. a few minutes) and may settle spontaneously or be relieved temporarily by sublingual glyceryl trinitrate, before recurring within a few hours.

3. An unprovoked and prolonged episode of chest pain, raising suspicion of AMI, but without definite ECG or laboratory evidence of AMI (see below).

In unstable angina, the ECG may:

   a) be normal;

   b) show evidence of acute myocardial ischaemia (usually ST segment depression);

   c) show non-specific abnormalities (e.g. T wave inversion).

In unstable angina, cardiac enzymes are usually normal (but remember that there are causes other than myocardial infarction for elevated muscle enzymes such as creatine kinase [CK]), and troponin release is absent. ECG abnormality, especially ST segment depression, is a marker of increased risk of further coronary events in patients with unstable angina. However, a normal ECG and absent troponin release does not necessarily mean that a patient with unstable angina is not at high risk of early further life-threatening coronary events. Only if the ECG and troponin concentration are normal, and further risk assessment (e.g. by exercise testing or non-invasive imaging) does not indicate evidence of reversible myocardial ischaemia, should other possible causes of acute chest pain be considered if the initial history suggested unstable angina.

Non-ST-segment-elevation myocardial infarction (NSTEMI)

Acute myocardial infarction typically presents with chest pain that is felt as a heaviness or tightness or indigestion-like discomfort in the chest or upper abdomen, usually sustained for at least 20 - 30 min, often longer. The chest pain/discomfort often radiates into the throat, into one or both arms, into the back or into the epigastrium. Some patients experience the discomfort predominantly in one or more of these other areas rather than in the chest. Sometimes it may be accompanied by belching and this may be misinterpreted as evidence of indigestion as the cause of the discomfort.

When patients present with chest pain suggestive of AMI, non-specific ECG abnormalities such as ST segment depression or T wave inversion (Figures 4.1 and 4.2) or occasionally a normal ECG, and laboratory tests showing release of troponin (with or without elevated plasma concentrations of cardiac enzymes) this indicates that myocardial damage has occurred. This is referred to as NSTEMI. In this situation it is less likely that there has been abrupt complete occlusion of the culprit artery than in ST-segment-elevation MI (STEMI).

The amount of troponin or cardiac enzyme released reflects the extent of myocardial damage. Some of these patients will be at high risk of progression to coronary occlusion, more extensive myocardial damage, and sudden arrhythmic death. The risk of this is highest in the first few hours, days and months after the index event and diminishes progressively with time.

NSTEMI and unstable angina are classified together as 'non-ST-segment-elevation ACS' because the treatment of the two is essentially the same and differs in some respects from the treatment of STEMI. Treatment is dictated largely by assessment of risk.

ST-segment-elevation myocardial infarction (STEMI)

A history of sustained acute chest pain typical of AMI, accompanied by acute ST segment elevation or new left bundle branch block (LBBB) on a 12-lead ECG is the basis for diagnosis of STEMI.

These findings almost always indicate on-going myocardial damage caused by acute complete occlusion of the 'culprit' coronary artery (after initial plaque

fissuring). Left untreated there is likely to be further myocardial damage in the territory of the occluded artery, usually reflected in the development of Q waves on the ECG. During the acute phase of STEMI there is a substantial risk of ventricular tachycardia (VT) and ventricular fibrillation (VF) and sudden death (Figure 4.3).

Diagnosis of acute coronary syndromes

History

An accurate history is a crucial first step in establishing a diagnosis, but there are potential sources of confusion. Some patients (e.g. the elderly, diabetics, patients during the peri-operative period) may develop an ACS with little or no chest discomfort. The pain of angina or myocardial infarction is often mistaken for indigestion both by patients and healthcare professionals. Symptoms such as belching, nausea or vomiting are not helpful in distinguishing cardiac pain from indigestion; all may accompany angina and myocardial infarction.

Clinical examination

Clinical examination is of limited benefit in the diagnosis of ACS. Severe pain of any source may provoke some of the clinical signs, such as sweating, pallor and tachycardia, which commonly accompany ACS. History and examination are essential in order to recognise alternative, obvious causes for chest pain (e.g. localised severe chest wall tenderness), or identify other life-threatening diagnoses (e.g. aortic dissection, pulmonary embolism).

Examination may identify other important abnormalities (e.g. a cardiac murmur or signs of heart failure) that will influence choices of investigation and treatment. In patients with acute chest pain remember also to check for evidence of aortic dissection, especially if fibrinolytic therapy is intended. The presence of aortic dissection may be suggested by clinical signs such as loss of a pulse or asymmetry of the pulses in the upper limbs, acute aortic regurgitation, or signs of stroke from carotid artery involvement. Suspect aortic dissection in any patient whose acute chest pain is accompanied by marked hypotension but no obvious ECG evidence of AMI. However, in a patient with a good history and typical ECG evidence of STEMI do not delay reperfusion therapy without strong clinical evidence to justify prior investigation of possible aortic dissection.

Initial examination also serves as an important baseline so that changes, due either to progression of the underlying condition or in response to treatment, may be detected.

Also suspect extensive right ventricular (RV) infarction in patients with inferior or posterior STEMI who have elevated jugular venous pressure but no evidence of pulmonary oedema. Kussmaul's sign may be positive (JVP increases on inspiration). These patients are often hypotensive.

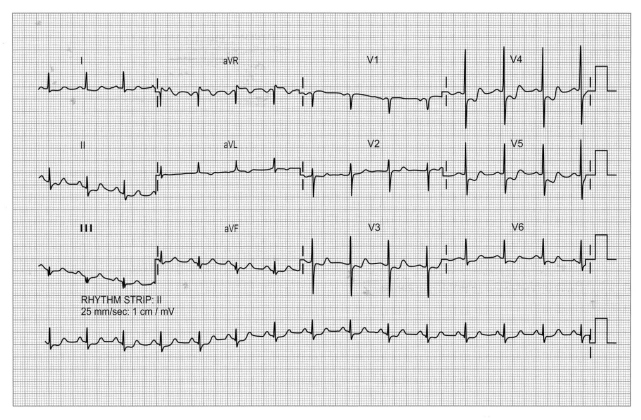

Figure 4.1 12-lead ECG showing acute ST-segment depression caused by myocardial ischaemia in a patient with a non-ST-segment ACS

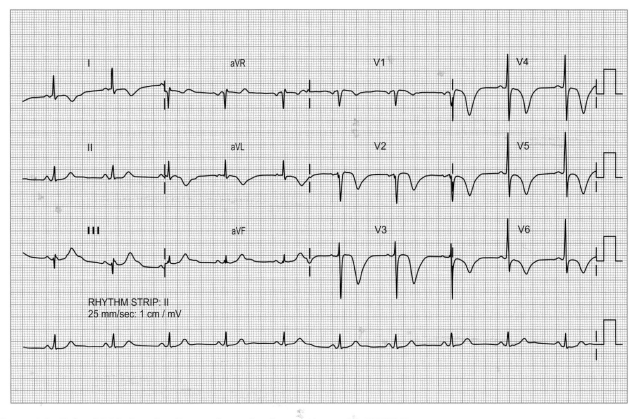

Figure 4.2 12-lead ECG showing T wave inversion in a patient with NSTEMI

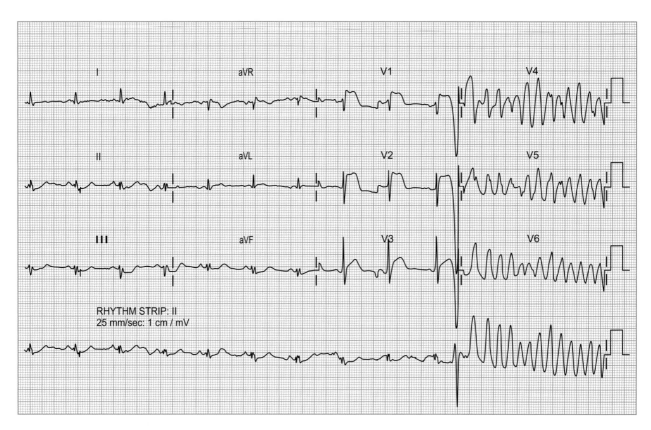

Figure 4.3 12-lead ECG showing onset of VF in a patient with an acute anteroseptal STEMI

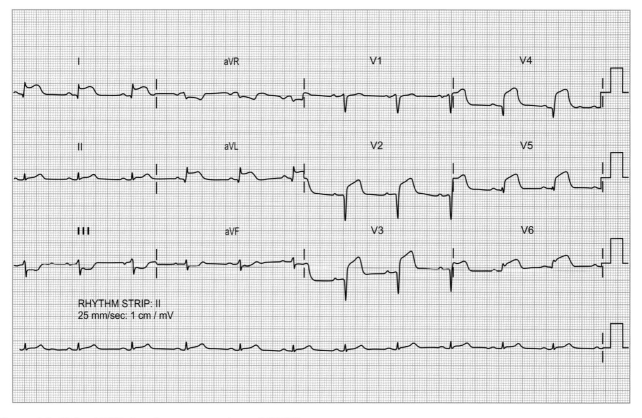

Figure 4.4 12-lead ECG showing an anterolateral STEMI

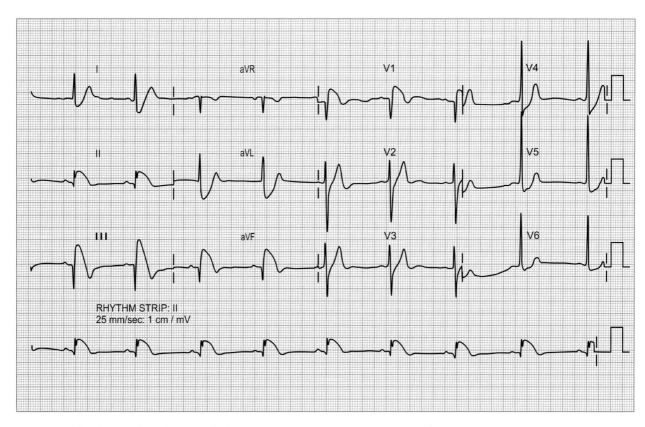

Figure 4.5 12-lead ECG showing an inferior STEMI

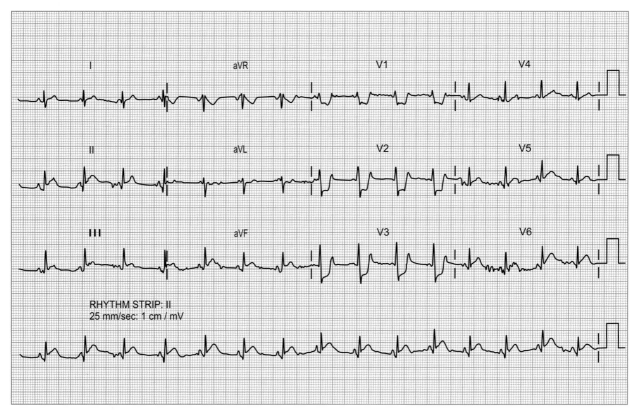

Figure 4.6 12-lead ECG showing a posterior STEMI

ALS

Investigations

The 12-lead ECG

Record a 12-lead ECG as soon as possible during the initial assessment and subsequently to assess progression of the ACS and the response to treatment. The presence of ECG abnormalities on the initial recording may support the clinical suspicion of ACS and indicate the appropriate treatment. A single normal 12-lead ECG does not exclude an ACS.

The ECG is a crucial component of risk assessment and planning of treatment. Acute ST segment elevation or new LBBB in a patient with a typical history of AMI is an indication for treatment to try to re-open an occluded coronary artery (reperfusion therapy), either by emergency percutaneous coronary intervention (PCI) or with fibrinolytic therapy. In contrast, ST segment depression suggests a low probability of benefit from fibrinolytic therapy, regardless of whether the ultimate diagnostic label is unstable angina or NSTEMI. In unstable angina, the presence of ST segment depression indicates a higher risk of further coronary events than if ST segment depression is absent. These higher-risk patients require immediate medical treatment (e.g. low-molecular-weight heparin, aspirin, clopidogrel, beta blockade, glycoprotein IIb/IIIa inhibitor), prompt investigation by coronary angiography, and often revascularisation by PCI, or coronary artery bypass surgery.

The ECG provides some information about the site and extent of myocardial damage in AMI particularly in STEMI. This is important since the site and extent of myocardial ischaemia or damage influences prognosis and, in some cases, the appropriate choice of treatment:

1. Anterior or anteroseptal infarction is seen usually in leads V1 - V4 and is almost always caused by a lesion in the left anterior descending (LAD) coronary artery. Extension to involve leads V5 - V6, I and aVL indicates an anterolateral infarct (Figure 4.4). An anterior MI has a worse prognosis and is more likely to cause substantial impairment of left ventricular function. Therefore these patients benefit more from immediate reperfusion therapy and early treatment with an angiotensin converting enzyme inhibitor (ACEI).

2. Inferior infarction is seen usually in leads II, III, and aVF (Figure 4.5), and is caused often by a lesion in the right coronary artery or, less commonly, the circumflex artery.

3. Lateral infarction is seen usually in leads V5 - V6 and/or leads I and aVL (sometimes aVL alone) and is caused often by a lesion in the circumflex artery or diagonal branch of the LAD artery.

4. Posterior myocardial infarction is usually recognised when there is a reciprocal change in the anterior chest leads (Figure 4.6). ST segment depression in these leads reflects posterior ST elevation, and development of a dominant R wave reflects posterior Q wave development. This is also most commonly due to a right coronary artery lesion but may be caused by a circumflex artery lesion in those people in whom this artery provides the main blood supply to the posterior part of the left ventricle and septum. Suspicion of a posterior infarction can be confirmed by repeating the ECG with posterior leads. These leads (V8, V9 and V10) are placed in a horizontal line around the chest, continuing from V6 (mid-axillary line) and V7 (posterior axillary line). V9 is placed to the left of the spine, V8 half way between V7 and V9 and V10 to the right of the spine.

Right ventricular (RV) infarction may be present in up to one third of patients with inferior and posterior STEMI. Extensive RV infarction may be seen on a conventional 12-lead ECG when ST segment elevation in lead V1 accompanies an inferior or posterior STEMI; use of right-sided precordial leads, especially V4R can also be useful in detecting RV infarction. In this case right-sided precordial leads, particularly V4R, may reveal RV infarction. Two-dimensional echocardiography is also very useful. A diagnosis of extensive RV infarction is suggested by fluid-responsive hypotension and signs of high CVP (as jugular venous distension) without pulmonary congestion. In these patients nitrates should be avoided.

The ST segment depression and T wave inversion that may occur in NSTEMI are less clearly related to the site of myocardial damage than the changes in STEMI. Remember also that use of modified limb leads for ECG recording may alter the morphology of the 12-lead ECG and in particular the modified inferior leads may not show true electrical activity from the inferior wall of the left ventricle.

Laboratory tests

The other important components of diagnosis and risk assessment are laboratory tests.

Cardiac troponins (troponin T and troponin I)

Cardiac-specific troponins are components of the contractile structure of myocardial cells. Because concentrations of troponin in the blood of healthy individuals are undetectably low, and cardiac-specific troponins measured by current assays do not arise from extra-cardiac sources, the troponins are very sensitive and specific markers of cardiac injury. In the context of a typical clinical presentation of ACS, troponin release provides evidence of myocardial damage and therefore indicates myocardial infarction rather than unstable angina. In addition troponin measurement provides useful assessment of risk. The greater the troponin concentration, the greater is the risk of a further event. A combination of ST segment depression on the ECG and raised troponin identifies a particularly high-risk group for subsequent MI and sudden cardiac death.

ALS

The release of troponin does not in itself indicate a diagnosis of ACS. Troponin release aids diagnosis and is a marker of risk when the history indicates a high probability of AMI. Troponin may be released in other life-threatening conditions presenting with chest pain, such as pulmonary embolism and aortic dissection, and also in myocarditis, acute or chronic heart failure, sustained tachyarrhythmia, renal failure and acute sepsis. As with all clinical evidence, it is essential that troponin results are interpreted in the context of the clinical history.

Creatine kinase (CK), aspartate transaminase (AST) and lactate dehydrogenase (LDH)

These enzymes are released from cardiac muscle when it is damaged; however, they are released also from skeletal muscle when it is damaged or during prolonged, vigorous exercise. To help clarify whether elevated CK concentrations in the blood originate from cardiac or skeletal muscle, the specific iso-enzyme of CK in cardiac muscle (CK-MB) can be measured. In many hospitals, measurement of CK-MB is not available routinely.

The amount of CK release from myocardium (e.g. when measured on sequential blood samples over three days) can serve as an approximate measure of the amount of myocardial damage.

Echocardiography

This can be useful in assessing the severity of LV impairment resulting from any AMI. It is particularly important and urgent in confirming RV dilatation and impairment when extensive RV infarction is suspected, and in identifying some complications of AMI, including acquired ventricular septal defect and severe mitral regurgitation, both of which may require urgent surgical correction.

Risk assessment

The choice of treatment is determined largely by the extent of myocardial damage and by the risk of early further coronary events. Accurate risk assessment in ACS enables early treatment to reduce risk and thereby prevent some instances of cardiac arrest and sudden death.

Immediate treatment

General measures in all acute coronary syndromes

Start with a rapid clinical assessment and record an ECG. Give immediate treatment to relieve symptoms, limit myocardial damage and reduce the risk of cardiac arrest. Immediate general treatment for ACS comprises:

- aspirin 300 mg, orally, crushed or chewed, as soon as possible;

- nitroglycerine, as sublingual glyceryl trinitrate (tablet or spray) unless patient is hypotensive or extensive

RV infarction is suspected;

- oxygen, to achieve an arterial blood oxygen saturation of 94 - 98% (or 88 - 92% in the presence of COPD);

- relief of pain is of paramount importance and intravenous morphine (or diamorphine) should be given, titrated to control symptoms but avoiding sedation and respiratory depression.

Most patients with cardiac ischaemic pain will be more comfortable sitting up. In some instances lying flat may provoke or worsen the pain. Give an anti-emetic with opiate analgesia or if the patient has nausea.

Treatment of STEMI (or AMI with new LBBB)

For patients presenting with STEMI within 12 h of symptom onset, mechanical or pharmacological reperfusion must be achieved without delay. The aim is to restore the blood supply to myocardium that has not yet been damaged irreversibly. Clinical trials have confirmed the effectiveness of reperfusion therapy in reducing infarct size, complications, and mortality from MI. Reperfusion therapy is most effective when undertaken early after the onset of myocardial infarction and the benefit diminishes progressively with delay.

The risk/benefit ratio for reperfusion therapy favours reperfusion therapy for those patients who are at highest risk of immediate major myocardial damage and death.

Beyond 12 h from the onset of chest pain, the risks of fibrinolytic therapy probably outweigh any small residual benefit, but emergency percutaneous coronary intervention (PCI) should be considered in this situation if there is ongoing clinical or ECG evidence of ischaemia.

Coronary reperfusion therapy

In STEMI, coronary reperfusion may be achieved in one of two ways:

- Percutaneous coronary intervention (PCI) may be used to re-open the occluded artery. This is referred to as primary PCI.

- Fibrinolytic therapy may be given in an attempt to dissolve the occluding thrombus that precipitated the MI.

Primary PCI

Primary PCI (PPCI) is the preferred treatment for STEMI if it can be performed by an experienced team in a timely manner. Coronary angiography is used to identify the occluded coronary artery, following which a guidewire is passed through the occluding thrombus, enabling a deflated balloon to be positioned at the site of occlusion and inflated to re-open the artery. Aspiration devices may be used to remove thrombus from the vessel and glycoprotein IIb/IIIa inhibitors may be injected intravenously or directly into the coronary artery. It is usual practice to insert a stent into the segment of previously occluded artery, to reduce the risk of re-occlusion at this point.

Primary PCI is the most reliable method of re-opening of the culprit artery in the majority of patients. Coronary artery patency can be confirmed, secured and maintained. There is a lower risk of major, particularly intracerebral, bleeding than with fibrinolytic therapy.

For PPCI to provide reliable, timely reperfusion a fully-equipped catheter laboratory staffed by an experienced team must be available 24-h a day. A fail-safe pathway of communication and care must be implemented in each region in order that patients in whom STEMI is diagnosed can access the service, ideally by direct transfer to this facility. Primary PCI can then be offered to patients for whom a 'call-to-balloon' time of 120 min can be achieved (National Infarct Angioplasty Project [NIAP]). In patients who present within 2 hours of onset of chest pain the time from first medical contact to reperfusion should be less than 90 min. Longer delays are associated with higher mortality.

Where PPCI is not available immediately, the need to achieve reperfusion as early as possible remains a high priority and for those patients initial treatment by fibrinolytic therapy may offer the best chance of achieving early reperfusion.

Platelet inhibition and anticoagulant therapy in PPCI

In addition to aspirin, give all patients being transferred for PPCI:

- clopidogrel as a 600 mg loading dose; or

- prasugrel as a 60 mg loading dose (not if >75 years, < 60 kg, history of bleeding or stroke).

Anticoagulation with unfractionated or low molecular weight heparin is given in the catheter laboratory often with a glycoprotein IIb/IIIa inhibitor. Bivalirudin, a direct thrombin inhibitor may be chosen as an alternative.

Typical indications for immediate reperfusion therapy for AMI

Presentation within 12 hours of onset of chest pain suggestive of AMI and:

- ST segment elevation > 0·2 mV in 2 adjacent chest leads, or > 0·1 mV in 2 or more 'adjacent' limb leads; or

- Dominant R waves and ST depression in V1 - V3 (posterior infarction); or

- New-onset (or presumed new-onset) LBBB.

Table 4.1 Typical indications for immediate reperfusion therapy for AMI

Typical contraindications to fibrinolytic therapy

Absolute

- Previous haemorrhagic stroke

- Ischaemic stroke during the previous 6 months

- Central nervous system damage or neoplasm

- Recent (within 3 weeks) major surgery, head injury or other major trauma

- Active internal bleeding (menses excluded) or gastro-intestinal bleeding within the past month

- Known or suspected aortic dissection

- Known bleeding disorder

Relative

- Refractory hypertension (systolic blood pressure >180 mmHg)

- Transient ischaemic attack in preceding 6 months

- Oral anticoagulant treatment

- Pregnancy or less than 1 week post-partum

- Non-compressible vascular puncture

- Active peptic ulcer disease

- Advanced liver disease

- Infective endocarditis

- Previous allergic reaction to the fibrinolytic drug to be used

Table 4.2 Typical contraindications to fibrinolytic therapy

Fibrinolytic therapy

Fibrinolytic therapy has been shown in large-scale clinical trials to provide substantial reduction in mortality from AMI when given during the first few hours after the onset of chest pain. One of the major advantages of fibrinolytic therapy is that it does not require a cardiac catheter laboratory or an operator skilled in angioplasty. Early reperfusion may be achieved by pre-hospital fibrinolytic therapy with resulting clinical benefit, particularly when transport times to hospital are very long. Early treatment may also be achieved by minimising door-to-needle time (time from arrival at hospital to administration of fibrinolytic therapy).

Fibrinolytic therapy carries a risk of bleeding, including cerebral haemorrhage, and not all patients can be given this treatment safely. Table 4.1 lists typical indications for reperfusion therapy and the typical contraindications to fibrinolytics are shown in Table 4.2. Most of these contra-indications are relative; the experienced clinician will decide whether the benefit from fibrinolytic therapy outweighs the risk to the individual patient or whether emergency angiography with a view to primary PCI would be more appropriate.

Figure 4.7 describes the options for reperfusion therapy for STEMI in the form of an algorithm.

Platelet inhibition and anticoagulant therapy with fibrinolytic therapy

Give all patients receiving a fibrinolytic agent for STEMI:

- aspirin 300 mg, and

- clopidogrel as a 600 mg loading dose, and

- antithrombin therapy: low molecular weight heparin (IV bolus then SC) or unfractionated heparin (full dose) or fondaparinux.

Rescue angioplasty

In 20 - 30% of patients receiving a fibrinolytic for STEMI, reperfusion is not achieved. Observe patients closely with cardiac monitoring during and after administration of a fibrinolytic. Record a 12-lead ECG at 60 - 90 min after giving fibrinolytic therapy. Failure of ST segment elevation to resolve by more than 50% compared with the pre-treatment ECG suggests that fibrinolytic therapy has failed to re-open the culprit artery. Symptoms are a less accurate guide to reperfusion because most patients will have received opiate analgesia. Even after initially successful thrombolysis there is a significant risk of re-occlusion and patients should be admitted to a coronary care unit with continuous ECG monitoring.

In cases of failed reperfusion or re-occlusion/re-infarction transfer the patient immediately to a cardiac catheter laboratory for mechanical reperfusion (PCI). In failed thrombolysis this is referred to as rescue PCI and has been shown to improve event-free survival and reduce heart failure when compared to conservative therapy or repeat fibrinolytic therapy. Again rescue PCI must be performed without any time-delay in order to be effective.

The role of 'facilitated PCI' in which initial fibrinolytic therapy is followed by immediate coronary angiography and PCI remains a subject of ongoing debate. So far there is insufficient evidence in support of this strategy but trials are ongoing.

Treatment of unstable angina and NSTEMI

The immediate treatment objectives in these syndromes are:

- To prevent new thrombus formation, which may occlude an artery and lead to, or extend, myocardial damage.

- To reduce myocardial oxygen demand, providing myocardial cells with a better chance of survival in the presence of a limited supply of oxygen and glucose.

Prevention of further thrombus formation

- Give subcutaneous low molecular weight heparin in therapeutic doses (weight-related, 12-hourly, dose reduction in renal impairment); or fondaparinux (once daily, contraindicated in severe renal impairment).

- Give aspirin 75 mg per day after the initial 300 mg loading dose.

- Start clopidogrel with a loading dose of at least 300 mg (consider 600 mg for rapid loading before urgent angiography), followed by 75 mg daily.

- In diabetic patients undergoing urgent PCI consider prasugrel (60 mg loading dose and then 10 mg daily) as a more effective alternative to clopidogrel.

- In high-risk patients, if early PCI is planned, consider starting a glycoprotein IIb/IIIa inhibitor (tirofiban or eptifibatide). The balance of ischaemic risk versus bleeding risk must be considered carefully.

Reduction in oxygen demand

- Start beta-adrenoceptor blockade (unless contra-indicated).

- Consider diltiazem if beta blockade contra-indicated.

- Avoid dihydropyridine calcium channel blockers (e.g. nifedipine).

- Consider intravenous or buccal nitrate if angina persists or recurs after sublingual nitrate.

- Consider early introduction of an ACEI, especially if there is left ventricular systolic impairment or heart failure.

- Treat complications such as heart failure or tachyarrhythmia promptly and effectively.

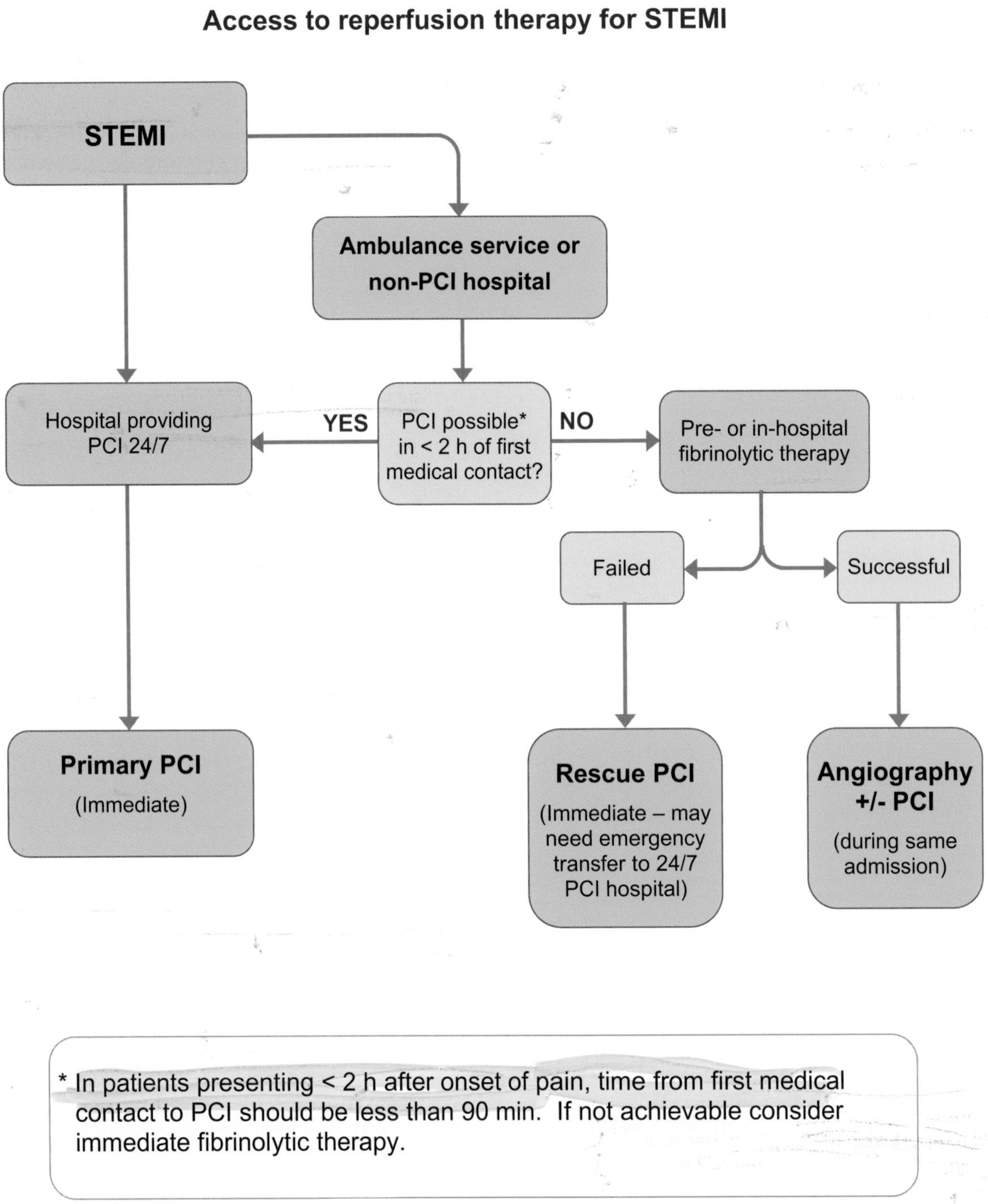

Access to reperfusion therapy for STEMI

Figure 4.7 Access to reperfusion therapy for STEMI

ALS

Subsequent management of patients with acute coronary syndromes

Suspected unstable angina – low risk patients

Patients with suspected unstable angina without a definite history of preceding angina of effort or myocardial infarction and without high-risk features at presentation (ECG and troponin levels normal after 6 - 8 h) should undergo early further risk assessment either by exercise testing or non-invasive imaging.

Suspected angina – high risk unstable angina and NSTEMI

Patients with unstable angina and high-risk features (e.g. resting ST segment depression, high-risk features on exercise test or non-invasive imaging) should be considered for early investigation by invasive coronary angiography

Patients with NSTEMI should be regarded as a high-risk group, requiring early assessment by coronary angiography during the same hospital admission in the majority of cases, ideally within 72 h.

Many patients in both these groups will benefit from revascularisation by PCI. A few may require coronary artery bypass grafts (CABG).

Formal risk-scoring systems such as GRACE (Global Registry of Acute Coronary Events) should be used to guide clinical management. Those patients at the highest risk derive the greatest benefit from early intervention in terms of reducing further major cardiac events.

STEMI

If fibrinolytic therapy has been used, many patients will be left with a severe stenosis or unstable plaque in the culprit coronary artery. PCI can stabilise this situation and reduce the risk of re-occlusion of the artery and resulting further myocardial infarction, cardiac arrest or sudden death. Coronary angiography and, if indicated, PCI should be undertaken early during the same hospital admission.

In patients with completed STEMI who have not been treated with reperfusion therapy (e.g. because of late presentation) it is usually recommended that coronary angiography is undertaken during the same hospital admission. Although the benefits of re-opening an occluded culprit artery late after STEMI are uncertain, there is often disease in other coronary vessels that can give rise to further major coronary events over subsequent months. Defining the severity and anatomy of such disease can help to identify those at highest risk, in whom early intervention may reduce that risk.

Ventricular arrhythmia complicating acute coronary syndromes

When ventricular arrhythmia complicates an acute coronary syndrome, interpret its significance in the context of the precise clinical setting and the time of onset of the arrhythmia. When VF/VT cardiac arrest occurs within the first 24 - 48 h after STEMI, and subsequent recovery is uncomplicated, the risk of another ventricular arrhythmia is relatively low and is determined by other factors, especially the severity of left ventricular impairment.

If VF/VT cardiac arrest occurs in the context of non-ST segment elevation ACS, there may be a continuing risk of further ventricular arrhythmia. If the arrhythmia has been caused by severe myocardial ischaemia, very urgent revascularisation is needed to prevent recurrence of the ischaemia and reduce the risk of resulting arrhythmia. If this is not achievable or if the arrhythmia has occurred without evidence of severe ischaemia, the patient will be at risk of recurrent ventricular arrhythmia and should be referred to a heart rhythm specialist with a view to insertion of an implantable cardioverter-defibrillator (ICD) **before discharge from hospital.**

Patients who have a VF/VT cardiac arrest as a late complication after myocardial infarction, or outside the context of an ACS, will be at risk of recurrent cardiac arrest and should be seen urgently by a heart rhythm specialist with a view to ICD implantation **before discharge from hospital.**

Other complications of ACS

Heart failure

Patients with heart failure complicating AMI or other ACS are at increased risk of deterioration, cardiac arrest and death: prompt, effective treatment of the heart failure is required to reduce risk. Give a loop diuretic (e.g. furosemide) and/or glyceryl trinitrate (sublingual and/or intravenous) for immediate symptomatic treatment. Give regular loop diuretic to maintain symptom control but review the need for this and the dose at least daily for the first few days. Ensure that angiotensin converting enzyme inhibitor (ACEI) treatment has been started and increase the dose as tolerated, until the target dose is achieved. In patients intolerant of ACEI, consider an angiotensin receptor blocker. Maintain beta blockade unless contraindicated or not tolerated. If more than mild LV systolic impairment is confirmed (ejection fraction 40% or less) consider addition of an aldosterone antagonist (e.g. eplerenone or spironolactone).

Cardiogenic shock

This consists of severe hypotension with poor peripheral perfusion, often accompanied by pulmonary oedema, drowsiness or mental confusion due to poor cerebral under-perfusion and oliguria caused by poor renal perfusion. The mortality is very high, but can be reduced by early revascularisation by PCI.

Some patients may improve with inotropic therapy (e.g. dobutamine) but this requires initiation and supervision by those experienced in its use. Other treatments such as intra-aortic balloon pumping may be of benefit in selected patients, but require expert supervision.

When cardiogenic shock develops in a patient after STEMI, seek early expert assessment with a view to possible emergency PCI as this may be life-saving for some patients in this setting.

Other cardiac arrhythmia

The treatment of other cardiac arrhythmia will be covered in more detail in Chapter 11.

When atrial fibrillation occurs in the context of an ACS it usually indicates some degree of left ventricular failure: treatment should address that as well as focusing on control of heart rate or rhythm.

When AV block occurs in the context of acute inferior wall myocardial infarction there is often excess vagal activity. QRS complexes are often narrow and heart rates may not be excessively slow. Treat symptomatic bradycardia in this setting with atropine and if necessary theophylline, and consider temporary cardiac pacing only if bradycardia and hypotension persist after atropine therapy. Complete AV block in this setting is usually transient and permanent cardiac pacing is often not necessary.

When AV block occurs in the context of acute anterior myocardial infarction this usually implies extensive myocardial injury and a poor prognosis. The QRS complexes are usually broad and the heart rate is usually slow and resistant to atropine. Temporary cardiac pacing is usually needed and should not be delayed. Many of those who survive this situation will require a permanent pacemaker.

Cardiac rehabilitation

In all patients after an ACS, an effective programme of cardiac rehabilitation can speed the return to normal activity and encourage measures that will reduce future risk (see below). There is evidence that effective cardiac rehabilitation reduces the need for readmission to hospital. Cardiac rehabilitation is a continuous process, beginning in the cardiac care unit and progressing through to a community-based approach to lifestyle modification and secondary prevention.

Secondary prevention

In patients with established coronary disease, general measures to reduce cardiovascular risk ('secondary prevention') can reduce the likelihood of future coronary events (including sudden cardiac death) and stroke.

Anti-thrombotic therapy

Continued platelet inhibition is appropriate in all patients. They should receive low-dose aspirin (75 mg daily) for life, unless they have or develop a contra-indication. Give clopidogrel 75 mg daily (or prasugrel 10 mg daily) to patients with high-risk ACS and all those undergoing PCI;

current guidelines recommend treatment for a minimum of one year. Clopidogrel alone may be used in patients who are intolerant of aspirin. In patients who develop atrial fibrillation as a complication of ischaemic heart disease, there is an additional risk of thromboembolism from the left atrium. Warfarin is more effective than aspirin or clopidogrel in preventing intra-cardiac thrombus formation, and should be considered in addition to, or instead of platelet inhibition.

Preservation of left ventricular function

Prognosis after AMI is determined partly by the severity of left ventricular impairment that results. Treatment after AMI with an ACEI can reduce the re-modelling that contributes to left ventricular dilatation and impairment, and where there is left ventricular systolic impairment, the use of ACEI therapy in adequate dose can reduce the risk and severity of subsequent heart failure, and the risk of future AMI and death. Echocardiographic examination of left ventricular function is appropriate during the first few days after an ACS to assess risk and identify those patients likely to benefit most from this treatment. The majority of patients should be considered for ACEI treatment during the first few days after AMI.

Beta-adrenoceptor blockade

Treatment with a beta blocker, started early after AMI and continued, was shown many years ago to reduce mortality, so beta blockade that has been started in the acute phase of treatment is usually continued, often indefinitely. There is evidence that prior treatment with beta blockade may reduce the size of subsequent myocardial infarction, so in patients with coronary disease this treatment may have a 'cardioprotective' effect, and it may help to protect against other complications such as arrhythmia. In patients with heart failure and left ventricular systolic impairment there is evidence of symptomatic and prognostic benefit from some beta blocking drugs (e.g. bisoprolol, carvedilol).

Reduction of cholesterol

Further reduction in risk can be achieved by effective suppression of cholesterol concentration in the blood; specifically, suppression of LDL cholesterol. Statins reduce the risk of most future coronary events by at least 30%. A low-fat, high-fibre diet and regular exercise will complement cholesterol suppression by drugs.

Avoidance of smoking

At least as important in reducing risk, is the removal of other avoidable risk factors such as smoking. Information, encouragement and support for patients to help them to stop smoking should begin at an early stage after presentation with an ACS.

Anti-hypertensive treatment

Effective control of raised blood pressure, using drugs as well as non-pharmacological methods, reduces the risk of stroke and of heart failure and contributes to some reduction in the risk of future coronary events.

Key learning points

- The acute coronary syndromes comprise unstable angina, non-ST-segment-elevation myocardial infarction, and ST-segment-elevation myocardial infarction.

- Give aspirin, nitroglycerine and morphine to patients presenting with acute coronary syndromes. Give oxygen to achieve SPO_2 of 94-98% (or 88-92% in the presence of COPD)

- Rapid initial assessment using the history, examination and 12-lead ECG will help to determine the diagnosis and immediate risk.

- Consider immediate reperfusion therapy in those patients with acute myocardial infarction accompanied by ST segment elevation or new LBBB.

- Effective assessment and immediate treatment of patients with acute coronary syndromes will reduce the risk of cardiac arrest and death.

Further reading

Arntz HR, Bossaert L, Danchin N, Nikolaou N. European Resuscitation Council Guidelines for Resuscitation 2010. Section 5. Initial Management of Acute Coronary Syndromes Resuscitation 2010;81:1353-63.

Bassand JP, Hamm CW, Ardissino D, et al. Guidelines for the diagnosis and treatment of non-ST-segment elevation acute coronary syndromes. Eur Heart J 2007;28:1598-660. www.escardio.org

Bossaert L, O'Connor RE, Arntz H-R, et al. 2010 International Consensus on Cardiopulmonary Resuscitation and Emergency Cardiovascular Care Science with Treatment Recommendations. Part 9: Acute Coronary Syndromes. Resuscitation 2010;81:e170-e207.

Department of Health 2008. Treatment of Heart Attack National Guidance. Final Report of the National Infarct Angioplasty Project (NIAP). www.dh.gov.uk

Silber S, Albertsson P, Aviles FF, et al. The Task Force for Percutaneous Coronary Interventions of the European Society of Cardiology. Guidelines for Percutaneous Coronary Interventions. European Heart Journal 2005;26:804-47. www.escardio.org

Thygesen K, Alpert JS, White HD. Universal definition of myocardial infarction. Eur Heart J 2007;28:2525-38. www.escardio.org

Van de Werf F, Bax J, Betriu A, et al. Management of acute myocardial infarction in patients presenting with persistent ST-segment elevation: the Task Force on the Management of ST-Segment Elevation Acute Myocardial Infarction of the European Society of Cardiology. Eur Heart J 2008;29:2909-45. www.escardio.org

CHAPTER 5

In-hospital Resuscitation

Learning outcomes

To understand:

▶ **How to start resuscitation in hospital**

▶ **How to continue resuscitation until more experienced help arrives**

▶ **The importance of high quality CPR with minimal interruption**

Introduction

After in-hospital cardiac arrest, the division between basic life support and advanced life support is arbitrary; in practice, the resuscitation process is a continuum. The public expect that clinical staff can undertake cardiopulmonary resuscitation (CPR). For all in-hospital cardiac arrests, ensure that:

- cardiorespiratory arrest is recognised immediately;

- help is summoned using a standard telephone number, e.g. 2222 in the UK;

- CPR is started immediately and, if indicated, defibrillation is attempted as soon as possible (within 3 min at the most).

This chapter is primarily for healthcare professionals who are first to respond to an in-hospital cardiac arrest, but may also be applicable to healthcare professionals working in other clinical settings.

Why is in-hospital resuscitation different?

The exact sequence of actions after in-hospital cardiac arrest depends on several factors including:

- location (clinical/non clinical area; monitored/unmonitored area);

- skills of the first responders;

- number of responders;

- equipment available;

- hospital response system to cardiac arrest and medical emergencies, e.g. medical emergency team (MET), resuscitation team.

Location

In patients who are being monitored closely, cardiorespiratory arrest is usually identified rapidly. Patients in many areas without facilities for close monitoring may have had a period of deterioration and can have an unwitnessed arrest. All patients who are at high risk of cardiac arrest should be cared for in a monitored area where facilities for immediate resuscitation are available. Patients, visitors or staff may also have a cardiac arrest in non-clinical areas (e.g. car parks, corridors). Victims of cardiac arrest may need to be moved to enable effective resuscitation. The Resuscitation Council (UK) has published guidance for safer handling during resuscitation in healthcare settings (http://www.resus.org.uk/pages/safehand.pdf).

Training of first responders

All healthcare professionals should be able to recognise cardiac arrest, call for help and start resuscitation. Staff should do what they have been trained to do. For example, staff in critical care and emergency medicine may have more advanced resuscitation skills and greater experience in resuscitation than those who are not involved regularly in resuscitation in their normal clinical role. Hospital staff who respond to a cardiac arrest may have different levels of skill to manage the airway, breathing and circulation. Rescuers must use the skills for which they are trained.

Number of responders

The single responder must always ensure that help is coming. Usually, other staff are nearby and several actions can be undertaken simultaneously. Hospital staffing tends to be at its lowest during the night and at weekends. This may influence patient monitoring, treatment and outcomes. Studies show that survival rates from in-hospital cardiac arrest are lower during nights and weekends.

Equipment available

Staff in all clinical areas should have immediate access to resuscitation equipment and drugs to facilitate rapid resuscitation of the patient in cardiorespiratory arrest. Ideally, the equipment used for cardiopulmonary resuscitation (including defibrillators) and the layout of equipment and drugs should be standardised throughout the hospital. You should be familiar with the resuscitation equipment used in your clinical area.

In-hospital Resuscitation

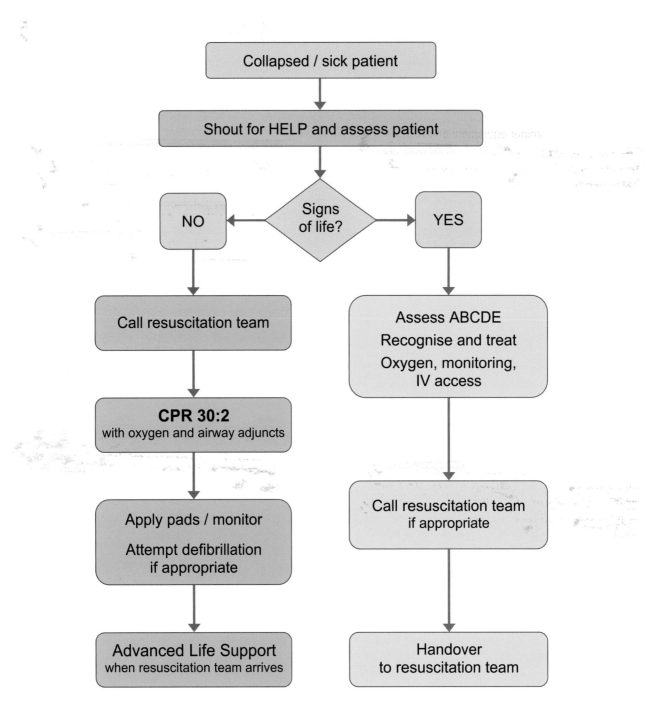

Figure 5.1 In-hospital resuscitation algorithm

A review by the Resuscitation Council (UK) of serious patient safety incidents associated with CPR and patient deterioration reported to the National Patient Safety Agency showed that equipment problems during resuscitation (e.g. equipment missing or not working) is common. All resuscitation equipment needs to be checked on a regular basis to ensure it is ready for use. AEDs should be considered for clinical and non-clinical areas where staff do not have rhythm recognition skills or rarely need to use a defibrillator.

After successful resuscitation, patients may need transferring to other clinical areas (e.g. intensive care unit) or other hospitals. Transfer equipment and drugs should be available to enable this. This should include waveform capnography for those patients have had tracheal intubation and are ventilated (see Chapter 7).

Resuscitation team

The resuscitation team may take the form of a traditional cardiac arrest team, which is called only when cardiac arrest is recognised. Alternatively, hospitals may have strategies to recognise patients at risk of cardiac arrest and summon a team (e.g. MET) before cardiac arrest occurs. The term resuscitation team reflects the range of response teams. In-hospital cardiac arrests are rarely sudden or unexpected. A strategy of recognising patients at risk of cardiac arrest may enable some of these arrests to be prevented or prevent futile resuscitation attempts in those who are unlikely to benefit from CPR (Chapter 3).

Resuscitation teams rarely have formal pre- and post event briefings (briefings and debriefings) to plan roles and actions during resuscitations. Resuscitation team members should meet for introductions and plan before they attend actual events. Team members should also debrief after each event based on what they actually did during the resuscitation. This should ideally be based on data collected during the event.

Sequence for collapsed patient in a hospital

An algorithm for the initial management of in-hospital cardiac arrest is shown in Figure 5.1.

1. Ensure personal safety

There are very few reports of harm to rescuers during resuscitation.

- Your personal safety and that of resuscitation team members is the first priority during any resuscitation attempt.

- Check that the patient's surroundings are safe.

- Put on gloves as soon as possible. Other protective measures, such as eye protection, aprons and face masks, may be necessary.

- The risk of infection is much lower than perceived. There are isolated reports of infections such as tuberculosis (TB), and severe acute respiratory distress syndrome (SARS). Transmission of HIV during CPR has never been reported.

- Wear full personal protective equipment (PPE) when the victim has a serious infection such as TB or SARS. Follow local infection control measures to minimise risks.

- Be careful with sharps; a sharps box must be available. Use safe handling techniques for moving victims during resuscitation.

- Take care with patients exposed to poisons. Avoid mouth-to-mouth ventilation and exhaled air in hydrogen cyanide or hydrogen sulphide poisoning.

- Avoid contact with corrosive chemicals (e.g. strong acids, alkalis, paraquat) or substances such as organophosphates that are easily absorbed through the skin or respiratory tract.

- There are no reports of infection acquired during CPR training. Nevertheless, take sensible precautions to minimise potential cross-infection from manikins. Clean manikins regularly and disinfect thoroughly after each use. Some manikins have disposable face pieces and airways to simplify cleaning.

2. Check the patient for a response

- If you see a patient collapse or find a patient apparently unconscious first shout for help, then assess if he is responsive (shake and shout). Gently shake his shoulders and ask loudly: "Are you all right?" (Figure 5.2).

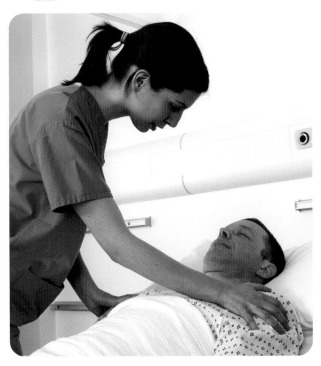

Figure 5.2 Shake and shout

- If other members of staff are nearby it will be possible to undertake actions simultaneously.

3A If he responds

- Urgent medical assessment is required. Call for help according to local protocols. This may be a resuscitation team (e.g. MET).

- While waiting for the team, assess the patient using the ABCDE (Airway, Breathing, Circulation, Disability, Exposure) approach.

- Give the patient oxygen - use pulse oximetry to guide oxygen therapy.

- Attach monitoring (minimum pulse oximetry, ECG and blood pressure) and record vital signs.

- Obtain venous access.

- Prepare for handover to team using SBAR (Situation, Background, Assessment, Recommendation) or RSVP (Reason, Story, Vital signs, Plan).

3B If he does not respond

- The exact sequence will depend on your training and experience in assessment of breathing and circulation in sick patients. Agonal breathing (occasional gasps, slow, laboured or noisy breathing) is common in the early stages of cardiac arrest and is a sign of cardiac arrest and should not be confused as a sign of life.

- Shout for help (if not already).

- Turn the patient on to his back.

- Open the airway using head tilt and chin lift (Figure 5.3).

- If there is a risk of cervical spine injury, establish a clear upper airway by using jaw thrust or chin lift in combination with manual in-line stabilisation (MILS) of the head and neck by an assistant (if enough personnel are available). If life-threatening airway obstruction persists despite effective application of jaw thrust or chin lift, add head tilt a small amount at a time until the airway is open; establishing a patent airway, oxygenation and ventilation takes priority over concerns about a potential cervical spine injury.

- Keeping the airway open, look, listen, and feel (Figure 5.4) to determine if the victim is breathing normally. This is a rapid check and should take **less than 10 seconds**:

  - Look for chest movement (breathing or coughing).

  - Look for any other movement or signs of life.

  - Listen at the victim's mouth for breath sounds.

  - Feel for air on your cheek.

- If the patient has no signs of life (based on lack of purposeful movement, normal breathing, coughing), start CPR until more help arrives or the patient shows signs of life.

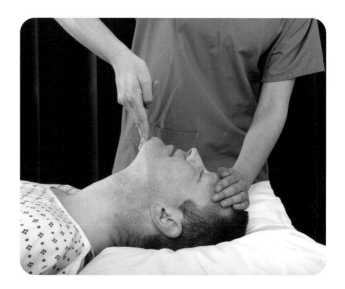

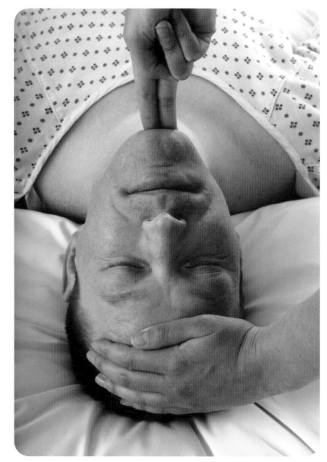

Figure 5.3 Head tilt and chin lift

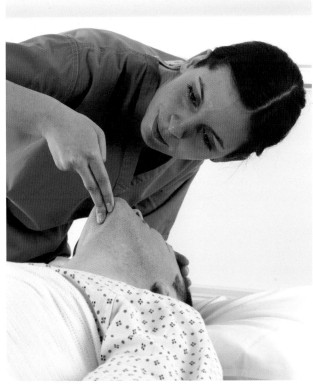

Figure 5.4 Looking for breathing and any other movement

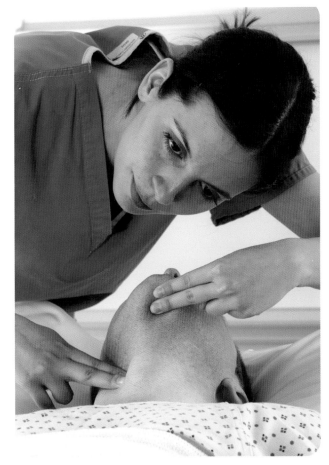

Figure 5.5 Simultaneous check for breathing and carotid pulse

- If trained and experienced in the assessment of sick patients, check for breathing and assess the carotid pulse at the same time (Figure 5.5).

- If the patient has no signs of life, no pulse, or if there is any doubt, start CPR immediately.

- If unsure, do not delay starting CPR. Delays in diagnosis of cardiac arrest and starting CPR will affect survival adversely and must be avoided. Several studies show that even trained healthcare staff cannot assess the breathing and pulse sufficiently reliably to confirm cardiac arrest. Agonal breathing (occasional gasps, slow, laboured or noisy breathing) is common in the early stages of cardiac arrest and is a sign of cardiac arrest and should not be confused as a sign of life/circulation. Agonal breathing can also occur during chest compressions as cerebral perfusion improves, but is not indicative of a return of spontaneous circulation. Starting CPR on a very sick patient with a low cardiac output is unlikely to be harmful and may be beneficial. However, delays in diagnosis of cardiac arrest and starting CPR will effect survival adversely and must be avoided.

- Assess the patient to confirm cardiac arrest even if the patient is monitored in a critical care area.

4A If there is a pulse or other signs of life

- Urgent medical assessment is required. Depending on the local protocols, this may take the form of a resuscitation team. While awaiting this team, assess the patient using the ABCDE approach, give oxygen, attach monitoring, and insert an intravenous cannula.

- Follow the steps in 3A above whilst waiting for the team.

- The patient is at high risk of further deterioration and cardiac arrest and needs continued observation until the team arrives.

4B If there is no pulse or signs of life

- Start CPR and get a colleague to call the resuscitation team (Figure 5.6) and collect the resuscitation equipment and a defibrillator.

- If alone, leave the patient to get help and equipment.

- Give 30 chest compressions followed by 2 ventilations.

- The correct hand position for chest compression is the middle of the lower half of the sternum (Figure 5.7).

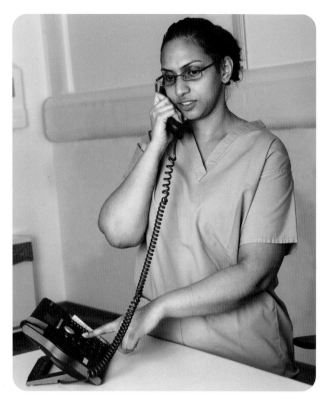

Figure 5.6 Call the resuscitation team

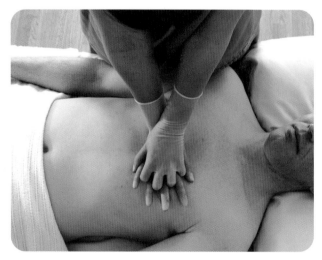

Figure 5.7 Hand position for chest compressions

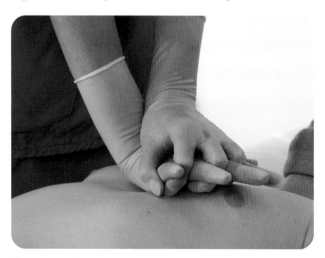

Figure 5.8 Hands placed in the middle of the lower half of the sternum

- This hand position can be found quickly if you have been taught to 'place the heel of one hand in the centre of the chest with the other hand on top' and your teaching included a demonstration of placing hands in the middle of the lower half of the sternum (Figure 5.8).

- Ensure high quality chest compressions:

  - Depth of 5 - 6 cm

  - Rate of 100 - 120 compressions min⁻¹

  - Allow the chest to recoil completely after each compression

  - Take approximately the same amount for compression and relaxation

  - Minimise any interruptions to chest compression (hands-off time)

- If available, use a prompt and/or feedback device to help ensure high quality chest compressions. Do not rely on a palpable carotid or femoral pulse to assess effective arterial flow.

- Each time compressions are resumed, place your hands without delay in the centre of the chest.

- The person doing chest compressions will get tired. If there are enough rescuers, this person should change about every 2 min or earlier if unable to maintain high quality chest compressions. This change should be done with minimal interruption to compressions.

- Use whatever equipment is available immediately for airway and ventilation. A pocket mask, which can be supplemented with an oral airway should be readily available (Figure 5.9). Alternatively, use a supraglottic airway device (e.g. laryngeal mask airway (LMA)) and self-inflating bag, or bag-mask, according to local policy.

- Tracheal intubation should be attempted only by those who are trained, competent and experienced in this skill. Waveform capnography should be routinely available for confirming tracheal tube placement (in the presence of a cardiac output) and subsequent monitoring of an intubated patient. Waveform capnography can also be used to monitor the quality of CPR.

- Use an inspiratory time of about 1 s and give enough volume to produce a visible chest rise. Add supplemental oxygen as soon as possible.

- Avoid rapid or forceful breaths.

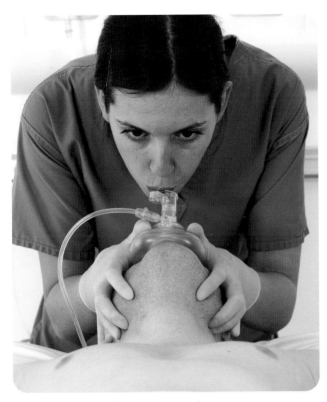

Figure 5.9 Use of the pocket mask

- Once the patient's trachea has been intubated, continue chest compressions uninterrupted (except for defibrillation or pulse checks when indicated), at a rate of 100 - 120 min⁻¹, and ventilate the lungs at approximately 10 breaths min⁻¹ (i.e. do not stop chest compressions for ventilation). Avoid hyperventilation (both excessive rate and tidal volume), which may worsen outcome. If a supraglottic airway (e.g. LMA) device has been inserted it may also be possible to ventilate the patient without stopping chest compressions.

L is that after 30 compression or ventilate 10 breaths.

- If airway and ventilation equipment are unavailable, consider mouth-to-mouth ventilation. If there are clinical reasons to avoid mouth-to-mouth contact, or you are unwilling or unable to do this, do chest compressions until help or airway equipment arrives. A pocket mask or bag-mask should be immediately available in all clinical areas. A pocket mask with filter, or a barrier device with one-way valve will minimise infection risk during rescue breathing.

- **When the defibrillator arrives**, apply self-adhesive defibrillation electrodes to the patient and analyse the rhythm. These should be applied whilst chest compressions are ongoing (Figure 5.10). The use of adhesive electrode pads will enable rapid assessment of heart rhythm compared with attaching ECG electrodes.

- If using an automated external defibrillator (AED) switch on the machine and follow the AED's audio-visual prompts.

- For manual defibrillation, minimise the interruption to CPR to deliver a shock (see Chapter 9 for a more detailed sequence of actions for manual defibrillation). Using a manual defibrillator, it is possible to reduce the pause between stopping and restarting of chest compressions to < 5 s.

- This means that safety issues should be addressed and planned for while chest compressions are ongoing. Plan what to do if the rhythm is shockable before CPR is stopped.

- Pause briefly to assess the heart rhythm. With a manual defibrillator, if the rhythm is ventricular fibrillation/pulseless ventricular tachycardia (VF/VT), charge the defibrillator and restart chest compressions. Once the defibrillator is charged and everyone apart from the person doing compressions is clear, pause the chest compressions, rapidly ensure that all rescuers are clear of the patient and then deliver the shock. Restart chest compressions immediately after shock delivery. This sequence should be planned before stopping chest compressions for the rhythm check.

- The length of the pre-shock pause, the interval between stopping chest compressions and delivering a shock, is inversely proportional to the chance of successful defibrillation. Every 5 s increase in the duration of the pre-shock pause almost halves the chance of successful defibrillation, therefore it is critical to minimise the pause. The lengthy 'top-to-toe' safety check (e.g. "head, middle, bottom, self, oxygen away") performed after the defibrillator has charged and before shock delivery, commonly taught and used in clinical practice, will therefore significantly diminish the chances of successful defibrillation.

- Rescuers should not compromise on safety. Actions should be planned before stopping chest compressions. If there are delays caused by

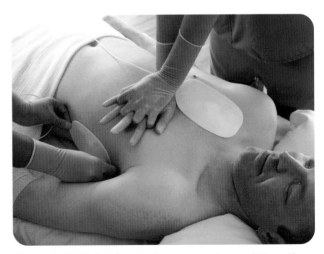

Figure 5.10 Maintain chest compressions while self-adhesive pads are applied

difficulties in rhythm analysis or if individuals are still in contact with the patient, chest compressions should be restarted whilst plans are made to decide what to do when compressions are next stopped. Rescuers should wear gloves during CPR attempts. If they are not immediately available this should not delay starting CPR. Wearing gloves may decrease the risk of accidental shocks to rescuers although this requires further study.

- Continue resuscitation until the resuscitation team arrives or the patient shows signs of life. Follow the advanced life support algorithm (see Chapter 6).

- Once resuscitation is underway, and if there are sufficient staff present, prepare intravenous cannulae and drugs likely to be used by the resuscitation team (e.g. adrenaline).

- Use a watch or clock for timing between rhythm checks. It is difficult to keep track of the number of 30:2 cycles. Any interruption to CPR should be planned before completing the cycle.

- The importance of uninterrupted chest compressions cannot be over emphasised. Even short interruptions to chest compressions are disastrous for outcome and every effort must be made to ensure that continuous, effective chest compression is maintained throughout the resuscitation attempt.

- Identify one person to be responsible for handover to the resuscitation team leader. Use a structured communication tool for handover (e.g. SBAR, RSVP). Locate the patient's records.

4C If he is not breathing and has a pulse (respiratory arrest)

- Ventilate the patient's lungs (as described above) and check for a pulse every 10 breaths (about every minute).

- This diagnosis can be made only if you are confident in assessing breathing and pulse or the patient has other signs of life (e.g. warm and well perfused, normal capillary refill).

- If there are any doubts about the presence of a pulse, start chest compressions until more experienced help arrives.

- All patients in respiratory arrest will develop cardiac arrest if the respiratory arrest is not treated rapidly and effectively.

5 If the patient has a monitored and witnessed cardiac arrest

If a patient has a monitored and witnessed cardiac arrest in the catheter laboratory or early after cardiac surgery:

- Confirm cardiac arrest and shout for help.

- If the initial rhythm is VF/VT, give up to three quick successive (stacked) shocks. Start chest compressions immediately after the third shock and continue CPR for 2 min. With respect to the ALS algorithm, these three quick, successive shocks are regarded as the first shock.

- This three-shock strategy may also be considered for an initial, witnessed VF/VT cardiac arrest if the patient is already connected to a manual defibrillator - these circumstances are rare.

- A precordial thump in these settings rarely works and may succeed only if given within seconds of the onset of a shockable rhythm. Delivery of a precordial thump must not delay calling for help or accessing a defibrillator. It is therefore appropriate therapy only when several clinicians are present at a witnessed, monitored arrest, and when a defibrillator is not immediately to hand. In practice, this is only likely to be in a critical care setting such as the emergency department or ICU.

National Cardiac Arrest Audit

All in-hospital cardiac arrests should be reviewed and audited. The National Cardiac Arrest Audit (NCAA) is a UK-wide database of in-hospital cardiac arrests and is supported by the Resuscitation Council (UK) and the Intensive Care National Audit & Research Centre (ICNARC). NCAA monitors and reports on the incidence of and outcome from, in-hospital cardiac arrests in order to inform practice and policy. It aims to identify and foster improvements in the prevention, care delivery and outcomes from cardiac arrest. Participating in NCAA means that your hospital is collecting and contributing to national, standardised data on cardiac arrest, enabling improvements in patient care.

Key learning points

- The exact sequence of actions after in-hospital cardiac arrest depends on the location, skills of the first responders, number of responders, equipment available, and the hospital response system to cardiac arrest and medical emergencies.

- Deliver high quality chest compressions with a depth of 5 - 6 cm, rate of 100 - 120 min^{-1}, and allow complete recoil between compressions.

- Minimise interruptions to chest compressions for other interventions – this means all interruptions must be planned before stopping compressions.

Further reading

Abella BS, Alvarado JP, Myklebust H, et al. Quality of cardiopulmonary resuscitation during in-hospital cardiac arrest. JAMA 2005;293:305-10.

Chan PS, Krumholz HM, Nichol G, Nallamothu BK. Delayed time to defibrillation after in-hospital cardiac arrest. N Engl J Med 2008;358:9-17.

Deakin CD, Nolan JP, Soar J, et al. European Resuscitation Council Guidelines for Resuscitation 2010. Section 4. Adult Advanced Life Support. Resuscitation 2010;81:1305-52.

Deakin CD, Nolan JP, Sunde K, Koster RW European Resuscitation Council guidelines for resuscitation 2010. Section 3. Electrical therapies: automated external defibrillators, defibrillation, cardioversion and pacing. Resuscitation 2010;81:1293-1304.

Edelson DP, Abella BS, Kramer-Johansen J, et al. Effects of compression depth and pre-shock pauses predict defibrillation failure during cardiac arrest. Resuscitation 2006;71:137-45.

Edelson DP, Litzinger B, Arora V, et al. Improving in-hospital cardiac arrest process and outcomes with performance debriefing. Arch Intern Med 2008;168:1063-9.

Gabbott D, Smith G, Mitchell S, et al. Cardiopulmonary resuscitation standards for clinical practice and training in the UK. Resuscitation 2005;64:13-9.

Koster RW, Baubin MA, Caballero A, et al. European Resuscitation Council Guidelines for Resuscitation 2010. Section 2. Adult basic life support and use of automated external defibrillators. Resuscitation 2010;81:1277-92.

Marshall S, Harrison J, Flanagan B. The teaching of a structured tool improves the clarity and content of interprofessional clinical communication. Qual Saf Health Care 2009;18:137-40.

Meaney PA, Nadkarni VM, Kern KB, Indik JH, Halperin HR, Berg RA. Rhythms and outcomes of adult in-hospital cardiac arrest. Crit Care Med 2010;38:101-8.

National Patient Safety Agency. Establishing a standard crash call telephone number in hospitals. Patient Safety Alert 02. London: National Patient Safety Agency; 2004.

O'Driscoll BR, Howard LS, Davison AG. BTS guideline for emergency oxygen use in adult patients. Thorax 2008;63 Suppl 6:vi1-68.

Peberdy MA, Ornato JP, Larkin GL, et al. Survival from in-hospital cardiac arrest during nights and weekends. JAMA 2008;299:785-92.

Resuscitation Council (UK). Guidance for safer handling during resuscitation in healthcare settings. November 2009. http://www.resus.org.uk/pages/safehand.pdf

Soar J, Mancini ME, Bhanji F, et al. 2010 International Consensus on Cardiopulmonary Resuscitation and Emergency Cardiovascular Care Science with Treatment Recommendations. Part 12: Education, Implementation, and Teams. Resuscitation 2010;81:e283-e325.

Advanced Life Support Algorithm

Introduction

Heart rhythms associated with cardiac arrest are divided into two groups: shockable rhythms (ventricular fibrillation / pulseless ventricular tachycardia (VF/VT)) and non-shockable rhythms (asystole and pulseless electrical activity (PEA)). The principle difference in the management of these two groups of arrhythmias is the need for attempted defibrillation in patients with VF/VT. Subsequent actions, including chest compressions, airway management and ventilation, venous access, injection of adrenaline and the identification and correction of reversible factors, are common to both groups.

The ALS algorithm (Figure 6.1) is a standardised approach to cardiac arrest management. This has the advantage of enabling treatment to be delivered expediently, without protracted discussion. It enables each member of the resuscitation team to predict and prepare for the next stage in the patient's treatment, further enhancing efficiency of the team. Although the ALS algorithm is applicable to most cardiac arrests, additional interventions may be indicated for cardiac arrest caused by special circumstances (see Chapter 12).

The interventions that unquestionably contribute to improved survival after cardiac arrest are prompt and effective bystander cardiopulmonary resuscitation (CPR), uninterrupted, high quality chest compressions, and early defibrillation for VF/VT. The use of adrenaline has been shown to increase return of spontaneous circulation (ROSC), but no resuscitation drugs or advanced airway interventions have been shown to increase survival to hospital discharge after cardiac arrest. Thus, although drugs and advanced airways are still included among ALS interventions, they are of secondary importance to high-quality, uninterrupted chest compressions and early defibrillation.

Shockable rhythms (VF/VT)

The first monitored rhythm is VF/VT in approximately 25% of cardiac arrests, both in- or out-of-hospital. VF/VT will also occur at some stage during resuscitation in about 25% of cardiac arrests with an initial documented rhythm of asystole or PEA.

Treatment of shockable rhythms (VF/VT)

1. Confirm cardiac arrest - check for signs of life or if trained to do so, breathing and pulse simultaneously.

2. Call resuscitation team.

3. Perform uninterrupted chest compressions while applying self-adhesive defibrillation/monitoring pads - one below the right clavicle and the other in the V6 position in the midaxillary line.

4. Plan actions before pausing CPR for rhythm analysis and communicate these to the team.

5. Stop chest compressions; confirm VF from the ECG.

6. Resume chest compressions immediately; simultaneously, the designated person selects the appropriate energy on the defibrillator (150 - 200 J biphasic for the first shock and 150 - 360 J biphasic for subsequent shocks) and presses the charge button (Figure 6.2).

7. While the defibrillator is charging, warn all rescuers other than the individual performing the chest compressions to "stand clear" and remove any oxygen delivery device as appropriate.

8. Once the defibrillator is charged, tell the rescuer doing the chest compressions to "stand clear"; when clear, give the shock (Figure 6.3).

9. Without reassessing the rhythm or feeling for a pulse, restart CPR using a ratio of 30:2, starting with chest compressions.

10. Continue CPR for 2 min; the team leader prepares the team for the next pause in CPR.

Adult Advanced Life Support

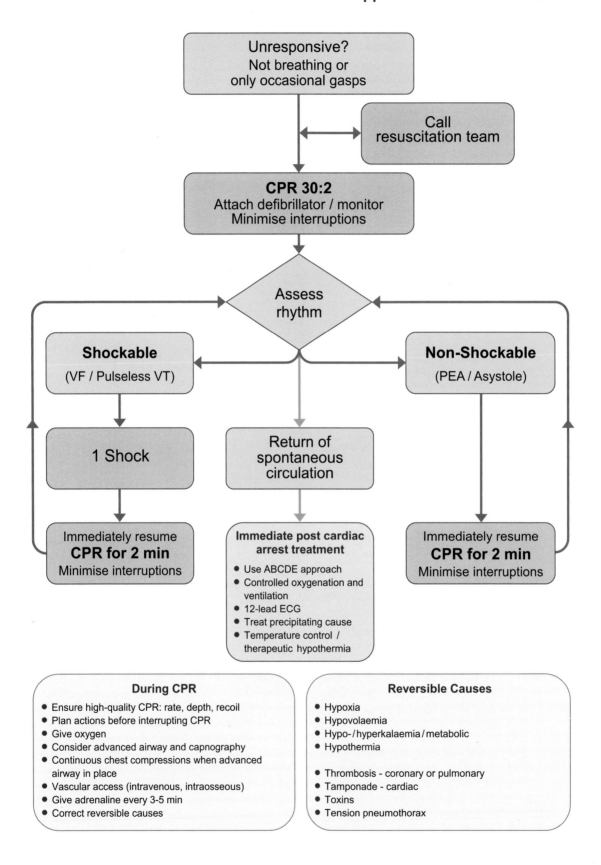

Figure 6.1 Adult advanced life support algorithm

11. Pause briefly to check the monitor.

12. If VF/VT, repeat steps 6 - 11 above and deliver a second shock.

13. If VF/VT persists repeat steps 6 - 8 above and deliver a third shock. Resume chest compressions immediately and then give adrenaline 1 mg IV and amiodarone 300 mg IV while performing a further 2 min CPR.

14. Repeat this 2 min CPR - rhythm/pulse check - defibrillation sequence if VF/VT persists.

15. Give further adrenaline 1 mg IV after alternate shocks (i.e., approximately every 3 - 5 min).

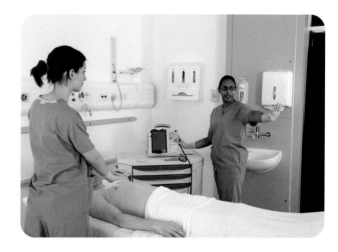

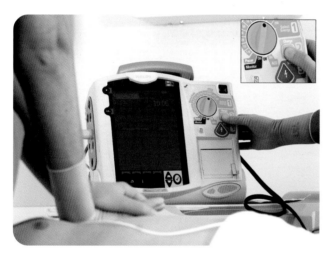

Figure 6.2 Continuing chest compressions during charging with a manual defibrillator

If organised electrical activity compatible with a cardiac output is seen during a rhythm check, seek evidence of ROSC:

- Check a central pulse and end-tidal (ETCO$_2$) trace if available

- If there is evidence of ROSC, start post-resuscitation care.

- If no signs of ROSC, continue CPR and switch to the non-shockable algorithm.

If asystole is seen, continue CPR and switch to the non-shockable algorithm.

The interval between stopping compressions and delivering a shock must be minimised and, ideally, should not exceed 5 s). Longer interruptions to chest compressions reduce the chance of a shock restoring a spontaneous circulation.

Chest compressions are resumed immediately after a shock without checking the rhythm or a pulse because

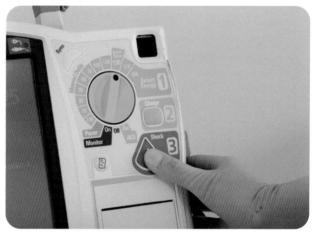

Figure 6.3 Shock delivery

even if the defibrillation attempt is successful in restoring a perfusing rhythm, it is very rare for a pulse to be palpable immediately after defibrillation and the delay in trying to palpate a pulse will further compromise the myocardium if a perfusing rhythm has not been restored. If a perfusing rhythm has been restored, giving chest compressions does not increase the chance of VF recurring. In the presence of post-shock asystole chest compressions may usefully induce VF.

Despite the widespread use of adrenaline during resuscitation, and several studies involving vasopressin, there is no placebo-controlled study that shows that the routine use of any vasopressor at any stage during human cardiac arrest increases neurologically intact survival to hospital discharge. Current evidence is insufficient to support or refute the routine use of any particular drug or sequence of drugs. Despite the lack of human data, the use of adrenaline is still recommended, based largely on animal data and increased short-term survival in humans.

The first dose of adrenaline is given immediately after delivery of the third shock; amiodarone 300 mg may also be given after the third shock. Do not stop CPR to check the rhythm before giving drugs unless there are clear signs of ROSC.

Subsequent doses of adrenaline are given after alternate 2-minute loops of CPR (which equates to every 3 - 5 min) for as long as cardiac arrest persists. If VF/VT persists, or recurs, a further dose of 150 mg amiodarone may be given. Lidocaine, 1 mg kg^{-1}, may be used as an alternative if amiodarone is not available, but do not give lidocaine if amiodarone has been given already.

When the rhythm is checked 2 min after giving a shock, if a non-shockable rhythm is present and the rhythm is organised (complexes appear regular or narrow), try to palpate a central pulse and look for other evidence of ROSC (e.g. sudden increase in ETCO$_2$ or evidence of cardiac output on any invasive monitoring equipment). Rhythm checks must be brief, and pulse checks undertaken only if an organised rhythm is observed. If an organised rhythm is seen during a 2-minute period of CPR, do not interrupt chest compressions to palpate a pulse unless the patient shows signs of life suggesting ROSC. If there is any doubt about the presence of a pulse in the presence of an organised rhythm, resume CPR. If the patient has ROSC, begin post-resuscitation care. If the patient's rhythm changes to asystole or PEA, see non-shockable rhythms below.

It is important in shock-refractory VF/VT to check the position and contact of the defibrillation pads. The duration of any individual resuscitation attempt is a matter of clinical judgement, and should take into account the perceived prospect of a successful outcome. If it was considered appropriate to start resuscitation, it is usually considered worthwhile continuing as long as the patient remains in identifiable VF/VT.

If there is doubt about whether the rhythm is asystole or very fine VF, do not attempt defibrillation; instead, continue chest compressions and ventilation. Very fine VF that is difficult to distinguish from asystole is unlikely to be shocked successfully into a perfusing rhythm. Continuing good-quality CPR may improve the amplitude and frequency of the VF and improve the chance of subsequent successful defibrillation to a perfusing rhythm. Delivering repeated shocks in an attempt to defibrillate what is thought to be very fine VF will increase myocardial injury both directly from the electric current and indirectly from the interruptions in coronary blood flow. If the rhythm is clearly VF, attempt defibrillation.

Precordial thump

A single precordial thump has a very low success rate for cardioversion of a shockable rhythm and is likely to succeed only if given within the first few seconds of the onset of a shockable rhythm. There is more success with pulseless VT than with VF. Delivery of a precordial thump must not delay calling for help or accessing a defibrillator. It is therefore appropriate therapy only when several clinicians are present at a witnessed, monitored arrest, and when a defibrillator is not immediately to hand.

A precordial thump should be undertaken immediately after confirmation of cardiac arrest and only by healthcare professionals trained in the technique. Using the ulnar edge of a tightly clenched fist, deliver a sharp impact to the lower half of the sternum from a height of about 20 cm, then retract the fist immediately to create an impulse-like stimulus. There are very rare reports of a precordial thump converting a perfusing to a non-perfusing rhythm.

Witnessed, monitored VF/VT in the cardiac catheter laboratory or after cardiac surgery

If a patient has a **witnessed** and **monitored** cardiac arrest in the catheter laboratory or early after cardiac surgery:

- Confirm cardiac arrest and shout for help.

- If the initial rhythm is VF/VT, give up to three quick successive (stacked) shocks. Start chest compressions immediately after the third shock and continue CPR for 2 min. With respect to the ALS algorithm, these three quick, successive shocks are regarded as the first shock.

This three-shock strategy may also be considered for an initial, witnessed VF/VT cardiac arrest if the patient is already connected to a manual defibrillator - these circumstances are rare. There are no data supporting a three-shock strategy in any of these circumstances, but it is unlikely that chest compressions will improve the already very high chance of ROSC when defibrillation occurs early in the electrical phase, immediately after onset of VF.

Non-shockable rhythms (PEA and asystole)

Pulseless electrical activity (PEA) is defined as organised cardiac electrical activity in the absence of any palpable pulses. These patients often have some mechanical myocardial contractions but they are too weak to produce a detectable pulse or blood pressure. PEA may be caused by reversible conditions that can be treated (see below). Survival following cardiac arrest with asystole or PEA is unlikely unless a reversible cause can be found and treated quickly and effectively.

Asystole is the absence of electrical activity on the ECG trace. During CPR, ensure the ECG pads are attached to the chest and the correct monitoring mode is selected. Ensure the gain setting is appropriate. Whenever a diagnosis of asystole is made, check the ECG carefully for the presence of P waves because in this situation ventricular standstill may be treated effectively by cardiac pacing. Attempts to pace true asystole are unlikely to be successful.

Treatment for PEA and asystole

- Start CPR 30:2.

- Give adrenaline 1 mg IV / IO as soon as intravascular access is achieved.

- Continue CPR 30:2 until the airway is secured - then continue chest compressions without pausing during ventilation.

- Recheck the rhythm after 2 min:

  - *If organised electrical activity is seen, check for a pulse and/or signs of life:*

    o If a pulse and/or signs of life are present, start post resuscitation care.

    o If no pulse and/or no signs of life are present (PEA):

      ▪ Continue CPR.

      ▪ Recheck the rhythm after 2 min and proceed accordingly.

      ▪ Give further adrenaline 1 mg IV every 3 - 5 min (during alternate 2-min loops of CPR).

  - *If VF/VT at rhythm check, change to shockable side of algorithm.*

  - *If asystole or an agonal rhythm is seen at rhythm check:*

    o Continue CPR.

    o Recheck the rhythm after 2 min and proceed accordingly.

    o Give further adrenaline 1 mg IV every 3 - 5 min (during alternate 2-min loops of CPR).

During CPR

During the treatment of persistent VF/VT or PEA / asystole, emphasis is placed on good quality chest compressions between defibrillation attempts, recognising and treating reversible causes (4 Hs and 4 Ts), obtaining a secure airway, and vascular access.

During CPR with a 30:2 ratio, the underlying rhythm may be seen clearly on the monitor as compressions are paused to enable ventilation. If VF is seen during this brief pause (whether on the shockable or non-shockable side of the algorithm), do not attempt defibrillation at this stage; instead, continue with CPR until the 2-minute period is completed. Knowing that the rhythm is VF, the team should be fully prepared to deliver a shock with minimal delay at the end of the 2-minute period of CPR.

Maintain high quality, uninterrupted chest compressions

The quality of chest compressions and ventilations are important determinants of outcome, yet are frequently performed poorly by healthcare professionals. Avoid interruptions in chest compressions because pauses cause coronary perfusion pressure to decrease substantially. Ensure compressions are of adequate depth (5 - 6 cm) and rate (100 - 120 min^{-1}), and release pressure from the chest completely between compressions.

As soon as the airway is secured, continue chest compressions without pausing during ventilation. To reduce fatigue, change the individual undertaking compressions every 2 min or earlier if necessary. Use CPR feedback / prompt devices when available. Be aware that some devices may fail to compensate for compression of the underlying mattress during CPR on a bed when providing feedback.

Airway and ventilation

A bag-mask, or preferably, a supraglottic airway device (e.g. laryngeal mask airway, i-gel) should be used in the absence of personnel skilled in tracheal intubation (Chapter 7). Once a supraglottic airway device has been inserted, attempt to deliver continuous chest compressions, uninterrupted during ventilation. Ventilate the lungs at 10 breaths min^{-1}; do not hyperventilate the lungs. If excessive gas leakage causes inadequate ventilation of the patient's lungs, chest compressions will have to be interrupted to enable ventilation (using a compression-ventilation ratio of 30:2).

No studies have shown that tracheal intubation increases survival after cardiac arrest. Incorrect placement of the tracheal tube is common in cardiac arrest if intubation is attempted by unskilled personnel. Tracheal intubation should be attempted **only** if the healthcare provider is properly trained and has regular, ongoing experience with the technique. Avoid stopping chest compressions during laryngoscopy and intubation; if necessary, a brief pause in chest compressions may be required as the tube is passed between the vocal cords, but this pause should not exceed 10 s. Alternatively, to avoid any interruptions in chest compressions, the intubation attempt may be deferred until after ROSC. After intubation, confirm correct tube position, ideally with waveform capnography, and secure it adequately. Once the patient's trachea has been intubated, continue chest compressions, at a rate of 100 - 120 min^{-1} without pausing during ventilation.

Vascular access

Obtain intravenous access if this has not been done already. Although peak drug concentrations are higher and circulation times are shorter when drugs are injected into a central venous catheter compared with a peripheral cannula, insertion of a central venous catheter requires interruption of CPR and is associated with several potential complications. Peripheral venous cannulation is quicker, easier, and safer. Drugs injected peripherally must be followed by a flush of at least 20 ml of fluid and elevation of the extremity for 10 - 20 s to facilitate drug delivery to the central circulation. If intravenous access cannot be established within the first 2 min of resuscitation, consider gaining intraosseous (IO) access (Figure 6.4). Tibial and humeral sites are readily accessible and provide equal flows for fluids. Intraosseous delivery of resuscitation drugs will achieve adequate plasma concentrations. Several studies indicate that IO access is safe and effective for fluid resuscitation and drug delivery.

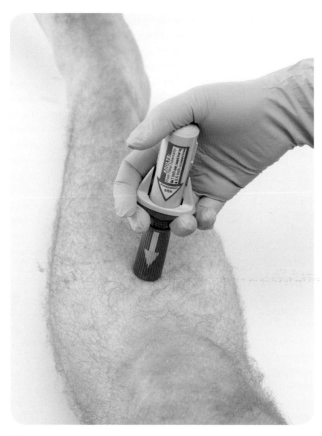

Figure 6.4 Intraosseous device

Reversible causes

Potential causes or aggravating factors for which specific treatment exists must be considered during any cardiac arrest. For ease of memory, these are divided into two groups of four based upon their initial letter - either H or T (Figure 6.5). More details on many of these conditions are covered in Chapter 12.

- Hypoxia

- Hypovolaemia

- Hyperkalaemia, hypokalaemia, hypoglycaemia, hypocalcaemia, acidaemia and other metabolic disorders

- Hypothermia

- Tension pneumothorax

- Tamponade

- Toxins

- Thrombosis (pulmonary embolism or coronary thrombosis)

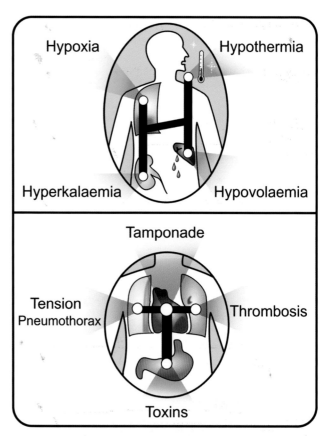

Figure 6.5 The four Hs and four Ts

The four Hs

Minimise the risk of **hypoxia** by ensuring that the patient's lungs are ventilated adequately with 100% oxygen. Make sure there is adequate chest rise and bilateral breath sounds. Using the techniques described in Chapter 7, check carefully that the tracheal tube is not misplaced in a bronchus or the oesophagus.

Pulseless electrical activity caused by **hypovolaemia** is due usually to severe haemorrhage. Evidence of haemorrhage may be obvious, e.g. trauma (Chapter 12), or occult e.g. gastrointestinal bleeding, or rupture of an aortic aneurysm. Intravascular volume should be restored rapidly with fluid and blood, coupled with urgent surgery to stop the haemorrhage.

Hyperkalaemia, hypokalaemia, hypoglycaemia, hypocalcaemia, acidaemia and other metabolic disorders are detected by biochemical tests or suggested by the patient's medical history e.g. renal failure (Chapter 12).

A 12-lead ECG may show suggestive features. Intravenous calcium chloride is indicated in the presence of hyperkalaemia, hypocalcaemia, and calcium channel-blocker overdose.

Suspect **hypothermia** in any drowning incident (Chapter 12); use a low reading thermometer.

The four Ts

A **tension pneumothorax** may be the primary cause of PEA and may follow attempts at central venous catheter insertion. The diagnosis is made clinically. Decompress rapidly by thoracostomy or needle thoracocentesis and then insert a chest drain.

Cardiac **tamponade** is difficult to diagnose because the typical signs of distended neck veins and hypotension cannot be assessed during cardiac arrest. Cardiac arrest after penetrating chest trauma or after cardiac surgery should raise strong suspicion of tamponade - the need for needle pericardiocentesis or resuscitative thoracotomy should be considered in this setting (Chapter 12).

In the absence of a specific history of accidental or deliberate ingestion, poisoning by therapeutic or **toxic** substances may be difficult to detect but in some cases may be revealed later by laboratory investigations (Chapter 12). Where available, the appropriate antidotes should be used but most often the required treatment is supportive. The commonest cause of **thromboembolic** or mechanical circulatory obstruction is massive pulmonary embolism. If pulmonary embolism is thought to be the cause cardiac arrest consider giving a thrombolytic drug immediately. Following fibrinolysis during CPR for acute pulmonary embolism, survival and good neurological outcome have been reported in cases requiring in excess of 60 min of CPR. If a fibrinolytic drug is given in these circumstances, consider performing CPR for at least 60 - 90 min before termination of resuscitation attempts.

Use of ultrasound during advanced life support

In skilled hands, ultrasound can be useful for the detection of potentially reversible causes of cardiac arrest (e.g. cardiac tamponade, pulmonary embolism, ischaemia (regional wall motion abnormality), aortic dissection, hypovolaemia, pneumothorax). The integration of ultrasound into advanced life support requires considerable training if interruptions to chest compressions are to be minimised. A sub-xiphoid probe position is recommended (Figure 6.6). Placement of the probe just before chest compressions are paused for a planned rhythm assessment enables a well-trained operator to obtain views within 10 s. The Focused Echocardiography Extended Life Support Course (FEEL-UK) provides a valuable introduction to echocardiography in this setting.

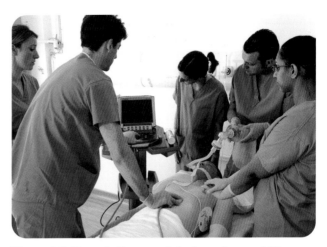

Figure 6.6 Use of ultrasound during advanced life support

Signs of life

If signs of life (such as regular respiratory effort, movement) or readings from patient monitors compatible with ROSC (e.g. sudden increase in exhaled carbon dioxide or arterial blood pressure waveform) appear during CPR, stop CPR briefly and check the monitor. If an organised rhythm is present, check for a pulse. If a pulse is palpable, continue post-resuscitation care and/or treatment of peri-arrest arrhythmias if appropriate. If no pulse is present, continue CPR. The use of waveform capnography may enable ROSC to be detected without pausing chest compressions. A significant increase in $ETCO_2$ during CPR may be seen when ROSC occurs.

Discontinuing resuscitation and diagnosing death

If attempts at obtaining ROSC are unsuccessful the cardiac arrest team leader should discuss stopping CPR with the resuscitation team. The decision to stop CPR requires clinical judgement and a careful assessment of the likelihood of achieving ROSC.

After stopping CPR, observe the patient for a minimum of 5 min before confirming death. The absence of mechanical cardiac function is normally confirmed using a combination of the following:

- absence of a central pulse on palpation;

- absence of heart sounds on auscultation.

One or more of the following can supplement these criteria:

- asystole on a continuous ECG display;

- absence of pulsatile flow using direct intra-arterial pressure monitoring;

- absence of contractile activity using echocardiography.

Any return of cardiac or respiratory activity during this period of observation should prompt a further 5 min observation from the next point of cardiorespiratory arrest. After 5 min of continued cardiorespiratory arrest, the absence of the pupillary responses to light, of the corneal reflexes, and of any motor response to supra-orbital pressure should be confirmed. The time of death is recorded as the time at which these criteria are fulfilled.

Key learning points

- The ALS algorithm provides a framework for the standardised resuscitation of all adult patients in cardiac arrest.

- The delivery of high quality chest compression with minimal interruptions and avoidance of hyperventilation are important determinants of outcome.

- Treatment depends on the underlying rhythm.

- Look for reversible causes and, if present, treat early.

- Whenever possible, secure the airway early to enable continuous chest compressions.

Further reading

Academy of Medical Royal Colleges. A code of practice for the diagnosis and confirmation of death. 2008. http://www.aomrc.org.uk

Deakin CD, Morrison LJ, Morley PT, et al. 2010 International Consensus on Cardiopulmonary Resuscitation and Emergency Cardiovascular Care Science with Treatment Recommendations. Part 8: Advanced Life Support. Resuscitation 2010;81:e93-e169.

Deakin CD, Nolan JP, Soar J, et al. European Resuscitation Council Guidelines for Resuscitation 2010. Section 4. Adult Advanced Life Support. Resuscitation 2010;81:1305-52.

Deakin CD, Nolan JP, Sunde K, Koster RW. European Resuscitation Council Guidelines for Resuscitation 2010. Section 3. Electrical Therapies: Automated External Defibrillators, Defibrillation, Cardioversion and Pacing. Resuscitation 2010;81:1293-1304.

Sunde K, Jacobs I, Deakin CD, et al. 2010 International Consensus on Cardiopulmonary Resuscitation and Emergency Cardiovascular Care Science with Treatment Recommendations. Part 6: Defibrillation. Resuscitation 2010;81:e71-e85.

Yeung J, Meeks R, Edelson D, Gao F, Soar J, Perkins GD. The use of CPR feedback/prompt devices during training and CPR performance: A systematic review. Resuscitation 2009;80:743-51.

Airway Management and Ventilation

CHAPTER 7

Section 1. Basic airway management and ventilation

Learning outcomes

To understand:

▶ **The causes and recognition of airway obstruction**

▶ **Techniques for airway management when starting resuscitation**

▶ **The use of simple adjuncts to maintain airway patency**

▶ **The use of simple devices for ventilating the lungs**

Introduction

Patients requiring resuscitation often have an obstructed airway, usually caused by loss of consciousness, but occasionally it may be the primary cause of cardiorespiratory arrest. Prompt assessment, with control of airway patency and provision of ventilation if required are essential. This will help to prevent secondary hypoxic damage to the brain and other vital organs. Without adequate oxygenation it may be impossible to restore an organised, perfusing cardiac rhythm. These principles may not apply to the witnessed primary cardiac arrest in the vicinity of a defibrillator; in this case, the priority is immediate defibrillation followed by attention to the airway.

Causes of airway obstruction

Obstruction of the airway may be partial or complete. It may occur at any level from the nose and mouth down to the level of the carina and bronchi. In the unconscious patient, the commonest site of airway obstruction is the pharynx. The precise cause of airway obstruction in the unconscious state has been identified by studying patients under general anaesthesia. Airway obstruction had previously been attributed to posterior displacement of the tongue caused by decreased muscle tone, with the tongue ultimately touching the posterior pharyngeal wall. These studies of anaesthetised patients have shown that the site of airway obstruction is more often at the soft palate and epiglottis and not the tongue. Obstruction may also be caused by vomit or blood, as a result of regurgitation of gastric contents or trauma, or by foreign bodies. Laryngeal obstruction may be caused by oedema from burns, inflammation or anaphylaxis. Upper airway stimulation or inhalation of foreign material may cause laryngeal spasm. Obstruction of the airway below the larynx is less common, but may be caused by excessive bronchial secretions, mucosal oedema, bronchospasm, pulmonary oedema, or aspiration of gastric contents. Extrinsic compression of the airway may also occur above or below the larynx e.g. trauma, haematoma or tumour.

Recognition of airway obstruction

Airway obstruction can be subtle and is often missed by healthcare professionals. Recognition is best achieved by the look, listen and feel approach.

- LOOK for chest and abdominal movements.

- LISTEN and FEEL for airflow at the mouth and nose.

In partial airway obstruction, air entry is diminished and usually noisy.

- Inspiratory stridor - caused by obstruction at the laryngeal level or above.

- Expiratory wheeze - suggests obstruction of the lower airways, which tend to collapse and obstruct during expiration.

- Gurgling - suggests the presence of liquid or semisolid foreign material in the upper airways.

- Snoring - arises when the pharynx is partially occluded by the tongue or palate.

- Crowing or stridor - is the sound of laryngeal spasm or obstruction.

Complete airway obstruction in a patient who is making respiratory efforts causes paradoxical chest and abdominal movement, described as 'see-saw breathing'. As the patient attempts to breathe in, the chest is drawn in and the abdomen expands; the opposite occurs in expiration. This is in contrast to the normal breathing pattern of synchronous movement of the abdomen upwards and outwards (pushed down by the diaphragm) with lifting of the chest wall. During airway obstruction, accessory muscles of respiration are used - the neck and the shoulder muscles contract to assist movement of the thoracic cage. There may also be intercostal and subcostal recession and a tracheal tug. Full examination of the neck, chest and abdomen should enable differentiation of the movements associated with complete airway obstruction from those of normal breathing. Listen for airflow: normal breathing should be quiet, completely obstructed breathing will be silent, and noisy breathing indicates partial airway obstruction.

During apnoea, when spontaneous breathing movements are absent, complete airway obstruction is recognised by failure to inflate the lungs during attempted positive pressure ventilation. Unless airway obstruction can be relieved to enable adequate lung ventilation within a few minutes it will cause injury to the brain and other vital organs, and cardiac arrest if this has not already occurred. Whenever possible, give high-concentration oxygen during the attempt to relieve airway obstruction. Arterial blood oxygen saturation (SaO_2) measurements (normally using pulse oximetry [SpO_2]) will guide further use of oxygen as airway patency improves. If airway patency remains poor and SaO_2 remains low, continue to give high inspired oxygen concentration. As airway patency improves, blood oxygen saturation levels will be restored more rapidly if the inspired oxygen concentration is initially high. Inspired oxygen concentrations can then be adjusted to maintain SaO_2 at 94% - 98%.

Patients with tracheostomies or permanent tracheal stomas

A patient with a tracheostomy tube or a permanent tracheal stoma (usually following a laryngectomy) may develop airway obstruction from blockage of the tracheostomy tube or stoma — airway obstruction cannot occur at the level of the pharynx in these patients. Remove any obvious foreign material from the stoma or tracheostomy tube. If necessary, remove the tracheostomy tube or, if present, exchange the tracheostomy tube liner. If a blocked tracheostomy tube is removed it should be possible to ventilate the patient's lungs by sealing the stoma and using a bag-mask applied to the face, or by intubating the trachea orally with a standard tracheal tube. In a patient with a permanent tracheal stoma, give oxygen and, if required, assist ventilation via the stoma, and not the mouth. The National Trachestomy and Safety Project in collaboration with the Resuscitation Council (UK) has produced emergency guidelines and resources that are available at www.tracheostomy.org.uk

Choking

Recognition

Foreign bodies may cause either mild or severe airway obstruction. The signs and symptoms enabling differentiation between mild and severe airway obstruction are summarised in Table 7.1.

Sequence for the treatment of adult choking

1. If the patient shows signs of mild airway obstruction (Figure 7.1):

    *   Encourage him to continue coughing, but do nothing else.

General signs of choking	
• Attack occurs while eating • Patient may clutch his neck	
Signs of severe airway obstruction	**Signs of mild airway obstruction**
Response to question 'Are you choking?' • Patient unable to speak • Patient may respond by nodding	*Response to question 'Are you choking?'* • Patient speaks and answers yes
Other signs • Patient unable to breathe • Breathing sounds wheezy • Attempts at coughing are silent • Patient may be unconscious	*Other signs* • Patient is able to speak, cough, and breathe

Table 7.1 Signs of choking

2. If the patient shows signs of severe airway obstruction and is conscious:

    *   Give up to 5 back blows.

        ○ Stand to the side and slightly behind the patient.

        ○ Support the chest with one hand and lean the patient well forwards.

        ○ Give **up to** 5 sharp blows between the scapulae with the heel of the other hand.

    *   Check to see if each back blow has relieved the airway obstruction.

    *   If 5 back blows fail to relieve the airway obstruction give up to 5 abdominal thrusts.

        ○ Stand behind the patient and put both arms round the upper part of his abdomen.

        ○ Place a clenched fist just under the xiphisternum; grasp this hand with your other hand and pull sharply inwards and upwards.

        ○ Repeat up to 5 times.

    *   If the obstruction is still not relieved, continue alternating 5 back blows with 5 abdominal thrusts.

3. If the patient becomes unconscious, call the resuscitation team and start CPR.

4. As soon as an individual with appropriate skills is present, undertake laryngoscopy and attempt to remove any foreign body with Magill's forceps.

ALS

Adult Choking Treatment Algorithm

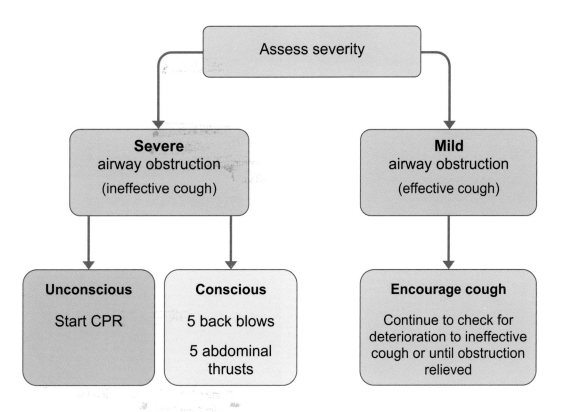

Figure 7.1 Adult choking algorithm

Basic techniques for opening the airway

Once airway obstruction is recognised, take immediate action to relieve the obstruction and maintain a clear airway. Three manoeuvres that can be used to relieve upper airway obstruction are:

- head tilt;

- chin lift;

- jaw thrust.

Head tilt and chin lift

Place one hand on the patient's forehead and tilt the head back gently; place the fingertips of the other hand under the point of the patient's chin, and gently lift to stretch the anterior neck structures (Figure 7.2).

Jaw thrust

Jaw thrust is an alternative manoeuvre for bringing the mandible forward and relieving obstruction by the tongue, soft palate and epiglottis (Figure 7.3). It is most successful when applied with a head tilt.

Procedure for jaw thrust

- Identify the angle of the mandible.

- With the index and other fingers placed behind the angle of the mandible, apply steady upwards and forward pressure to lift the mandible.

- Using the thumbs, slightly open the mouth by downward displacement of the chin.

ALS

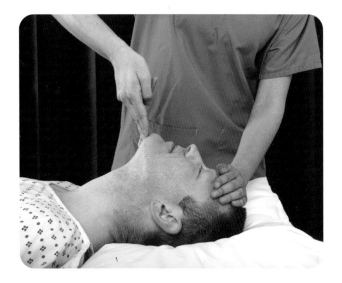

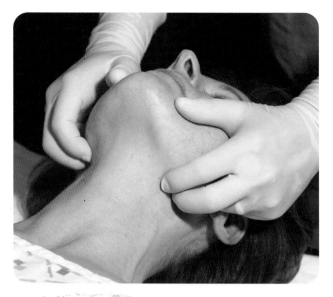

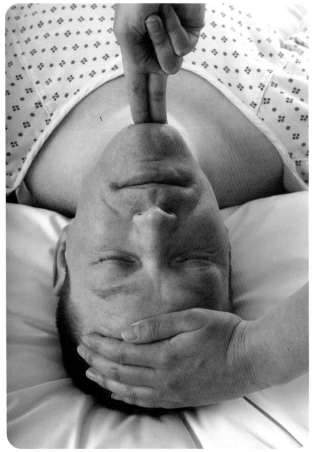

Figure 7.2 Head tilt and chin lift

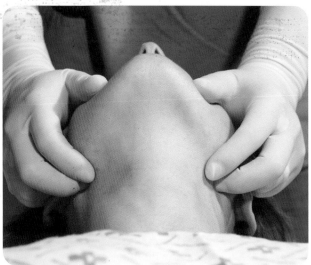

Figure 7.3 Jaw thrust

Airway manoeuvres in a patient with suspected cervical spine injury

If spinal injury is suspected (e.g. if the victim has fallen, been struck on the head or neck, or has been rescued after diving into shallow water) maintain the head, neck, chest, and lumbar region in the neutral position during resuscitation. Excessive head tilt could aggravate the injury and damage the cervical spinal cord; however, this complication remains theoretical and the relative risk is unknown. When there is a risk of cervical spine injury, establish a clear upper airway by using jaw thrust or chin lift in combination with manual in-line stabilisation (MILS) of the head and neck by an assistant. If life-threatening airway obstruction persists despite effective application of jaw thrust or chin lift, add head tilt a small amount at a time until the airway is open; establishing a patent airway takes priority over concerns about a potential cervical spine injury.

These simple positional methods are successful in most cases where airway obstruction is caused by loss of muscle tone in the pharynx. After each manoeuvre, check for success using the look, listen and feel sequence. If a clear airway cannot be achieved, look for other causes of airway obstruction. Use a finger sweep to remove any solid foreign material visible in the mouth. Remove broken or displaced dentures but leave well-fitting dentures in place as they help to maintain the contours of the mouth, facilitating a good seal for ventilation by mouth-to-mask or bag-mask techniques.

Adjuncts to basic airway techniques

Simple airway adjuncts are often helpful, and sometimes essential to maintain an open airway, particularly when resuscitation is prolonged. The position of the head and neck must be maintained to keep the airway aligned. Oropharyngeal and nasopharyngeal airways are designed to overcome soft palate obstruction and backward tongue displacement in an unconscious patient, but head tilt and jaw thrust may also be required.

Oropharyngeal airway

The oropharyngeal or Guedel airway is a curved plastic tube, flanged and reinforced at the oral end with a flattened shape to ensure that it fits neatly between the tongue and hard palate (Figure 7.4). It is available in sizes suitable for small and large adults. An estimate of the size required may be obtained by selecting an airway with a length corresponding to the vertical distance between the patient's incisors and the angle of the jaw (Figure 7.5). The most common sizes are 2, 3 and 4 for small, medium and large adults respectively. An oropharyngeal airway that is slightly too big will be more beneficial than one that is slightly too small.

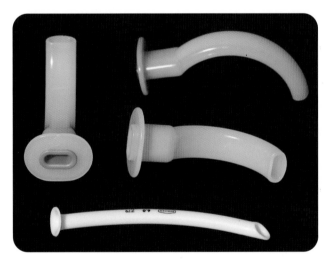

Figure 7.4 Oropharyngeal and nasopharyngeal airways

During insertion of an oropharyngeal airway, the tongue can occasionally be pushed backwards, exacerbating obstruction instead of relieving it. The oropharyngeal airway may lodge in the vallecula, or the epiglottis may obstruct the lumen. Ensuring a correct insertion technique should avoid this problem. Attempt insertion only in unconscious patients: vomiting or laryngospasm may occur if glossopharyngeal or laryngeal reflexes are present.

Technique for insertion of an oropharyngeal airway:

- Open the patient's mouth and ensure that there is no foreign material that may be pushed into the larynx (if there is any, then use suction to remove it).

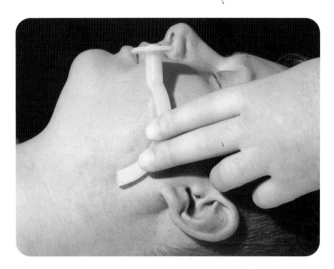

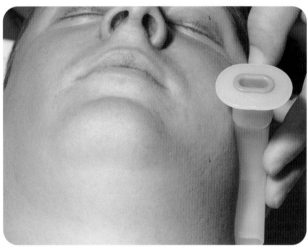

Figure 7.5 Sizing an oropharyngeal airway

- Insert the airway into the oral cavity in the 'upside-down' position as far as the junction between the hard and soft palate and then rotate it through 180° (Figure 7.6). Advance the airway until it lies within the pharynx. This rotation technique minimises the chance of pushing the tongue backwards and downwards. Remove the airway if the patient gags or strains. Correct placement is indicated by an improvement in airway patency and by the seating of the flattened reinforced section between the patient's teeth or gums (if edentulous). A jaw thrust may further aid final placement of the airway as it is finally pushed into the correct position

After insertion, maintain head-tilt/chin-lift or jaw thrust, and check the patency of the airway and ventilation using the look, listen and feel technique. Where there is suspicion of an injury to the cervical spine, maintain alignment and immobilisation of the head and neck. Suction is usually possible through an oropharyngeal airway using a fine bore flexible suction catheter.

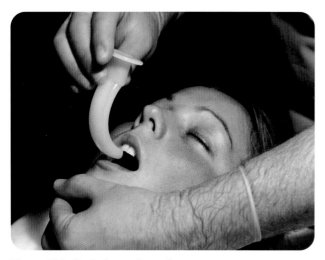

Figure 7.6 Oral airway insertion

Nasopharyngeal airway

This is made from soft malleable plastic, bevelled at one end and with a flange at the other (Figure 7.4). In patients who are not deeply unconscious, it is tolerated better than an oropharyngeal airway. It may be life-saving in patients with clenched jaws, trismus or maxillofacial injuries.

Inadvertent insertion of a nasopharyngeal airway through a fracture of the skull base and into the cranial vault is possible, but extremely rare. In the presence of a known or suspected basal skull fracture an oral airway is preferred, but if this is not possible, and the airway is obstructed, gentle insertion of a nasopharyngeal airway may be life-saving (i.e. the benefits may far outweigh the risks).

The tubes are sized in millimetres according to their internal diameter, and the length increases with diameter. The traditional methods of sizing a nasopharyngeal airway (measurement against the patient's little finger or anterior nares) do not correlate with the airway anatomy and are unreliable. Sizes 6 - 7 mm are suitable for adults. Insertion can cause damage to the mucosal lining of the nasal airway, resulting in bleeding in up to 30% of cases. If the tube is too long it may stimulate the laryngeal or glossopharyngeal reflexes to produce laryngospasm or vomiting.

Technique for insertion of a nasopharyngeal airway

- Check for patency of the right nostril.

- Some designs require a safety pin to be inserted through the flange to provide an extra precaution against the airway disappearing beyond the nares. The safety pin should be inserted BEFORE inserting the airway.

- Lubricate the airway thoroughly using water-soluble jelly.

- Insert the airway bevel end first, vertically along the floor of the nose with a slight twisting action (Figure 7.7). The curve of the airway should direct it towards the patient's feet. If any obstruction is met, remove the tube and try the left nostril.

- Once in place, use the look, listen and feel technique to check the patency of the airway and adequacy of ventilation. Chin lift or jaw thrust may still be required to maintain airway patency. Where there is suspicion of an injury to the cervical spine, maintain correct alignment and immobilisation of the head and neck.

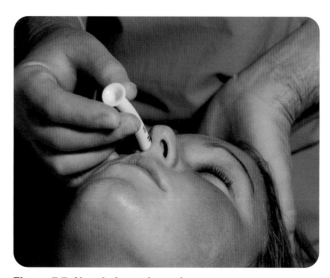

Figure 7.7 Nasal airway insertion

Oxygen

In the absence of data indicating the optimal SaO_2 during CPR, ventilate the lungs with 100% until return of spontaneous circulation (ROSC) is achieved. After ROSC is achieved and in any acutely ill, or unconscious patient, give high-flow oxygen until the SaO_2 can be measured reliably. There are some registry data indicating an association between hyperoxaemia after ROSC and worse outcome. A standard oxygen mask will deliver up to 50%, providing the flow of oxygen is high enough. Initially, give the highest possible oxygen concentration - a mask with reservoir bag (non-rebreathing mask) can deliver an inspired oxygen concentration of 85% at flow rates of 10 l min⁻¹. Monitor the SpO_2 or arterial blood gases to enable titration of the inspired oxygen concentration. When blood oxygen saturation can be measured reliably, SpO_2 should be maintained at 94% - 98%; or 88% - 92% if the patient has COPD.

Suction

Use a wide-bore rigid sucker (Yankauer) to remove liquid (blood, saliva and gastric contents) from the upper airway (Figure 7.8). Use the sucker cautiously if the patient has an intact gag reflex – it can provoke vomiting. Fine-bore flexible suction catheters may be required in patients with limited mouth opening. These suction catheters can also be passed through oropharyngeal or nasopharyngeal airways.

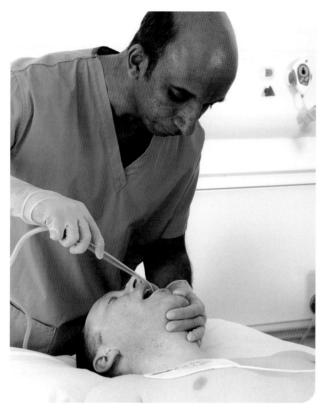

Figure 7.8 Suctioning

Ventilation

Artificial ventilation is started as soon as possible in any patient in whom spontaneous ventilation is inadequate or absent. Expired air ventilation (rescue breathing) is effective but the rescuer's expired oxygen concentration is only 16 - 17%; so it must be replaced as soon as possible by ventilation with oxygen-enriched air. Although mouth-to-mouth ventilation has the benefit of not requiring any equipment, the technique is aesthetically unpleasant, particularly when vomit or blood is present, and the rescuer may be reluctant to place themselves in intimate contact with the victim who may be unknown to them.

There are only isolated reports of individuals acquiring infections after providing CPR, e.g. tuberculosis and severe acute respiratory distress syndrome (SARS). Transmission of HIV during provision of CPR has never been reported. Simple adjuncts are available to enable direct person-to-person contact to be avoided; some of these devices may reduce the risk of cross infection between patient and rescuer.

The pocket resuscitation mask is used widely. It is similar to an anaesthetic face mask and enables mouth-to-mask

ventilation. It has a unidirectional valve, which directs the patient's expired air away from the rescuer. The mask is transparent so that vomit or blood from the patient can be seen. Some masks have a port for the addition of oxygen. When using masks without an oxygen port, supplemental oxygen can be given by placing oxygen tubing underneath one side and ensuring an adequate seal. Use a two-hand technique to maximise the seal with the patient's face (Figure 7.9).

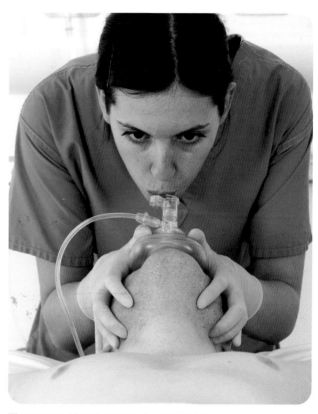

Figure 7.9 Mouth-to-mask ventilation

High airway pressures can be generated if the tidal volumes or inspiratory flows are too great, predisposing to gastric inflation and subsequent risk of regurgitation and pulmonary aspiration. As gastric inflation occurs, lung compliance is further reduced making ventilation more difficult. The possibility of gastric inflation is increased by:

- malalignment of the head and neck, and an obstructed airway;

- an incompetent oesophageal sphincter (present in all patients with cardiac arrest);

- a high inflation pressure.

Tidal volumes in the region of 6 - 7 ml kg^{-1} will provide adequate oxygenation and ventilation, and will reduce the risk of gastric inflation. If inspiratory flow is too low, inspiratory time will be prolonged and the time available to give chest compressions is reduced. Deliver each breath over approximately 1 s and give a volume that corresponds to normal visible chest movement; this represents a compromise between giving an adequate volume, minimising the risk of gastric inflation, and allowing adequate time for chest compressions. During CPR with an unprotected airway, give 2 ventilations after each sequence of 30 chest compressions.

Technique for mouth-to-mask ventilation

- Place the patient supine with the head in a 'sniffing' position i.e. neck slightly flexed on a pillow with the head extended (tilted backwards) on the neck.

- Apply the mask to the patient's face using the thumbs of both hands.

- Lift the jaw into the mask with the remaining fingers by exerting pressure behind the angles of the jaw (jaw thrust). At the same time, press the mask onto the face with the thumbs to make a tight seal (Figure 7.9).

- Blow gently through the inspiratory valve and watch the chest rise normally.

- Stop inflation and observe the chest falling.

- Any leaks between the face and mask can be reduced by adjusting the contact pressure, altering the position of the fingers and thumbs, or increasing jaw thrust.

- If oxygen is available, add it via the port at a flow of 10 l min-1.

Self-inflating bag

The self-inflating bag can be connected to a face mask, tracheal tube, or supraglottic airway device. As the bag is squeezed, the contents are delivered to the patient's lungs. On release, the expired gas is diverted to the atmosphere via a one-way valve; the bag then refills automatically via an inlet at the opposite end. When used without supplemental oxygen, the self-inflating bag ventilates the patient's lungs with only ambient air (oxygen concentration 21%). This is increased to around 45% by attaching high-flow oxygen directly to the bag adjacent to the air intake. An inspired oxygen concentration of approximately 85% is achieved if a reservoir system is attached and the oxygen flow is maximally increased. As the bag re-expands it fills with oxygen from both the reservoir and the continuous flow from the attached oxygen tubing.

Although the bag-mask apparatus enables ventilation with high concentrations of oxygen, its use by a single person requires considerable skill. When used with a face mask, it is often difficult to achieve a gas-tight seal between the mask and the patient's face, and maintain a patent airway with one hand whilst squeezing the bag with the other. Any significant leak will cause hypoventilation and if the airway

is not patent, gas may also be forced into the stomach. This will reduce ventilation further and greatly increase the risk of regurgitation and aspiration. There is a natural tendency to try to compensate for a leak by excessive compression of the bag, which causes high peak airway pressures and forces more gas into the stomach. Some self-inflating bags have flow restrictors that limit peak airway pressure with the aim of reducing gastric inflation. Cricoid pressure can reduce the risk of gastric inflation but requires the presence of a trained assistant. Poorly applied cricoid pressure may make it more difficult to ventilate the patient's lungs.

The two-person technique for bag-mask ventilation is preferable (Figure 7.10). One person holds the face mask in place using a jaw thrust with both hands and an assistant squeezes the bag. In this way, a better seal can be achieved and the patient's lungs can be ventilated more effectively and safely.

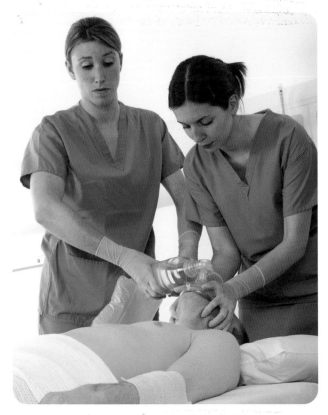

Figure 7.10 The two-person technique for bag-mask ventilation

Key learning points

- Airway patency and ventilating the lungs are important components of CPR.

- Use of simple airway manoeuvres, with or without basic adjuncts, will often achieve a patent airway.

- Give all patients high-concentration oxygen until the arterial oxygen saturation is measurable.

Introduction

Effective bag-mask ventilation requires a reasonable level of skill and experience: the inexperienced are likely to achieve ineffective tidal volumes and cause gastric inflation with risk of regurgitation and pulmonary aspiration. In comparison with bag-mask ventilation, use of supraglottic airway devices (SADs) may enable more effective ventilation and reduce the risk of gastric inflation. Furthermore, SADs are easier to insert than a tracheal tube and, unlike tracheal intubation, they can generally be positioned without interrupting chest compressions.

Without adequate training and experience, the incidence of complications associated with attempted tracheal intubation is unacceptably high. Unrecognised oesophageal intubation is disastrous and prolonged attempts at tracheal intubation are harmful: the pause in chest compressions during this time will severely compromise coronary and cerebral perfusion. Alternative airway devices should be used if attempted tracheal intubation by those highly skilled to perform the technique has failed or by all other personnel not skilled in regular intubation of the trachea.

There are no data supporting the routine use of any specific approach to airway management during cardiac arrest. The best technique is dependent on the precise circumstances of the cardiac arrest and the competence of the rescuer.

Laryngeal mask airway

The laryngeal mask airway (LMA) consists of a wide-bore tube with an elliptical inflated cuff designed to seal around the laryngeal opening (Figure 7.11). It was introduced into anaesthetic practice in the middle of the 1980s and is a reliable and safe device, which can be introduced easily, with a high success rate after a short period of training. Ventilation using the LMA is more efficient and easier than with a bag-mask apparatus; provided high inflation pressures (>20 cmH₂O) are avoided, gastric inflation is minimised. When an LMA can be inserted without delay it is preferable to avoid bag-mask ventilation altogether: the risk of gastric inflation and regurgitation is reduced. Though not guaranteeing protection of the airway from gastric contents, pulmonary aspiration during use of the LMA is uncommon. The LMA does protect against sources of aspiration from above the larynx. Use of the LMA by nursing, paramedical and medical staff during resuscitation has been studied and reported to be effective. Like tracheal intubation, it requires the patient to be deeply unconscious. The LMA is particularly valuable if attempted intubation by skilled personnel has failed and bag-mask ventilation is impossible (the cannot ventilate, cannot intubate scenario). The conventional LMA (LMA Classic™) can be reused up to 40 times after sterilisation. The practical limitations imposed by having to resterilise the LMA Classic™ make the single-use versions of the LMA more suitable for prehospital use and for cardiac arrests in hospital. However, some of the single-use LMAs are of a slightly different design and material to the LMA Classic™ and their performance has not been validated in the CPR setting.

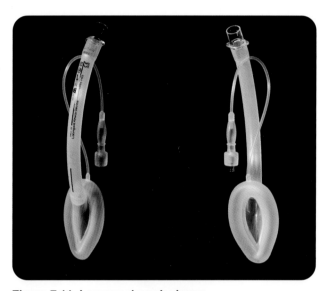

Figure 7.11 Laryngeal mask airway

Technique for insertion of a laryngeal mask airway

- Try to maintain chest compressions throughout the insertion attempt; if it is necessary to stop chest compressions during the insertion attempt, limit this pause in chest compressions to a maximum of 10 s.

- Select a LMA of an appropriate size for the patient and deflate the cuff fully. A size 5 will be correct for most men and a size 4 for most women. Lubricate the outer face of the cuff area (the part that will not be in contact with the larynx) with water-soluble gel.

- Flex the patient's neck slightly and extend the head (try to maintain neutral alignment of the head and neck if there is suspicion of cervical spine injury).

- Holding the LMA like a pen, insert it into the mouth (Figure 7.12). Advance the tip behind the upper incisors with the upper surface applied to the palate until it reaches the posterior pharyngeal wall. Press the mask backwards and downwards around the corner of the pharynx until a resistance is felt as it locates in the back of the pharynx. If possible, get an assistant to apply a jaw thrust after the LMA has been inserted into the mouth - this increases the space in the posterior pharynx and makes successful placement easier. A slight 45 degree twist will often aid placement if initial attempts at insertion beyond the pharynx are proving difficult.

- Connect the inflating syringe and inflate the cuff with air (40 ml for a size 5 LMA and 30 ml for a size 4 LMA); alternatively, inflate the cuff to a pressure of 60 cmH$_2$O. If insertion is satisfactory, the tube will lift 1 - 2 cm out of the mouth as the cuff finds its correct position and the larynx is pushed forward.

- If the LMA has not been inserted successfully after 30 s, oxygenate the patient using a pocket mask or bag-mask before reattempting LMA insertion.

- Confirm a clear airway by listening over the chest during inflation and observing bilateral chest movement. A large, audible leak suggests malposition of the LMA, but a small leak is acceptable provided chest rise is adequate.

- Insert a bite block alongside the tube if available and secure the LMA with a bandage or tape.

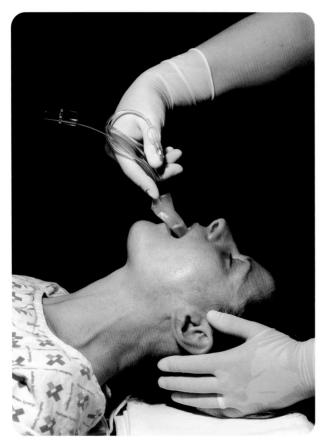

Figure 7.12 Insertion of a laryngeal mask airway

Limitations of the LMA

- In the presence of high airway resistance or poor lung compliance (pulmonary oedema, bronchospasm, chronic obstructive pulmonary disease) there is a risk of a significant leak around the cuff causing hypoventilation. Most of the gas leaking around the cuff normally escapes through the patient's mouth but some gastric inflation may occur.

- There are no data demonstrating whether or not it is possible to provide adequate ventilation via an LMA without interruption of chest compressions. Uninterrupted chest compressions are likely to cause at least some gas leak from the LMA cuff when ventilation is attempted. Attempt continuous compressions initially but abandon this if persistent leaks and hypoventilation occur.

- There is a theoretical risk of aspiration of stomach contents because the LMA does not sit within the larynx like a tracheal tube; however, this complication has not been documented widely in clinical practice.

- If the patient is not deeply unconscious, insertion of the LMA may cause coughing, straining or laryngeal spasm. This will not occur in patients in cardiorespiratory arrest.

- If an adequate airway is not achieved, withdraw the LMA, deflate the cuff and attempt reinsertion ensuring a good alignment of the head and neck.

- Uncommonly, airway obstruction may be caused by the epiglottis folding down to cover the laryngeal inlet. Withdraw the LMA, deflate the cuff and attempt reinsertion.

To become proficient in the insertion of an LMA requires practice on patients and this should be achieved under the supervision of an appropriately experienced person (e.g. anaesthetist) in a controlled environment.

The ProSeal LMA

The ProSeal LMA (PLMA) is a modified version of the original LMA. It has an additional posterior cuff and a gastric drain tube (Figure 7.13). The device has been studied extensively in anaesthetised patients, but there are no studies of its function and performance during CPR. It has several attributes that, in theory, make it more suitable than the original LMA for use during CPR: improved seal with the larynx enabling ventilation at higher airway pressures (commonly up to 35 - 40 cmH$_2$O), the inclusion of a gastric drain tube enabling venting of liquid regurgitated gastric contents from the upper oesophagus and passage of a gastric tube to drain liquid gastric contents, and the inclusion of a bite block. The higher seal pressures achieved with the PLMA may enable ventilation volume to be maintained during uninterrupted chest compressions.

Potential weaknesses of the PLMA as an airway device for CPR are that it is slightly more difficult to insert than the original LMA, it is relatively expensive and that solid, regurgitated gastric contents could block the gastric drain tube. Recently a disposable form of the PLMA has become available - the LMA Supreme. It has a more rigid shape and lacks a posterior inflatable cuff. Apart from two case reports, there are few data on the use of this device in CPR at present.

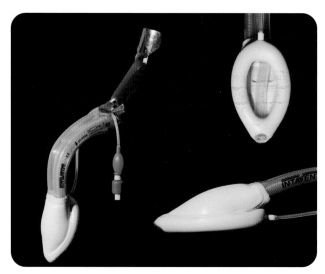

Figure 7.13 Proseal LMA

i-gel airway

The i-gel is a relatively new supraglottic airway. The cuff is made of thermoplastic elastomer gel and does not require inflation; the stem of the i-gel incorporates a bite block and a narrow oesophageal drain tube (Figure 7.14). It is easy to insert, requiring only minimal training and a laryngeal seal pressure of 20 - 24 cmH$_2$O can be achieved. In two manikin studies, insertion of the i-gel was significantly faster than several other airway devices. The ease of insertion of the i-gel and its favourable leak pressure make it theoretically very attractive as a resuscitation airway device for those inexperienced in tracheal intubation. Use

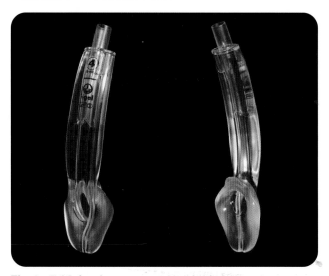

Figure 7.14 i-gel

of the i-gel during cardiac arrest has been reported but more data on its use in this setting are awaited.

Laryngeal tube

The laryngeal tube (LT) is another of the new supraglottic airway devices that have been developed. It is a single-lumen tube with both an oesophageal and pharyngeal cuff (Figure 7.15). A single pilot balloon inflates both cuffs simultaneously and it is available in a variety of sizes. Successful insertion and airway pressures generated are comparable to the LMA when performed by non-anaesthetists. There are several observational studies that document successful use of the LT by nurses and paramedics during prehospital cardiac arrest. A double lumen LT with an oesophageal vent and a disposable version (LT-D) are available.

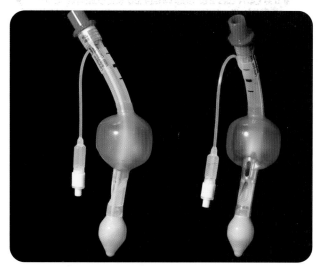

Figure 7.15 Laryngeal tube

Key learning points

- Supraglottic airway devices are good alternatives to the bag-mask and should be used instead of the bag-mask technique wherever possible.

- Supraglottic airway devices should be used instead of tracheal intubation unless individuals highly skilled in intubation are immediately available. They should also be used if attempted intubation is unsuccessful.

Section 3. Tracheal intubation and cricothyroidotomy

Learning outcomes

To understand:

▶ **The advantages and disadvantages of tracheal intubation during cardiopulmonary resuscitation**

▶ **Some simple aids to tracheal intubation**

▶ **Some methods for confirming correct placement of a tracheal tube**

▶ **The role of needle and surgical cricothyroidotomy**

Tracheal intubation

There is insufficient evidence to support or refute the use of any specific technique to maintain an airway and provide ventilation in adults with cardiorespiratory arrest. Despite this, tracheal intubation is perceived as the optimal method of providing and maintaining a clear and secure airway. It should be used only when trained personnel are available to carry out the procedure with a high level of skill and competence. A systematic review of randomised controlled trials (RCTs) of tracheal intubation versus alternative airway management in acutely ill and injured patients has identified just three trials: two were RCTs of the Combitube versus tracheal intubation for out-of-hospital cardiac arrest which showed no difference in survival. The third study was a RCT of prehospital tracheal intubation versus management of the airway with a bag-mask in children requiring airway management for cardiac arrest, primary respiratory disorders and severe injuries. There was no overall benefit for tracheal intubation; on the contrary, of the children requiring airway management for a respiratory problem, those randomised to intubation had a lower survival rate than those in the bag-mask group. The Ontario Prehospital Advanced Life Support (OPALS) study has also documented no increase in survival to hospital discharge when the skills of tracheal intubation and injection of cardiac supporting drugs were added to an optimised basic life support-automated external defibrillator system.

The perceived advantages of tracheal intubation over bag-mask ventilation include maintenance of a patent airway which is protected from aspiration of gastric contents or blood from the oropharynx, ability to provide an adequate tidal volume reliably even when chest compressions are uninterrupted, the potential to free the rescuers hands for other tasks and the ability to suck-out airway secretions. Use of a bag-mask is more likely to cause gastric distension, which, theoretically, is more likely to cause

regurgitation and the risk of aspiration. This theoretical risk has yet to be proven in randomised clinical trials.

The perceived disadvantages of tracheal intubation over bag-mask ventilation include the risk of an unrecognised misplaced tracheal tube (which is as high as 17% in some studies of out-of-hospital cardiac arrest), a prolonged time without chest compressions while tracheal intubation is attempted (tracheal intubation attempts accounted for almost 25% of all CPR interruptions in one prehospital study) and a comparatively high failure rate. Tracheal intubation success rates correlate with the intubation experience attained by the rescuer. Rates for failure to intubate the trachea are as high as 50% in prehospital systems with a low patient volume and providers who do not perform intubation frequently. The cost of training prehospital staff to undertake tracheal intubation should also be considered. Healthcare personnel who undertake prehospital intubation should do so only within a structured, monitored program, which should include comprehensive competency-based training and regular opportunities to refresh skills.

Rescuers must therefore weigh the risks and benefits of tracheal intubation against the need to provide effective chest compressions. The intubation attempt will require some interruption of chest compressions but, once an advanced airway is in place, ventilation will not require further interruption of chest compressions. Personnel skilled in advanced airway management should be able to undertake laryngoscopy without stopping chest compressions; a brief pause in chest compressions will be required only as the tube is passed through the vocal cords. Alternatively, to avoid any interruptions in chest compressions, the intubation attempt may be deferred until ROSC. No tracheal intubation attempt should interrupt chest compressions for more than 10 s; if intubation is not achievable within these constraints, recommence bag-mask or bag-supraglottic airway device ventilation. After tracheal intubation, tube placement must be confirmed and the tube secured adequately. If there is any doubt about the correct position of the tube, remove it and re-oxygenate the patient before making another attempt.

In some cases, laryngoscopy and attempted intubation may prove impossible or cause life-threatening deterioration in the patient's condition. Such circumstances include acute epiglottitis, pharyngeal pathology, head injury (where coughing or straining may cause further increase in intracranial pressure), or in patients with cervical spine injury. In these circumstances, specialist skills such as the use of anaesthetic drugs or flexible fibreoptic laryngoscopy may be required. Such techniques require a high level of skill and training.

Essential equipment for tracheal intubation

- Laryngoscope - generally a curved Macintosh blade. Several sizes are available, but a size 3 will be adequate for most patients. Check the light source and battery regularly and just before use, and ensure that spares are immediately available.

- Cuffed tracheal tubes - a selection should be available appropriate to the size of the patient. An 8 mm internal diameter tube is suitable for an adult male and a 7 mm internal diameter tube for a female.

- Sizes 6, 7 and 8 mm will generally cover the immediate needs of all adults. Availability of smaller tracheal tubes will be helpful for patients with conditions causing narrowing of the upper airway.

- Syringe for cuff inflation.

- Equipment for confirming correct placement of the tracheal tube.

- Extras:

  o water-soluble lubricating jelly;

  o Magill's forceps;

  o introducers: either a gum elastic bougie or a semi-rigid stylet;

  o tape or bandage to secure tube in position;

  o suction apparatus with a wide-bore rigid suction end (e.g. Yankauer) and a range of smaller flexible catheters.

Post-intubation procedures

- After successful intubation, connect the tracheal tube (via a catheter mount if necessary) to a ventilating device, e.g. self-inflating bag, and ventilate with the highest oxygen concentration available.

- Inflate the cuff of the tracheal tube just sufficiently to stop an air leak during inspiration.

- Confirm correct placement of the tracheal tube using clinical assessment AND a technique for secondary confirmation - waveform capnography is the most reliable secondary technique (see below).

- Continue ventilation with a high concentration of oxygen until ROSC and oxygen saturations are recordable.

- Secure the tube with a bandage or tie. Adhesive tape is not reliable if the face is moist.

- An oropharyngeal airway may be inserted alongside the tracheal tube to maintain the position of the tube, and prevent damage from biting when consciousness returns.

Confirmation of correct tracheal tube placement

Unrecognised oesophageal intubation is the most serious complication of attempted tracheal intubation. Routine use of primary and secondary techniques to confirm correct placement of the tracheal tube will reduce this risk.

Clinical assessment

Primary assessment includes observation of chest expansion bilaterally, auscultation over the lung fields bilaterally in the axillae (breath sounds should be equal and adequate) and over the epigastrium (breath sounds should not be heard). Clinical signs of correct tube placement (condensation in the tube, chest rise, breath sounds on auscultation of lungs, and inability to hear gas entering the stomach) are not completely reliable. The reported sensitivity (proportion of tracheal intubations correctly identified) and specificity (proportion of oesophageal intubations correctly identified) of clinical assessment varies.

Secondary confirmation of tracheal tube placement by an exhaled carbon dioxide or oesophageal detection device should reduce the risk of unrecognised oesophageal intubation but the performance of the available devices varies considerably. Furthermore, none of the secondary confirmation techniques will differentiate between a tube placed in a main bronchus and one placed correctly in the trachea.

Oesophageal detector device

The oesophageal detector device creates a suction force at the tracheal end of the tracheal tube, either by pulling back the plunger on a large syringe or releasing a compressed flexible bulb. Air is aspirated easily from the lower airways through a tracheal tube placed in the cartilage-supported rigid trachea. When the tube is in the oesophagus, air cannot be aspirated because the oesophagus collapses when aspiration is attempted. The oesophageal detector device may be misleading in patients with morbid obesity, late pregnancy or severe asthma or when there are copious tracheal secretions; in these conditions the trachea may collapse when aspiration is attempted.

Carbon dioxide detectors

Carbon dioxide (CO_2) detector devices measure the concentration of exhaled carbon dioxide from the lungs. The persistence of exhaled CO_2 after six ventilations indicates placement of the tracheal tube in the trachea or a main bronchus. Confirmation of correct placement

ALS

above the carina will require auscultation of the chest bilaterally in the mid-axillary lines. Broadly, there are three types of carbon dioxide detector device:

1. Disposable colorimetric end-tidal carbon dioxide ($ETCO_2$) detectors use a litmus paper to detect CO_2, and these devices generally give readings of purple ($ETCO_2$ <0.5%), tan ($ETCO_2$ 0.5 - 2%) and yellow ($ETCO_2$ > 2%). In most studies, tracheal placement of the tube is considered verified if the tan colour persists after a few ventilations. Although colorimetric CO_2 detectors identify placement quite well in patients with good perfusion, these devices are less accurate than clinical assessment in cardiac arrest patients because pulmonary blood flow may be so low that there is insufficient exhaled carbon dioxide. Furthermore, if the tracheal tube is in the oesophagus, six ventilations may lead to gastric distension, vomiting and aspiration.

2. Non-waveform electronic digital $ETCO_2$ devices generally measure $ETCO_2$ using an infrared spectrometer and display the results with a number; they do not provide a waveform graphical display of the respiratory cycle on a capnograph.

3. End-tidal CO_2 detectors that include a waveform graphical display (capnograph) are the most reliable for verification of tracheal tube position during cardiac arrest. Studies of waveform capnography to verify tracheal tube position in victims of cardiac arrest demonstrate 100% sensitivity and 100% specificity in identifying correct tracheal tube placement.

Waveform capnography is the most sensitive and specific way to confirm and continuously monitor the position of a tracheal tube in victims of cardiac arrest and should supplement clinical assessment (auscultation and visualisation of tube through cords). Waveform capnography will not discriminate between tracheal and bronchial placement of the tube - careful auscultation is essential. Existing portable monitors make capnographic initial confirmation and continuous monitoring of tracheal tube position feasible in almost all settings, including out-of-hospital, emergency department, and in-hospital locations where tracheal intubation is performed. Furthermore, waveform capnography may be a sensitive indicator of ROSC. Such waveform analysis may prove useful in PEA cardiac arrests.

In the absence of a waveform capnograph it may be preferable to use a supraglottic airway device when advanced airway management is indicated.

Potential problems during tracheal intubation

Anatomical and pathological variations that may make intubation difficult or impossible include receding lower jaw, short neck, poor movement at the atlanto-axial joint, prominent incisors, narrow mouth, stiff neck and trismus. If the vocal cords cannot be seen, do not make any attempts to insert the tube blindly. Often a gum-elastic bougie can be inserted through the glottis more easily than a tracheal tube and once in place the tube may be placed over the bougie and guided (rail-roaded) into the trachea. The intubating stylet may also be used to stiffen and pre-form the curvature of the tube or to guide it into the larynx. Problems during intubation may be caused by:

-   Facial burns and trauma - it may be impossible to use BLS techniques or intubate patients with severe facial trauma or thermal injury to the upper airway. In such cases it may be necessary to establish a surgical airway, e.g. cricothyroidotomy (see below).

-   Upper airway pathology e.g. tumours, infection, swelling from anaphylaxis, etc.

-   Insecure/loose teeth or dental prosthesis - these may be damaged or loosened if undue pressure is placed on them. Good intubation technique should reduce this risk.

-   Gastric regurgitation - always have a functioning suction device and wide-bore suction to hand. Cricoid pressure may prevent passive regurgitation and pulmonary aspiration.

-   Clenching of teeth - in the early stages of resuscitation good CPR may prevent the profound level of unconsciousness required for tracheal intubation. In this case, use basic airway and ventilation techniques.

-   Oesophageal intubation - this should not go unrecognised if the recommended protocols are followed, particularly if tracheal tube placement is confirmed with an oesophageal detector device and/or capnometry and capnography. If in doubt, take the tube out and re-oxygenate the lungs using a bag-mask.

-   Possible cervical spine injury - suspect this in all patients who have a history of major blunt trauma. Use manual inline stabilisation (MILS) of the head and neck and ensure an experienced operator undertakes the intubation.

Cricoid pressure

In non-arrest patients cricoid pressure may offer some measure of protection to the airway from aspiration but it may also impede ventilation or interfere with tracheal intubation. The role of cricoid pressure during cardiac arrest has not been studied. Application of cricoid pressure during bag-mask ventilation reduces gastric inflation. Studies in anaesthetised patients, however, show that cricoid pressure impairs ventilation in many patients, increases peak inspiratory pressures and causes

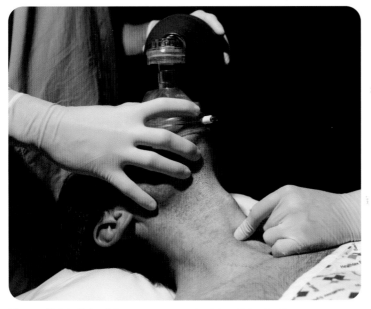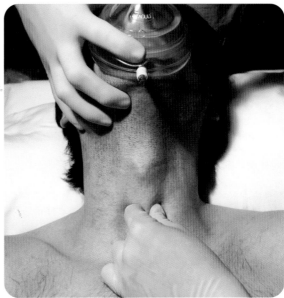

Figure 7.16 Cricoid pressure

complete obstruction in up to 50% of patients depending on the amount of cricoid pressure (in the range of recommended effective pressure) that is applied. Do not use cricoid pressure routinely in cardiac arrest. If cricoid pressure is used during cardiac arrest, adjust, relax or release the pressure if it impedes ventilation or tracheal tube placement.

The cricoid cartilage is immediately below the thyroid cartilage, where it forms a complete ring at the upper end of the trachea. A pressure of 30 N (3 kg) is applied anteroposteriorly, forcing the cricoid ring backwards, which compresses the oesophagus against the vertebral column (Figure 7.16). Do not apply cricoid pressure if there is active vomiting: it could cause oesophageal rupture.

Aids to intubation

Alternative laryngoscope blade

The Macintosh blade is a good general-purpose blade and a size 3 blade is suitable for most adults. Occasionally, a longer, size 4 blade is better for very large, long-necked patients. The McCoy levering laryngoscope has a hinged tip, and will often improve the view at laryngoscopy. A variety of new videolaryngoscopes are also now available but these are expensive and unlikely to be available in most cardiac arrest settings. A new disposable light assisted laryngoscope (Airtraq) which permits direct visualisation of the larynx via a viewing screen may prove more useful in cardiac arrest settings but, in this context, has been studied only in manikins.

Introducers

If visualisation is difficult, a gum-elastic bougie may be helpful to guide the tracheal tube into the larynx. It is best inserted into the larynx separately - the tube is then passed over it into the trachea. When correctly placed,

free passage of the bougie is stopped by the smaller airways of the bronchial tree; a bougie placed accidentally in the oesophagus can be inserted completely, without obvious resistance. Ultimately, when ventilation and intubation are impossible and alternatives, e.g. a supraglottic airway device, are not effective, it will be necessary to perform a cricothyroidotomy (see below).

Whilst descriptions of the advanced airway techniques above have been included, these descriptions are not intended as a substitute for practice on manikins, or on anaesthetised patients under the direction of an anaesthetist. Tracheal intubation during cardiac arrest should be attempted only by those undertaking this procedure regularly.

Suction

Use a wide-bore rigid suction end (Yankauer) to remove liquid (blood, saliva and gastric contents) from the upper airway. This is done best under direct vision during intubation but must not delay achieving a definitive airway. Apply suction to the trachea as briefly as possible and ventilate the lungs with 100% oxygen before and after the procedure. Use fine-bore suction catheters for tracheal suction and pass them directly down the tracheal tube.

Cricothyroidotomy

Occasionally it will be impossible to ventilate an apnoeic patient with a bag-mask, or to pass a tracheal tube or other airway device. This may occur in patients with extensive facial trauma or laryngeal obstruction caused by oedema, e.g. anaphylaxis, or foreign material. In these circumstances, it will be necessary to create a surgical airway below the level of the obstruction. A tracheostomy is contraindicated in an emergency because it is time consuming, hazardous and requires considerable surgical skill and equipment. Substantial bleeding can occur.

Surgical cricothyroidotomy provides a definitive airway that can be used to ventilate the patient's lungs until semi-elective intubation or tracheostomy is performed. Needle cricothyroidotomy is a much more temporary procedure providing only short-term oxygenation. It requires a wide-bore, non-kinking cannula, a high-pressure oxygen source and may cause serious barotrauma. It is also prone to failure because of kinking of the cannula, and is unsuitable for patient transfer.

Surgical cricothyroidotomy

Unlike needle cricothyroidotomy, the surgical technique will result in an airway that is protected by a cuffed tube. Higher airway pressures can be generated and tracheal suction is possible. Surgical cricothyroidotomy enables ventilation of the lungs despite complete airway obstruction at, or above, the glottis.

Procedure for surgical cricothyroidotomy

- Place the patient supine with the head extended if possible.

- Identify the cricothyroid membrane as the recess just above the cricoid cartilage and below the thyroid cartilage.

- Incise the skin over the membrane and extend the incision through the cricothyroid membrane. Make a vertical incision in the skin and a horizontal one into the cricothyroid membrane; this avoids the superiorly positioned cricothyroid artery.

- Use the reversed handle of a scalpel or tissue expanding forceps to open up the incision in the cricothyroid membrane.

- Insert a suitably sized tracheal tube into the trachea and inflate the cuff. Do not insert the tube too far into the trachea: the carina is not far from here.

- Ventilate the lungs with a standard self-inflating bag attached to high-flow oxygen. Exhalation occurs directly through the tracheal tube and tracheal suction is also now possible.

- Confirm correct tube placement by auscultation and capnography.

Key learning points

- When undertaken by someone with appropriate skills and experience, tracheal intubation is an effective airway management technique during cardiopulmonary resuscitation.

- In unskilled hands, prolonged interruptions of chest compressions, and the high risk of failure and other complications (e.g. unrecognised oesophageal intubation) make tracheal intubation attempts potentially harmful.

Section 4. Basic mechanical ventilation

Learning outcomes

To understand:

▶ **The role of automatic ventilators in the peri-arrest period**

There are very few studies that address specific aspects of ventilation during advanced life support. There are some data indicating that the ventilation rates delivered by healthcare personnel during cardiac arrest are excessive. Various small portable automatic ventilators may be used during resuscitation. They are usually gas powered. If an oxygen cylinder is used, both to supply the patient with oxygen and to power the ventilator, the contents may be used up rapidly. Most automatic resuscitators provide a constant flow of gas to the patient during inspiration; the volume delivered is dependent on the inspiratory time (a longer time provides a greater tidal volume). Because pressure in the airway rises during inspiration, these devices are often pressure-limited to protect the lungs against barotrauma. Expiration occurs passively into the atmosphere.

Set an automatic resuscitator initially to deliver a tidal volume of 6 - 7 ml kg^{-1} at 10 breaths min^{-1}. Some ventilators have co-ordinated markings on the controls to facilitate easy and rapid adjustment for patients of different sizes, and others are capable of sophisticated variation in respiratory pattern. In the presence of a spontaneous circulation, the correct setting will be determined by checking the patient's arterial blood gas values. If a tracheal tube or supraglottic airway has not been inserted, do not attempt chest compressions during the inspiratory phase. Once a tracheal tube has been inserted it is unnecessary to interrupt chest compressions during inspiration. If a supraglottic airway is inserted it may be necessary to synchronise chest compressions with the ventilator if an excessive leak is occurring.

Automatic resuscitators provide many advantages over alternative methods of ventilation.

- In unintubated patients, the rescuer has both hands free for mask and airway alignment.

- Cricoid pressure can be applied with one hand while the other seals the mask on the face.

- In intubated patients they free the rescuer for other tasks.

- Once set, they provide a constant tidal volume, respiratory rate and minute ventilation; thus, they may help to avoid excessive ventilation.

Certain professional first responders (e.g. police, fire, and sports rescue personnel) may use simple automatic resuscitators provided that they have been trained adequately.

Passive oxygen delivery

In the presence of a patent airway, chest compressions alone may result in some ventilation of the lungs. Oxygen can be delivered passively, either via an adapted tracheal tube or with the combination of an oropharyngeal airway and standard oxygen mask with non-rebreather reservoir. There is insufficient evidence to support or refute the use of passive oxygen delivery during CPR to improve outcome when compared with oxygen delivery by positive pressure ventilation and until further data are available, passive oxygen delivery without ventilation is not currently recommended for routine use during CPR.

Key learning points

- Automatic resuscitators may be a useful adjunct during cardiopulmonary resuscitation, although there are limited data on their use. Their safe use requires appropriate training.

Further reading

Deakin CD, Morrison LJ, Morley PT, et al. 2010 International Consensus on Cardiopulmonary Resuscitation and Emergency Cardiovascular Care Science with Treatment Recommendations. Part 8: Advanced Life Support. Resuscitation 2010;81:e93-e169.

Deakin CD, Nolan JP, Soar J, et al. European Resuscitation Council Guidelines for Resuscitation 2010. Section 4. Adult Advanced Life Support. Resuscitation 2010;81:1305-52.

Nolan JP, Soar J. Airway techniques and ventilation strategies. Curr Opin Crit Care 2008;14:279-86.

Wang HE, Simeone SJ, Weaver MD, Callaway CW. Interruptions in cardiopulmonary resuscitation from paramedic endotracheal intubation. Ann Emerg Med 2009;54:645-52.

Cardiac Monitoring, Electrocardiography, and Rhythm Recognition

CHAPTER 8

Learning outcomes

To understand:

▶ **The reasons for ECG monitoring**

▶ **How to monitor the ECG**

▶ **The origin of the ECG**

▶ **The importance of recording the ECG**

▶ **The cardiac rhythms associated with cardiac arrest**

▶ **How to identify other common arrhythmias**

Introduction

During cardiac arrest, identification of the cardiac rhythm will help to determine the correct treatment. Establish cardiac monitoring as soon as possible during cardiac arrest. In many patients who have been resuscitated from cardiac arrest there is a substantial risk of further arrhythmia and cardiac arrest. Maintain cardiac monitoring in people who have been resuscitated from cardiac arrest until you are confident that the risk of recurrence is very low.

Some patients present with an arrhythmia that may lead to cardiac arrest or other serious deterioration in their condition. Early detection and treatment of the arrhythmia may prevent cardiac arrest in some patients and prevent life-threatening deterioration in others. Patients at risk include those with persistent arrhythmia associated with structural heart disease, chest pain, heart failure, reduced conscious level or shock. In all patients with persistent cardiac arrhythmia at risk of deterioration, establish cardiac monitoring and whenever possible record a good-quality 12-lead ECG. Monitoring alone will not always allow accurate rhythm recognition and it is important to document the arrhythmia for future reference if required.

Some people experience symptoms (usually syncope) caused by an intermittent cardiac arrhythmia that, if not documented and treated, could lead to cardiac arrest or sudden death. However, the arrhythmia may not be present at the time of initial assessment. In people who present with syncope undertake careful clinical assessment and record a 12-lead ECG. People who have experienced uncomplicated faints, situational syncope (such as cough syncope or micturition syncope) or syncope due to orthostatic hypotension do not require cardiac monitoring and do not usually require hospital admission. In those who have had unexplained syncope, especially during exercise, those who have had syncope and have evidence of structural heart disease, and those who have had syncope and have an abnormal ECG (especially a prolonged QT interval) start cardiac monitoring and arrange further expert cardiovascular assessment.

Single-lead ECG monitoring is not a reliable technique for detecting evidence of myocardial ischaemia (ST segment depression). Record serial 12-lead ECGs in people experiencing chest pain suggestive of an acute coronary syndrome.

During cardiac arrest, recognition of ventricular fibrillation/pulseless ventricular tachycardia (VF/VT) as shockable rhythms is crucial to the delivery of effective treatment. Automated external defibrillators (AEDs) and shock advisory defibrillators (SADs) can identify these rhythms reliably by electronic analysis. If a shockable rhythm is present, the defibrillator will charge to the appropriate energy level and instruct the operator that a shock is required. The introduction of AEDs has enabled resuscitation from VF/VT to be achieved by people who do not have skill in rhythm recognition, both in hospitals and in the community.

The accurate analysis of some cardiac rhythm abnormalities requires experience and expertise; however, the non-expert can interpret most rhythms sufficiently to identify the appropriate treatment. The main priority is to recognise that the rhythm is abnormal and that the heart rate is inappropriately slow or fast. Use the structured approach to rhythm interpretation, described in this chapter, to avoid errors. The need for immediate treatment will be determined largely by the effect of the arrhythmia on the patient rather than by the nature of the arrhythmia. When an arrhythmia is present, first assess the patient (use the ABCDE approach), and then interpret the rhythm as accurately as possible. Treat the patient, not the ECG!

Techniques for ECG monitoring

Cardiac monitors

Cardiac monitors display the ECG on a screen in real time. The signal is obtained from adhesive electrodes on the patient's skin and transmitted to the monitor either by wires or by telemetry. Many monitor systems have other features, such as the ability to print samples of the ECG rhythm display or to store samples of the ECG. Most monitors include a display of heart rate, and some have alarms that can be programmed to provide an alert when the heart rate goes below or exceeds preset limits.

Many systems enable monitoring of other values such as blood pressure and oxygen saturation, which are important in the assessment of patients at risk. Digital processing of the ECG offers the potential for electronic analysis of the cardiac rhythm. If a patient requires monitoring, make sure that the monitor is being observed so that immediate action can be taken if necessary, should the rhythm change.

How to attach the monitor

Attach ECG electrodes to the patient using the positions shown in Figure 8.1. These will enable monitoring using 'modified limb leads' I, II and III. Make sure that the skin is dry, not greasy (use an alcohol swab and/or abrasive pad to clean), and either place the electrodes on relatively hair-free skin or shave off dense hair. Place electrodes over bone rather than muscle, to minimise interference from muscle artefact in the ECG signal. Different electrode positions may be used when necessary (e.g. trauma, recent surgery, skin disease).

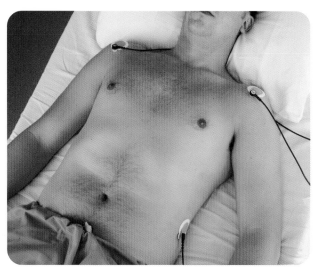

Figure 8.1 Position of electrode for monitoring the ECG using modified limb leads

Most leads are colour-coded to help with correct connection. The usual scheme (except in the United States) uses **R**ed for the **R**ight arm lead, ye**LL**ow for the **L**eft arm lead, **G**reen for the le**G** lead (usually placed on the abdomen or lower left chest wall) for modified limb leads.

Begin by monitoring in modified lead II as this usually displays good amplitude sinus P waves and good amplitude QRS complexes, but switch to another lead if necessary to obtain the best ECG signal. Try to minimise muscle and movement artefact by explaining to patients what the monitoring is for and by keeping them warm and relaxed.

Emergency monitoring

In an emergency, such as a collapsed patient, assess the cardiac rhythm as soon as possible by applying adhesive defibrillator pads, which can be used for monitoring and hands-free shock delivery (Figure 8.2). Apply the pads in the conventional positions, beneath the right clavicle and in the left mid-axillary line. Use anterior and posterior positions as an alternative if the conventional positions cannot be used (e.g. permanent pacemaker in right pectoral position, chest wall trauma). The rapid application of manual defibrillator paddles also enables the cardiac rhythm to be determined rapidly, but in most healthcare environments these paddles have been replaced with hands-free adhesive defibrillator pads.

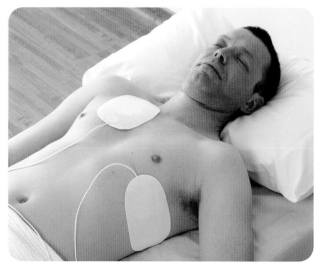

Figure 8.2 Defibrillator pads

Diagnosis from cardiac monitors

Use the displays and printouts from cardiac monitors only for rhythm recognition; do not attempt to interpret ST segment abnormalities or other more sophisticated elements of the ECG from monitors. When an arrhythmia is detected on a monitor, record a rhythm strip whenever possible.

If the arrhythmia persists for long enough, record a 12-lead ECG. It is not always possible to identify an arrhythmia from a single lead ECG recording. The heart is a three-dimensional organ and the 12-lead ECG examines the electrical signals from the heart in three dimensions. Sometimes, features that enable precise identification of cardiac rhythm are visible in only one or two leads of the 12-lead ECG and would not be seen on a single-lead recording of any other lead (Figure 8.3).

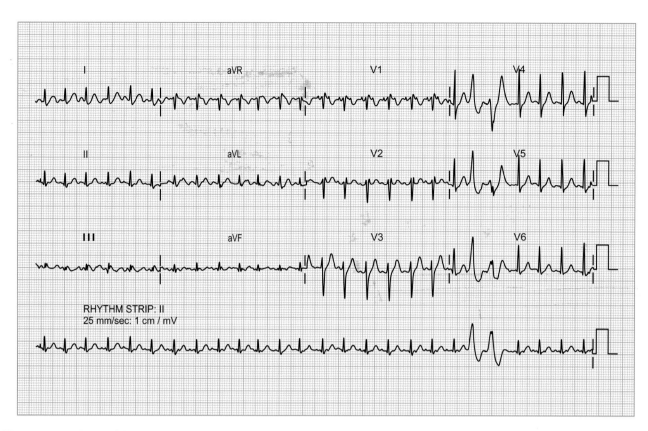

Figure 8.3 12-lead ECG showing atrial tachycardia, which is seen clearly only in lead V1

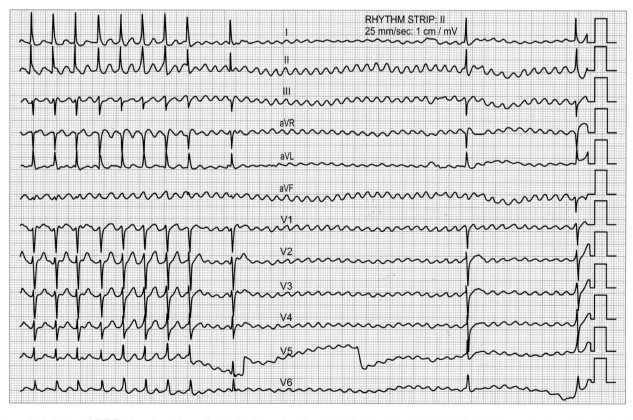

Figure 8.4 12-lead ECG showing the effect of adenosine in atrial flutter. Transient AV block demonstrates clearly that this regular narrow-complex tachycardia was atrial flutter with 2:1 AV conduction

These recordings may assist with rhythm interpretation at the time but are also useful for later examination and planning of treatment in the longer term. Therefore effective management of any arrhythmia, including a cardiac arrest arrhythmia, includes good quality ECG recording, as well as interpretation and treatment at the time.

Valuable information about the nature and origin of a tachyarrhythmia can also be obtained by recording the response to treatment (e.g. carotid sinus massage, adenosine). Whenever possible, the effect of any such intervention should be recorded on a continuous ECG recording, if possible using multiple leads (Figure 8.4).

Basic electrocardiography

At rest, the cells of the cardiac conducting system and myocardium are polarised. A potential difference of approximately 90 mV is present between the inside of the cell (which is negatively charged) and the extracellular space. A sudden shift of ions across the cell membrane triggers depolarisation, generating the electrical signal that travels through the conducting system and triggers contraction of myocardial cells.

In normal sinus rhythm, depolarisation begins in a group of specialised 'pacemaker' cells, called the sino-atrial (SA) node, located close to the entry of the superior vena cava into the right atrium. A wave of depolarisation then spreads from the SA node through the atrial myocardium.

This is seen on the ECG as the P wave (Figure 8.5). Atrial contraction is the mechanical response to this electrical impulse.

The transmission of this electrical impulse to the ventricles occurs through specialised conducting tissue (Figure 8.6).

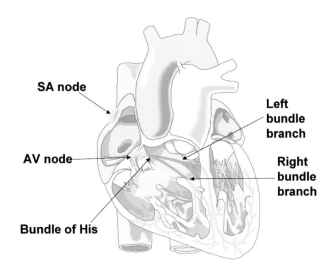

Figure 8.6 Electrical conduction in the heart

Firstly, there is slow conduction through the atrioventricular (AV) node, followed by rapid conduction to the ventricular myocardium by specialised conducting tissue (Purkinje fibres). The bundle of His carries these fibres from the AV node and then divides into right and left bundle branches, spreading out through the right and left ventricles respectively. Rapid conduction down these fibres ensures that the ventricles contract in a co-ordinated fashion.

Depolarisation of ventricular myocardium is seen on the ECG as the QRS complex (Figure 8.5). Ventricular contraction is the mechanical response to this electrical impulse.

Between the P wave and QRS complex is a small isoelectric segment, which largely represents the delay in transmission through the AV node. The normal sequence of atrial depolarisation followed by ventricular depolarisation (P wave followed by QRS complex) is sinus rhythm (Rhythm Strip 1).

The T wave, which follows the QRS complex, represents recovery of the resting potential in the cells of the conducting system and ventricular myocardium (ventricular repolarisation).

Because the normal conducting system transmits the depolarising impulse rapidly to both ventricles, the normal QRS complex is of relatively short duration (normally < 0.12 s).

When one of the bundle branches is diseased or damaged, rapid conduction to the corresponding ventricle is prevented. The depolarising impulse travels more rapidly down the other bundle branch to its ventricle and then more slowly, through ordinary ventricular myocardium to the other ventricle. This situation is called bundle branch block. Because depolarisation of both ventricles takes longer than normal it is seen on the ECG as a broad QRS complex (0.12 s or longer).

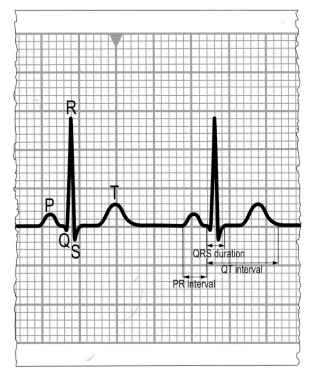

Figure 8.5 Components of the normal ECG signal

How to read a rhythm strip

Experience and expertise may be needed to identify some rhythm abnormalities with complete precision. However, a simple, structured approach to interpreting the rhythm on any ECG recording will define any rhythm in sufficient detail to enable the most appropriate treatment to be chosen.

Apply the following 6-stage system to the analysis of any rhythm on an ECG:

1. Is there any electrical activity?

2. What is the ventricular (QRS) rate?

3. Is the QRS rhythm regular or irregular?

4. Is the QRS complex width normal or prolonged?

5. Is atrial activity present?

6. Is atrial activity related to ventricular activity and, if so, how?

Any cardiac rhythm can be described accurately (e.g. irregular narrow complex tachycardia, regular broad-complex bradycardia, etc.) and managed safely and effectively using the first four steps.

Is there any electrical activity?

If you cannot see any electrical activity, check that the gain control is not too low and that the electrodes and leads are connected to both the patient and the monitor.

Check the patient: is a pulse present? If the patient is pulseless and there is still no activity on the ECG this is asystole (Rhythm Strip 2). Atrial and ventricular asystole are often both present, resulting in a line with no deflections. A completely straight line indicates usually that a monitoring lead has become disconnected. During asystole the ECG usually shows slight undulation of the baseline, and may show electrical interference due to respiratory movement, or chest compression.

Atrial activity (usually P waves but occasionally atrial fibrillation (AF) or atrial flutter) may continue for a short time after the onset of ventricular asystole. The ECG will show the atrial activity but no QRS complexes - ventricular standstill (Rhythm Strip 3). Recognition of this is important because pacing is more likely to achieve a cardiac output in this situation than in most cases of complete asystole (Chapter 10).

If the patient is pulseless and electrical activity is present, decide whether recognisable QRS complexes are present. If not, and the ECG shows rapid, bizarre, irregular deflections of random frequency and amplitude, this is VF (Rhythm Strip 4). In VF all co-ordination of electrical activity is lost, and there is no effective ventricular contraction, and no detectable cardiac output.

Ventricular fibrillation is sometimes classified as coarse (Rhythm Strip 4) or fine (Rhythm Strip 5) depending on the amplitude of the complexes; If there is doubt about whether the rhythm is asystole or fine VF, do not attempt defibrillation; instead, continue chest compressions and ventilation. Fine VF that is difficult to distinguish from asystole is unlikely to be shocked successfully into a rhythm that produces a cardiac output. Continuing good-quality CPR may improve the amplitude and frequency of the VF and improve the chance of subsequent successful defibrillation and return of spontaneous circulation. Delivering repeated shocks in an attempt to defibrillate what is thought to be fine VF will increase myocardial injury both directly from the electric current and indirectly from the interruptions in coronary blood flow (Chapter 6).

If electrical activity is present and contains recognisable QRS complexes, continue with the following steps in rhythm analysis.

If the patient is pulseless and there are recognisable complexes on the ECG that would be expected to produce a pulse, this is pulseless electrical activity (PEA) and requires immediate CPR. Do not delay CPR whilst the cardiac rhythm is analysed further.

What is the ventricular (QRS) rate?

The normal heart rate (ventricular rate) at rest is 60 - 100 beats min⁻¹. A bradycardia has a heart rate slower than 60 min⁻¹. A tachycardia has a rate faster than 100 min⁻¹. ECG paper is calibrated in mm, with bolder lines every 5 mm. Standard paper speed in the UK is 25 mm s⁻¹. One second is represented by 5 large squares (25 small squares).

The best way of estimating the heart rate is to count the number of cardiac cycles that occur in 6 s (30 large squares) and multiply by 10. This provides an estimate of heart rate, even when the rhythm is somewhat irregular. For example, if 20 cardiac cycles occur in 30 large squares the rate is 200 min⁻¹ (Figure 8.7). For shorter rhythm strips count the number of cardiac cycles in 3 s (15 large squares) and multiply by 20.

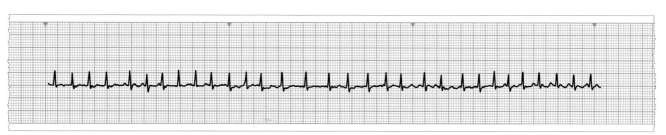

Figure 8.7 Calculation of heart rate from a rhythm strip (20 cardiac cycles occur in 30 large squares = 200 min⁻¹).

Is the QRS rhythm regular or irregular?

This is not always as easy as it seems; at faster heart rates beat-to-beat variation during some irregular rhythms appears less obvious. Some rhythms may be regular in places but intermittent variation in R-R interval makes them irregular. Inspect an adequate length of rhythm strip carefully, measuring out each R-R interval and comparing it to others to detect any irregularity that is not obvious at first glance. Dividers are very useful for comparing the R-R intervals. Alternatively, the position of two adjacent identical points in the cardiac cycle (such as the tips of the R waves) can be marked on a strip of paper; this can then be moved to another section of the rhythm strip. If the rhythm is regular the marks will align precisely with each pair of R waves.

If the QRS rhythm is irregular, decide:

- Is this totally irregular, with no recognisable pattern of R-R interval?

- Is the basic rhythm regular, with intermittent irregularity?

- Is there a recurring cyclical variation in the R-R intervals?

If there is a cyclical pattern, the relationship between the QRS waves and the P wave requires careful analysis, as described below. If the R-R intervals are totally irregular (irregularly irregular) and the QRS complex is of constant morphology, the rhythm is most likely to be AF (Rhythm Strip 6).

A regular underlying rhythm may be made irregular by extrasystoles (ectopic beats). Extrasystoles can arise from the atria or the ventricles, and the position or focus from which they arise will determine their morphology on an ECG.

If the QRS complex of ectopic beats is narrow (< 0.12 s), the beat is likely to have come from above the ventricular myocardium (i.e. from atrial muscle or the AV node).

Broad-complex ectopic beats may be of ventricular origin or may be supraventricular ectopic beats with bundle branch block.

Broad-complex atrial premature beats can sometimes be identified by a preceding ectopic P wave. Ventricular ectopic beats can be accompanied by a P wave occurring shortly after the QRS complex, caused by retrograde conduction from the ventricles to the atria.

Ectopic beats that occur early (that is before the next regular sinus beat was due to occur) are referred to as premature beats (Rhythm Strip 7).

A beat that arises from the AV node or from ventricular myocardium after a long pause, for example during sinus bradycardia or after sinus arrest, is referred to as an escape beat (Rhythm Strip 8). This implies that the focus in the AV node or ventricle that generates this beat is acting as a back-up pacemaker, because the normal pacemaker function of the sinus node is too slow or absent. Ectopic beats may occur singly, in pairs (couplets) or in threes (triplets). If more than three ectopic beats occur in rapid succession, this is regarded as a tachyarrhythmia.

An arrhythmia that occurs intermittently, interspersed with periods of normal sinus rhythm, is described as paroxysmal.

When ectopic beats occur alternately with sinus beats for a sustained period this is called bigeminy. It may be referred to as atrial bigeminy or ventricular bigeminy, depending on whether the ectopic beats are atrial or ventricular in origin.

Is the QRS complex width normal or prolonged?

The upper limit of normal for the QRS interval is 0.12 s (3 small squares). If the QRS width is less than this, the rhythm originates from above the bifurcation of the bundle of His and may be from the SA node, atria or AV node, but not from the ventricular myocardium. If the QRS duration is 0.12 s or more the rhythm may be coming from ventricular myocardium or may be a supraventricular rhythm, transmitted with aberrant conduction (i.e. bundle branch block).

Is atrial activity present?

Having defined the rhythm in terms of rate, regularity and QRS width, examine the ECG carefully for evidence of atrial activity. This may be difficult or impossible to identify, either because it is not visible or because atrial activity is partly or completely obscured by QRS complexes or T waves. Do not guess or try to convince yourself that you can identify atrial activity unless you are completely sure.

Depending on the nature of the arrhythmia and the ECG lead being examined, P waves may be present as positive deflections, negative deflections or biphasic deflections. When present, U waves may be mistaken for P waves. P waves may coincide with and cause distortion or variation of QRS complexes, ST segments, or T waves. Whenever possible, recording of a 12-lead ECG may enable P waves to be identified in one or more leads, even if they cannot be seen clearly in the initial monitoring lead. Lead V1 is often useful for clear demonstration of some types of atrial activity including sinus P waves and AF. Sinus P waves are usually seen clearly in lead II.

Other types of atrial activity may be present. During atrial flutter, atrial activity is seen as flutter waves - an absolutely regular repetitive deflection with a 'saw-tooth' appearance, often at a rate of about 300 min^{-1}. This is usually seen best in the inferior leads (II, III, aVF) (Figure 8.4).

During AF, circuits and waves of depolarisation travel randomly through both atria. There are no P waves. Atrial fibrillation waves may be seen as rapid deviations from the baseline of varying amplitude and duration, usually seen best in lead V1. In some patients this may be of such low amplitude that no atrial activity can be seen.

During a sustained tachycardia atrial activity may not be visible between the QRS complexes. If the rhythm is of atrial origin (e.g. atrial flutter or AF) it may be possible to reveal atrial activity by slowing the ventricular rate whilst recording an ECG, preferably in multiple leads. For example, if a regular tachycardia of 150 min^{-1} is due to atrial flutter with 2:1 conduction it may not be possible to identify flutter waves with confidence. A transient increase in AV block by vagal stimulation or by an intravenous bolus of adenosine will demonstrate the flutter waves and identify the rhythm accurately (Figure 8.4).

The shape and direction of P waves help to identify the atrial rhythm. For example, sinus P waves are upright in leads II and aVF. If retrograde activation of the atria is taking place from the region of the AV node (i.e. the rhythm is junctional or ventricular in origin), the P waves will be inverted in leads II and aVF because atrial depolarisation travels in the opposite direction to normal.

P wave rate and regularity (and flutter wave rate) are assessed in the same way as the rate and regularity of QRS complexes.

Is atrial activity related to ventricular activity and, if so, how?

If there is a consistent interval between each P wave and the following QRS complex, it is likely that conduction between atrium and ventricle is intact and that ventricular depolarisation is triggered by atrial depolarisation. Examine a long rhythm strip to make sure that subtle variation in the PR interval is not missed. Occasionally conduction between atria and ventricles is reversed (i.e. ventricular depolarisation is followed by retrograde conduction through the AV node and then by atrial depolarisation); the P wave occurs soon after the QRS complex. It may sometimes be difficult to distinguish between this situation and the presence of a very long PR interval.

In other circumstances careful inspection will detect no relationship between the timing of P waves and of QRS complexes. This will indicate that atrial and ventricular depolarisation is arising independently, sometimes referred to as atrioventricular dissociation. Examples of this include:

- Complete (third degree) AV block, where a normal sinus rate in the atria is accompanied by a regular bradycardia arising below the AV node.

- Some examples of VT in which regular broad QRS complexes are present and regular P waves can be seen at a different, slower rate, out of phase with the QRS complexes.

Difficulty may arise when the relationship between the P waves and the QRS complexes varies in a recurring pattern. This may be misinterpreted as atrioventricular dissociation. This is seen most commonly in one form of second degree AV block (called Wenkebach or Mobitz I AV block). Examine a long rhythm strip carefully for recurring patterns and plot and compare the timing of P waves and QRS complexes. In complete AV block, the QRS rhythm is usually completely regular.

In AF, the atrial activity is completely irregular, so there is no identifiable relationship between this atrial activity and the irregular ventricular rhythm that results from it. If AF is accompanied by a completely regular, slow ventricular rhythm this is likely to be due to complete AV block in the presence of AF in the atria.

In atrial flutter there may be a consistent relationship between the flutter waves and the QRS complexes, giving rise to 1:1, 2:1, 3:1 conduction etc. In some instances, there is a constantly varying relationship, producing an irregular QRS rhythm; this is atrial flutter with variable AV block.

Cardiac arrest rhythms

The rhythms present during cardiac arrest can be classified into 3 groups:

- ventricular fibrillation (VF) and some cases of ventricular tachycardia (VT);

- asystole;

- pulseless electrical activity (PEA).

Extreme bradycardia and rarely very fast supraventricular tachyarrhythmia may also cause such a severe fall in cardiac output to effectively cause cardiac arrest.

Ventricular fibrillation

The characteristic appearance of VF (Rhythm Strip 4) is usually easy to recognise, and this is the only rhythm that does not need the systematic rhythm analysis described earlier in this chapter. When a monitor appears to show VF check the patient immediately to establish whether this is VF requiring immediate defibrillation, or whether the appearance is due to artefact. If the patient has a pulse, the rhythm is not VF.

Two rhythm abnormalities may resemble VF in some circumstances, since both produce an irregular, broad-complex, fast rhythm:

One is polymorphic VT (Rhythm Strip 12). This may cause cardiac arrest, and when it does so the immediate treatment is the same as for VF, so failure to distinguish this immediately from VF would not lead to inappropriate treatment. However, it is important to document polymorphic VT and to recognise it following immediate resuscitation, so that the causes can be identified and corrected and appropriate treatment given to prevent recurrence.

The second possible source of confusion is pre-excited AF. This occurs in the presence of an accessory pathway connecting atrial and ventricular muscle in the Wolff-Parkinson-White (WPW) syndrome. Some of these accessory pathways can conduct very rapidly, transmitting atrial impulses to the ventricles, sometimes at 300 min^{-1} or faster. This produces an irregular broad complex tachycardia (Figure 8.8) that does not usually resemble VF but might be mistaken for polymorphic VT. Left untreated, this rhythm may lead to VT or VF causing cardiac arrest. If AF with WPW syndrome itself caused clinical cardiac arrest, the correct treatment would be immediate defibrillation (as for any broad-complex pulseless tachycardia) so misinterpretation as VT or VF would not lead to inappropriate treatment. Again, the importance of documenting and recognising the rhythm is to ensure that the patient receives immediate appropriate specialist referral for treatment to protect them against the risk of recurrence of this potentially dangerous arrhythmia.

Ventricular tachycardia

Ventricular tachycardia (VT) may cause loss of cardiac output resulting in cardiac arrest, particularly at faster rates or in the presence of structural heart disease (e.g. impaired left ventricular function, severe left ventricular hypertrophy, aortic stenosis). VT may degenerate suddenly into VF. Pulseless VT is treated in the same way as VF by immediate defibrillation.

In the presence of a cardiac output (i.e. palpable pulse), treatment of VT should follow the broad complex tachycardia algorithm described in Chapter 11.

The QRS morphology may be monomorphic or polymorphic. In monomorphic VT (Rhythm Strip 10), the rhythm is regular (or almost regular). The rate during VT may be anything from 100 to 300 min^{-1}, rarely faster. It is unusual to see more than slight variation in heart rate during any single episode of VT (other than in response to anti-arrhythmic drug therapy). Atrial activity may continue independently of ventricular activity; the identification of P waves, dissociated from QRS complexes during broad complex tachycardia, identifies the rhythm as VT. Occasionally these atrial beats may be conducted to the ventricles, causing capture beats or fusion beats (Rhythm Strip 11). A capture beat produces a single normal-looking QRS complex during monomorphic VT, without otherwise interrupting the arrhythmia. In a fusion beat, a wave of depolarisation travelling down from the AV node occurs simultaneously with a wave of depolarisation travelling up from the ventricular focus producing the arrhythmia. This results in a hybrid QRS complex caused by fusion of the normal QRS complex with the complex of the monomorphic VT.

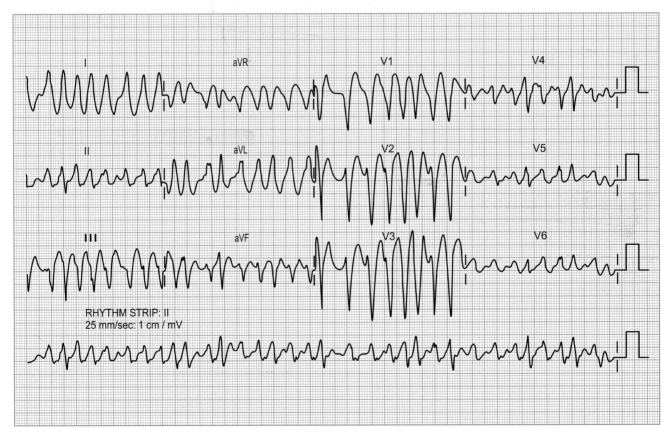

Figure 8.8 12-lead ECG showing pre-excited atrial fibrillation in a patient with Wolff-Parkinson-White syndrome

In the presence of bundle branch block, a supraventricular tachycardia (SVT) will produce a broad complex tachycardia. After myocardial infarction, most broad complex tachycardia will be ventricular in origin. The safest approach is to regard all broad complex tachycardia as VT until, or unless, proved otherwise.

One important type of polymorphic VT is torsade de pointes (TDP) in which the axis of the electrical activity changes in a rotational way so that the overall appearance of the ECG on a rhythm strip produces a sinusoidal pattern (Rhythm Strip 12). This arrhythmia usually arises in patients with a prolonged QT interval. This can occur as an inherited phenomenon in some families (long QT syndromes). In some people it is caused by drugs, including some anti-arrhythmic drugs, and it may occur less commonly as a manifestation of myocardial ischaemia. Many patients with TDP VT are also hypokalaemic and/or hypomagnesaemic. It is important to recognise TDP VT, because effective treatment (prevention of recurrent episodes) will require removal of any predisposing causes (i.e. drugs), treatment with intravenous magnesium and/or potassium, and may also require the use of overdrive pacing. Drugs that prolong QT interval (including amiodarone) should be avoided in patients with TDP VT. This arrhythmia can itself cause cardiac arrest (in which case it is treated by defibrillation) and it can also degenerate into VF.

Asystole

The appearance of asystole has been described already (Rhythm Strip 2). Sometimes it is not clear whether the observed rhythm is asystole or very fine VF. In this situation, immediate treatment is to provide high quality CPR. If fine VF was present, good CPR may increase the amplitude and frequency of the VF, making that diagnosis clear and increasing the probability of successful defibrillation.

Pulseless electrical activity

The term pulseless electrical activity (PEA) does not refer to a specific cardiac rhythm. It defines the clinical absence of cardiac output despite electrical activity that would normally be expected to produce a cardiac output. It generally has a poor prognosis especially when it is caused by a very large acute myocardial infarction. Potentially more treatable causes include massive pulmonary embolism, tension pneumothorax, cardiac tamponade and acute severe blood loss.

Peri-arrest arrhythmias

These are defined according to heart rate (bradyarrhythmia, tachyarrhythmia or arrhythmia with a normal rate), as this will dictate initial treatment (Chapter 11). In the unstable patient, concentrate on early treatment to prevent deterioration, rather than on prolonged attempts to identify the precise rhythm.

Bradyarrhythmia

A bradycardia is present when the ventricular (QRS) rate is < 60 min⁻¹ (Rhythm Strip 13). Bradycardia may be a physiological state in very fit people or during sleep, or may be an expected result of treatment (e.g. with a beta-blocker). Pathological bradycardia may be caused by malfunction of the SA node or from partial or complete failure of atrioventricular conduction. Some patients with these rhythm abnormalities may need treatment with an implanted pacemaker (Rhythm Strip 14).

The emergency treatment of most bradycardia is with atropine and/or cardiac pacing. Occasionally it may be necessary to use sympathomimetic drugs such as isoprenaline or adrenaline. The need for treatment depends on the haemodynamic effect of the arrhythmia and the risk of developing asystole, rather than the precise ECG classification of the bradycardia. Extreme bradycardia may sometimes precede cardiac arrest and this may be prevented by prompt and appropriate treatment. In this context the most important bradyarrhythmia is acquired complete heart block (see below).

Heart block: first degree atrioventricular block

The PR interval is the time between the onset of the P wave and the start of the QRS complex (whether this begins with a Q wave or R wave). The normal PR interval is between 0.12 and 0.20 s. First degree atrioventricular (AV) block is present when the PR interval is > 0.20 s and is a common finding (Rhythm Strip 15). It represents a delay in conduction through the AV junction (the AV node and bundle of His). In some instances this may be physiological (for example in trained athletes). There are many other causes of first degree AV block, including primary disease (fibrosis) of the conducting system, various types of structural heart disease, ischaemic heart disease and use of drugs that delay conduction through the AV node. First degree AV block rarely causes any symptoms and as an isolated finding rarely requires treatment.

Heart block: second degree atrioventricular block

Second degree AV block is present when some, but not all, P waves are conducted to the ventricles, resulting in absence of a QRS complex after some P waves. There are two types:

Mobitz Type I AV block (also called Wenckebach AV block)

The PR interval shows progressive prolongation after each successive P wave until a P wave occurs without a resulting QRS complex. Usually the cycle is then repeated (Rhythm Strip 16).

Any condition that delays AV conduction can produce Wenkebach AV block. In some situations this may be physiological, for example in highly trained athletes with high vagal tone. Outside that setting Wenckebach AV block is usually pathological. Its many causes include acute myocardial infarction (especially inferior infarction). If asymptomatic, this rhythm does not usually require immediate treatment. The need for treatment is dictated by the effect of the bradyarrhythmia on the patient and the risk of developing more severe AV block or asystole.

Mobitz Type II AV block

There is a constant PR interval in the conducted beats but some of the P waves are not followed by QRS complexes. This may occur randomly, without any consistent pattern. People with Mobitz II AV block have an increased risk of progression to complete AV block and asystole.

2:1 and 3:1 AV block

The term 2:1 AV block describes the situation in which alternate P waves are followed by a QRS complex (Rhythm Strip 17). 2:1 AV block may be due to Mobitz I or Mobitz II AV block and it may be difficult to distinguish which it is from the ECG appearance. If bundle branch block is present as well as 2:1 block (broad QRS complexes) this is likely to be Mobitz II block. 3:1 AV block (Rhythm strip 18) is less common and is a form of Mobitz II AV block. Immediate decisions about treatment of these rhythms (see algorithm for treatment of bradycardia - Chapter 11) will be determined by the effect of the resulting bradycardia on the patient. After identifying and providing any necessary immediate treatment continue cardiac monitoring and arrange expert cardiological assessment.

Heart block: third degree atrioventricular block

In third degree (complete) AV block, there is no relationship between P waves and QRS complexes; atrial and ventricular depolarisation arises independently from separate 'pacemakers' (Rhythm Strip 19). The site of the pacemaker stimulating the ventricles will determine the ventricular rate and QRS width. A pacemaker site in the AV node or proximal bundle of His may have an intrinsic rate of 40 - 50 min⁻¹ or sometimes higher and may produce a narrow QRS complex. A pacemaker site in the distal His-Purkinje fibres or ventricular myocardium will produce broad QRS complexes, often have a rate of 30 - 40 min⁻¹ or less, and is more likely to stop abruptly, resulting in asystole.

Escape rhythms

If the normal cardiac pacemaker (SA node) fails, or operates abnormally slowly, cardiac depolarisation may be initiated from a 'subsidiary' pacemaker in atrial myocardium, AV node, conducting fibres or ventricular myocardium. The resulting escape rhythm will be slower

than the normal sinus rate. As indicated above, subsidiary pacemakers situated distally in the conducting system tend to produce slower heart rates than those situated more proximally. Thus a ventricular escape rhythm will usually be slower than a 'junctional' rhythm arising from the AV node or bundle of His.

The term idioventricular rhythm is used to describe a rhythm arising from ventricular myocardium. This includes ventricular escape rhythms seen in the presence of complete AV block. The term accelerated idioventricular rhythm is used to describe an idioventricular rhythm with a normal heart rate (usually faster than the sinus rate but not fast enough to be VT). This type of rhythm is observed quite frequently after successful thrombolysis (or primary percutaneous coronary intervention) for acute myocardial infarction (a 'reperfusion arrhythmia'). Accelerated idioventricular rhythms do not influence prognosis unless they cause haemodynamic compromise or develop into VT or VF, which is uncommon. The QRS complex of an idioventricular rhythm will be broad (i.e. 0.12 s or greater), whereas a junctional rhythm may be narrow or broad, depending on whether conduction to the ventricles occurs normally, or with bundle branch block.

Agonal rhythm

Agonal rhythm occurs in dying patients. It is characterised by the presence of slow, irregular, wide ventricular complexes, often of varying morphology (Rhythm Strip 20). This rhythm is seen commonly during the later stages of unsuccessful resuscitation attempts. The complexes slow inexorably and often become progressively broader before all recognisable activity is lost.

Tachyarrhythmia

A pathological tachycardia may arise from atrial myocardium, the AV junction or ventricular myocardium. Sinus tachycardia is not an arrhythmia and usually represents a response to some other physiological or pathological state (e.g. exercise, anxiety, blood loss, fever etc).

Narrow-complex tachycardia

When a tachycardia arises from tissue situated above the bifurcation of the bundle of His, it is described as supraventricular (Rhythm Strip 21). The QRS complexes will be narrow if ventricular depolarisation occurs normally, but will be broad if bundle branch block is present. QRS complexes may be regular in many rhythms or may be irregular in the presence of atrial fibrillation or variably conducted atrial flutter. Most tachycardia with narrow QRS complexes has a favourable prognosis, but the outlook will vary with individual clinical circumstances. These rhythms may be tolerated poorly by patients with structural heart disease and may provoke angina, especially in patients with coronary artery disease.

Atrial fibrillation

Atrial fibrillation is the most common arrhythmia encountered in clinical practice. It is characterised by disorganised electrical activity in the atria. No recognisable P waves or co-ordinated atrial activity can be seen in any lead (Rhythm Strip 6). The baseline is irregular and chaotic atrial activity is best seen in lead V1 where the atrial waveform is irregular in both amplitude and frequency. The QRS rhythm is irregularly irregular (i.e. there is no consistent R-R interval from beat to beat). The ventricular rate will depend on the refractory period of the AV junction. In the absence of drug treatment or pre-existing disease affecting the AV node, the resulting ventricular rate will be rapid, usually 120 - 180 min^{-1} or faster.

Common causes of AF include hypertension, obesity, alcohol excess and structural heart disease. In coronary heart disease AF usually results from left ventricular impairment (acute or chronic) and not as a direct result of ischaemia of the atrial myocardium.

Atrial flutter

In atrial flutter, atrial activity is seen on the ECG as flutter or F waves at a rate of about 300 min^{-1} (Rhythm Strip 22). These are best seen in the inferior leads II, III and aVF where they have a 'saw-tooth' appearance (Figure 8.4). The ventricular rate depends on AV conduction but there is often 2:1 (Rhythm Strip 9) or 3:1 conduction (often referred to as atrial flutter with 2:1 or 3:1 block). If conduction is constant the ventricular rhythm will be regular, but variable conduction causes an irregular ventricular rhythm. Like atrial fibrillation, atrial flutter is often, but not always, associated with underlying disease. Atrial flutter usually arises in the right atrium so is a recognised complication of diseases that affect the right heart, including chronic obstructive pulmonary disease, major pulmonary embolism, complex congenital heart disease and chronic congestive heart failure of any cause.

Broad-complex tachycardia

Broad-complex tachycardia may be:

- a tachycardia arising in the ventricle below the bifurcation of the bundle of His, i.e. VT (Rhythm Strip 10); or

- a supraventricular tachycardia conducted aberrantly (right or left bundle branch block) to the ventricles.

The clinical consequences depend on:

- heart rate during the arrhythmia;

- the presence or absence of structural heart disease or coronary disease;

- duration of the arrhythmia.

Ventricular tachycardia may degenerate into VF, especially if the VT is very fast (e.g. 200 min^{-1} or faster) or if the heart is unstable as a consequence of acute ischaemia or infarction, or in the presence of electrolyte abnormality (hypokalaemia or hypomagnesaemia).

Treat all broad-complex tachycardia as ventricular tachycardia unless there is good evidence that it is supraventricular in origin.

Patients with WPW syndrome have accessory pathways connecting atrial and ventricular myocardium. Some atrioventricular conduction occurs through these pathways as well as through the AV node. This results in widening of the QRS complexes by so-called delta waves. In the presence of such an accessory pathway that bypasses the AV node, AF may result in a ventricular rate that is so fast that cardiac output decreases dramatically. The ECG appearances are of a very rapid, irregular, broad complex tachycardia that usually shows variability in the width of QRS complexes. This rhythm may be misdiagnosed as irregular VT or possibly as VF. Overall the rhythm is more organised than ventricular fibrillation and lacks the random chaotic activity of variable amplitude.

The QT interval

When identifying and treating rhythm abnormalities it is important to recognise likely underlying causes that may influence choice of effective treatment. These may be identified from clinical assessment (e.g. myocardial infarction), laboratory tests (e.g. electrolyte abnormality) or from the ECG. Prolongation of the QT interval predisposes people to ventricular arrhythmia, in particular TDP VT and VF.

The QT interval is measured from the start of the QRS complex to the end of the T wave. It can be difficult to measure accurately, mainly because it may be difficult to identify the end of the T wave. This may be especially difficult when prominent U waves are present, merging with the end of the T wave. U waves can be a feature of some abnormalities (e.g. hypokalaemia) but may be present in some healthy people with normal hearts.

The length of the QT interval may also vary between different leads of the same ECG. This may partly reflect variation in amplitude and direction of the T wave, making it more difficult to measure in some leads than others. Variation in the QT interval (QT dispersion) has also been shown to be associated with an increased risk of death in patients with ischaemic heart disease, but this finding has not been developed into a useful measurement for use in clinical practice.

The QT interval varies with age, with gender and in particular with heart rate. The QT interval shortens as the heart rate increases. A correction can be made to allow for this, using the measured QT interval and heart rate to

ALS

calculate the corrected QT interval (QTc). The upper end of the normal range for QTc is 0.42 s. Many modern ECG machines measure the QT and other intervals and calculate the QTc automatically. These measurements are accurate only if the ECG recording is of good quality. Most ECG machines cannot distinguish between T waves and U waves. Always look at the recording and make sure that the quoted measurements are not obviously inaccurate. If in doubt seek expert help with interpretation.

Abnormality of the QT interval can be seen in various situations. A shortened QT interval may be seen with hypercalcaemia and digoxin treatment. Hypokalaemia, hypomagnesaemia, hypocalcaemia, hypothermia, myocarditis and in some instances myocardial ischaemia can all cause QT prolongation. There is also a long list of drugs that may prolong the QT interval, including class I and class III anti-arrhythmic drugs.

There are several genetic abnormalities in which the QT interval is abnormal or there is abnormality of ventricular repolarisation (principally the long QT, short QT and Brugada syndromes). The abnormality of repolarisation places them at risk of ventricular arrhythmia and sudden death. These people require expert assessment to identify whether treatment is needed to reduce this risk. For some the only effective treatment is an implantable cardioverter-defibrillator to treat VF or VT immediately, if it occurs. It is especially important that patients with long QT syndromes are not given any drug that may cause further QT prolongation.

Further reading

Blomstrom-Lundqvist C, Scheinmann M M (Co-Chairs). American College of Cardiology/American Heart Association Task Force and the European Society of Cardiology Committee for Practice Guidelines. ACC/AHA/ESC Guidelines for the Management of Patients With Supraventricular Arrhythmias. European Heart Journal 2003;24:1857-1897. www.escardio.org

Fuster V, Ryden L E, Cannom DS, et al. ACC/AHA/ESC 2006 Guidelines for the Management of Patients with Atrial Fibrillation: a report of the American College of Cardiology/American Heart Association Task Force on Practice Guidelines and the European Society of Cardiology Committee for Practice Guidelines (Writing Committee to Revise the 2001 Guidelines for the Management of Patients With Atrial Fibrillation): developed in collaboration with the European Heart Rhythm Association and the Heart Rhythm Society. Circulation 2006;114:e257-354. www.escardio.org

Zipes DP, Camm AJ, Borggrefe M, et al. ACC/AHA/ESC 2006 guidelines for management of patients with ventricular arrhythmias and the prevention of sudden cardiac death: a report of the American College of Cardiology/American Heart Association Task Force and the European Society of Cardiology Committee for Practice Guidelines (Writing Committee to Develop Guidelines for Management of Patients With Ventricular Arrhythmias and the Prevention of Sudden Cardiac Death) J Am Coll Cardiol 2006;48:e247-e346. www.escardio.org

Key learning points

- A systematic approach to ECG rhythm analysis enables accurate assessment of any rhythm abnormality sufficiently to enable safe, effective treatment.

- Recordings of any rhythm abnormality and of the ECG in sinus rhythm provide valuable diagnostic information and help the correct choice of longer-term treatment.

- Accurate monitoring of the cardiac rhythm is essential for any patient at high risk of developing life-threatening arrhythmia.

- Accurate monitoring of the cardiac rhythm is essential in the management of cardiac arrest.

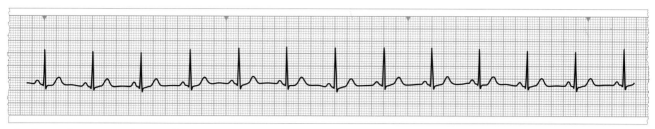

Rhythm Strip 1. Normal sinus rhythm

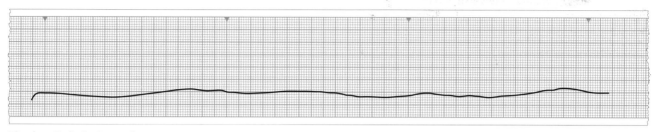

Rhythm Strip 2. Asystole

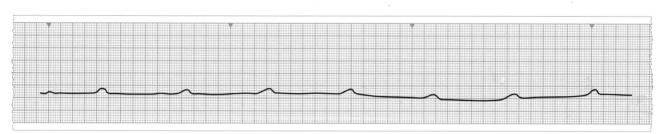

Rhythm Strip 3. P-wave asystole

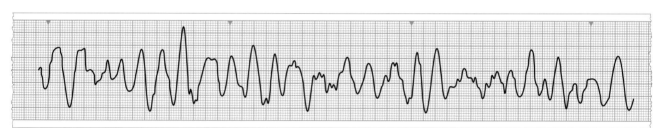

Rhythm Strip 4. Coarse ventricular fibrillation

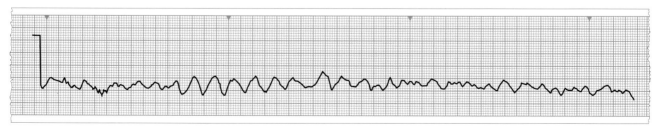

Rhythm Strip 5. Fine ventricular fibrillation

ALS

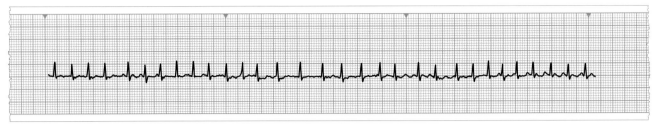

Rhythm Strip 6. Atrial fibrillation

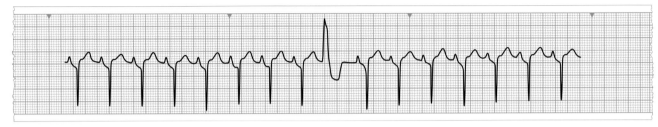

Rhythm Strip 7. Premature ventricular beat

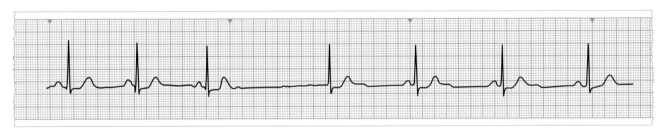

Rhythm Strip 8. Junctional escape beat

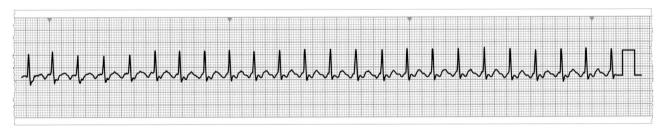

Rhythm Strip 9. Atrial flutter with 2:1 atrioventricular block

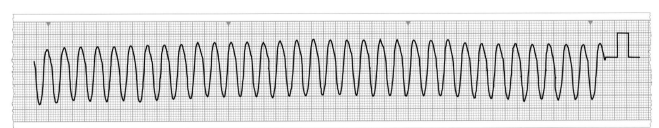

Rhythm Strip 10. Monomorphic ventricular tachycardia

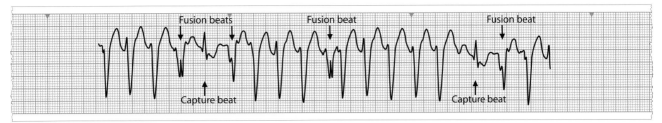

Rhythm Strip 11. Ventricular tachycardia with capture and fusion beats

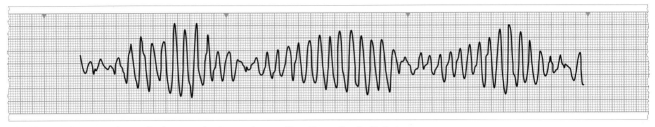

Rhythm Strip 12. Polymorhpic ventricular tachycardia - Torsade de Pointe

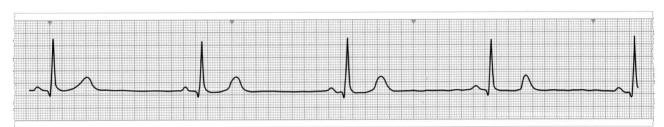

Rhythm Strip 13. Sinus bradycardia

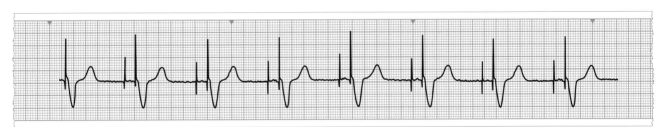

Rhythm Strip 14. Paced rhythm

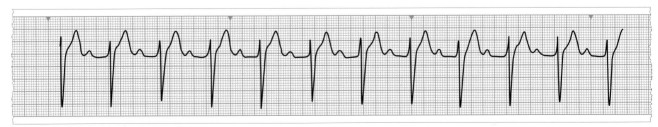

Rhythm Strip 15. First degree atrioventricular block

ALS

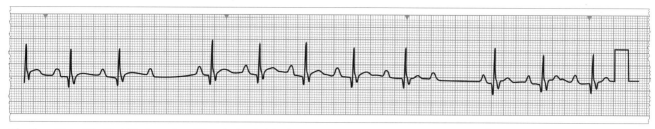

Rhythm Strip 16. Mobitz type I or Wenckebach block

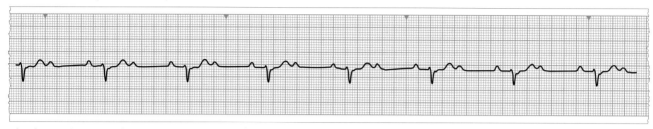

Rhythm Strip 17. Mobitz type II second degree atrioventricular block (2:1)

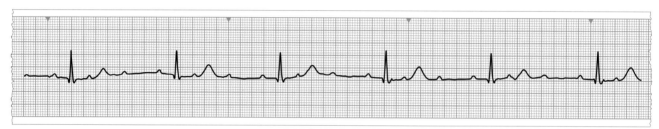

Rhythm Strip 18. Mobitz type II second degree atrioventricular block (3:1)

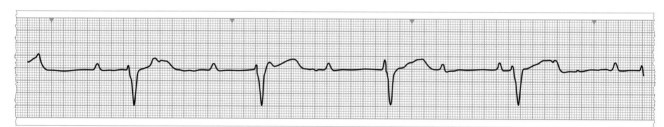

Rhythm Strip 19. Third degree (complete) atrioventricular block

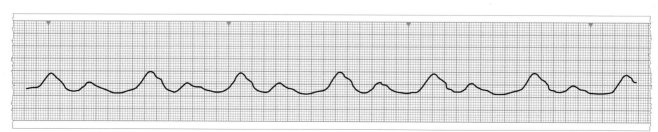

Rhythm Strip 20. Agonal rhythm

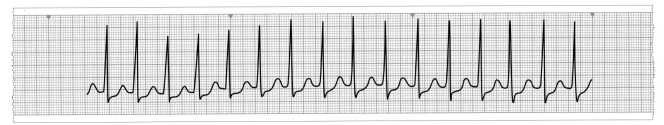

Rhythm Strip 21. Supraventricular tachycardia

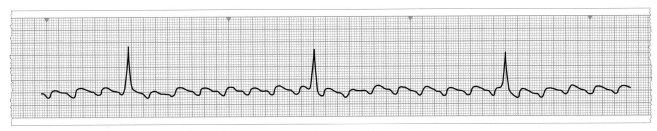

Rhythm Strip 22. Atrial flutter with a high degree of atrioventricular block

Defibrillation

Learning outcomes

To understand:

▶ **The mechanism of defibrillation**

▶ **The factors affecting defibrillation success**

▶ **The importance of minimising interruptions to chest compressions during defibrillation**

▶ **How to deliver a shock safely using either a manual or automated external defibrillator (AED)**

Introduction

Following the onset of ventricular fibrillation or pulseless ventricular tachycardia (VF/VT), cardiac output ceases and cerebral hypoxic injury starts within 3 min. If complete neurological recovery is to be achieved, early successful defibrillation with a return of spontaneous circulation (ROSC) is essential. Defibrillation is a key link in the chain of survival and is one of the few interventions that has been shown to improve outcome from VF/VT cardiac arrest. The probability of successful defibrillation declines rapidly with time; therefore early defibrillation is one of the most important factors in determining survival from cardiac arrest. In the absence of bystander CPR, for every minute that passes between collapse and attempted defibrillation, mortality increases 10 - 12%. **The shorter the interval between the onset of VF/VT and delivery of the shock, the greater the chance of successful defibrillation and survival.** Although defibrillation is key to the management of patients in VF/VT, continuous, uninterrupted chest compressions are also required to optimise the chances of successful resuscitation. Clinical studies have demonstrated that even short interruptions in chest compressions (to deliver rescue breaths or perform rhythm analysis) reduce significantly the chances of successful defibrillation. Animal studies show that even if defibrillation is successful, these short interruptions are associated with post-resuscitation myocardial dysfunction and reduced survival. Analysis of CPR performance during out-of-hospital and in-hospital cardiac arrest has shown that significant interruptions are common and every effort should be made to minimise interruptions. The aim should be to ensure that chest compressions are performed continuously throughout the resuscitation attempt, pausing only to enable specific interventions.

Another factor that is critical in determining the success of defibrillation is the duration of the interval between stopping chest compressions and delivering the shock: the pre-shock pause. The duration of the pre-shock pause is related inversely to the chance of successful defibrillation; every 5-second increase in the pre-shock pause almost halves the chance of successful defibrillation (defined by the absence of VF 5 s after shock delivery). Consequently, defibrillation must always be performed quickly and efficiently in order to maximise the chances of successful resuscitation.

If there is any delay in obtaining a defibrillator, and while the defibrillator is applied, start chest compressions and ventilation immediately. When bystander CPR is given, the decrease in survival is more gradual and averages 3 - 4% per minute from collapse to defibrillation. Bystander CPR can double survival from witnessed cardiac arrest.

Mechanism of defibrillation

Defibrillation is the passage of an electrical current of sufficient magnitude across the myocardium to depolarise a critical mass of cardiac muscle simultaneously, enabling the natural pacemaker tissue to resume control. To achieve this, all defibrillators have three features in common: a power source capable of providing direct current, a capacitor that can be charged to a pre-determined energy level and two electrodes which are placed on the patient's chest, either side of the heart, across which the capacitor is discharged. Successful defibrillation is defined scientifically as the absence of VF/VT at 5 s after shock delivery, although the ultimate goal is ROSC.

Factors affecting defibrillation success

Defibrillation success depends on sufficient current being delivered to the myocardium. However, the delivered current is difficult to determine because it is influenced by transthoracic impedance (electrical resistance) and electrode position. Furthermore, much of the current is diverted along non-cardiac pathways in the thorax and, as a result, as little as 4% reaches the heart.

Transthoracic impedance

Current flow is inversely proportional to transthoracic impedance. Defibrillation technique must be optimised to minimise the transthoracic impedance in order to maximise delivery of current to the myocardium. In adults, impedance is normally in the range 70 - 80 ohm, but in the presence of poor technique may rise to 150 ohm, reducing the current delivered and thereby decreasing the chance of successful defibrillation. Transthoracic impedance is influenced by; electrode-to-skin contact, electrode size and phase of ventilation. Modern biphasic defibrillators can measure the transthoracic impedance and adjust the energy delivered to compensate and are therefore less susceptible to higher transthoracic impedance (impedance compensation).

The presence of a transdermal drug patch on the patient's chest may prevent good contact and may cause arcing and burns if self-adhesive pads are placed over them; if removing them and wiping the area dry before applying the electrodes is likely to delay defibrillation, place the pads in an alternative position that avoids the patch.

Shaving the chest

It may be difficult to obtain good electrode-to-skin contact in patients with very hairy chests. This increases impedance, reduces defibrillation efficacy and may cause burns to the patient's chest. If a patient has a very hairy chest, and if a razor is available immediately, use it to remove excessive hair from the area where the electrodes are placed. However, defibrillation should not be delayed if a razor is not to hand immediately. In very hairy patients, a bi-axillary electrode position may enable more rapid defibrillation.

Electrode size

The optimal electrode size is unknown. Current recommendations are that the sum of the electrode area should be a minimum of 150 cm^2. Self-adhesive pads 8 - 12 cm in diameter are widely used and function well. In practice the self-adhesive pads recommended by the manufacturer for the specific defibrillator should be used.

Ventilatory phase

Transthoracic impedance varies during ventilation and is minimal at end expiration. Therefore if possible, defibrillation should be attempted at this point. Positive end-expiratory pressure (PEEP) increases impedance and where possible should be minimised during defibrillation. During severe asthma, gas trapping within the lungs generates auto-PEEP that may result in the need for higher energy levels for defibrillation.

Electrode position

No human studies have evaluated the electrode position as a determinant of ROSC or survival from cardiac arrest due to a shockable rhythm. Transmyocardial current during defibrillation is likely to be maximal when the electrodes are placed so that the area of the heart that is fibrillating lies directly between them (i.e. ventricles in VF/VT, atria in atrial fibrillation (AF)). Therefore, the optimal electrode position may not be the same for ventricular and atrial arrhythmias.

When attempting to defibrillate a patient in VF/VT, the standard procedure is to place one electrode to the right of the upper sternum below the clavicle. The apical pad is placed in the mid-axillary line, approximately level with the V6 ECG electrode or female breast. This position should be clear of any breast tissue. It is important that this electrode is placed sufficiently laterally (Figure 9.1). Although the electrodes are marked positive and negative, each can be placed in either position. Other acceptable pad positions include:

- One electrode anteriorly, over the left precordium, and the other electrode on the back behind the heart, just inferior to the left scapula (antero-posterior).

- One electrode placed in the mid-axillary line, approximately level with the V6 ECG electrode or female breast and the other electrode on the back, over the right scapula (postero-lateral).

- Each electrode on the lateral chest walls, one on the right and the other on the left side (bi-axillary).

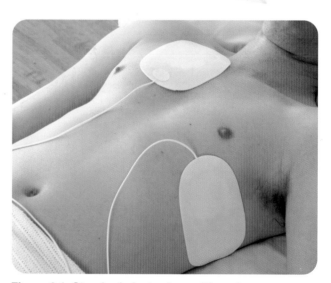

Figure 9.1 Standard electrode positions for defibrillation

CPR or defibrillation first?

In any unwitnessed cardiac arrest, those responding should provide high quality, uninterrupted CPR while a defibrillator is retrieved, attached and charged. Defibrillation must be performed as soon as possible, and a specific period of CPR (e.g. 2 - 3 min) before rhythm analysis and shock delivery is no longer recommended.

Shock sequence

Clinical studies have demonstrated improved defibrillation success and increased survival to hospital discharge when using a single-shock defibrillation protocol compared to a three-stacked-shock protocol for VF cardiac arrest.

With first-shock efficacy of biphasic waveforms generally exceeding 90%, failure to cardiovert VF successfully suggests the need for a period of CPR to perfuse the myocardium, rather than a further shock. Thus, immediately after giving a single shock, and without reassessing the rhythm or feeling for a pulse, resume CPR (30 compressions:2 ventilations) for 2 min before delivering another shock (if indicated - see below). Even if the defibrillation attempt is successful in restoring a perfusing rhythm, it is very rare for a pulse to be palpable immediately after defibrillation and the delay in trying to palpate a pulse will further compromise the myocardium if a perfusing rhythm has not been restored. If a perfusing rhythm has been restored, giving chest compressions does not increase the chance of VF recurring. In the presence of post-shock asystole, chest compressions may induce VF.

Witnessed, monitored VF/VT in the cardiac catheter laboratory or after cardiac surgery

If a patient has a **witnessed** and **monitored** cardiac arrest in the catheter laboratory or early after cardiac surgery:

- Confirm cardiac arrest and shout for help.

- If the initial rhythm is VF/VT, give up to three quick successive (stacked) shocks. Start chest compressions immediately after the third shock and continue CPR for 2 min. With respect to the ALS algorithm, these three quick, successive shocks are regarded as the first shock.

This three-shock strategy may also be considered for an initial, witnessed VF/VT cardiac arrest if the patient is already connected to a manual defibrillator - these circumstances are rare. There are no data supporting a three-shock strategy in any of these circumstances, but it is unlikely that chest compressions will improve the already very high chance of ROSC when defibrillation occurs early in the electrical phase, immediately after onset of VF.

Shock energy and waveforms

The optimal energy levels for defibrillation are unknown and the recommendations below are based on a consensus following a review of the current scientific literature. The aim is to achieve defibrillation and ROSC while minimising myocardial injury by using the lowest effective energy and reducing the number of repetitive shocks.

Although 'energy' levels are selected for defibrillation, it is the transmyocardial current flow that achieves defibrillation. Current correlates well with successful defibrillation and cardioversion. Transthoracic electrical current during defibrillation using biphasic waveforms is in the range of 15 - 20 A for approximately 10 ms.

Historically, defibrillators have delivered a monophasic pulse of current, i.e. one direction of flow between the pads/paddles. These devices are no longer manufactured,

having been superseded by biphasic defibrillators, but it is likely that many will remain in clinical use for several years.

Biphasic defibrillators

Biphasic waveforms deliver current that flows in a positive direction for a specified duration before reversing to a negative direction for the remainder of the electrical discharge. There are two main types of biphasic waveform: the biphasic truncated exponential (BTE) (Figure 9.2) and rectilinear biphasic (RLB) (Figure 9.3). Most biphasic defibrillators compensate for the wide variations in transthoracic impedance by electronically adjusting the waveform magnitude and duration. Biphasic defibrillation requires less energy than monophasic defibrillation; thus biphasic defibrillators have smaller capacitors and need less battery power, and the waveform shape can be controlled by solid-state circuitry. Consequently they are smaller, lighter and easily portable.

Biphasic waveforms are more effective at terminating ventricular arrhythmias at lower energy levels and have a greater first-shock efficacy than monophasic waveforms, particularly for long duration VF/VT (85 - 98% compared with 54 - 91%). Hence the use of biphasic waveforms is recommended whenever possible. Biphasic waveforms are also superior for the elective cardioversion of atrial fibrillation, using less energy and thereby reducing the severity of cutaneous burns. Biphasic waveforms are currently the waveform of choice for this procedure.

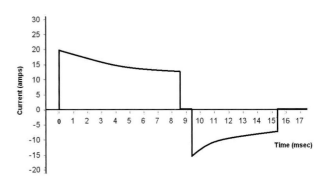

Figure 9.2 Biphasic truncated exponential waveform

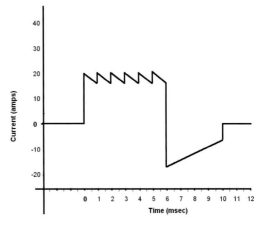

Figure 9.3 Rectilinear biphasic waveform

There is no evidence that either of the two most commonly used biphasic waveforms is more effective. Although the initial biphasic shock energy should be no lower than 120 J for a RLB waveform or 150 J for BTE waveforms, it is recommended that the initial biphasic shock should be at least 150 J for simplicity, irrespective of the biphasic waveform.

If the provider is unaware of the type of defibrillator (monophasic or biphasic) or its effective dose range, use the highest available energy for the first and subsequent shocks. If the first shock is unsuccessful, second and subsequent shocks can be delivered using either fixed or escalating energies of between 150 - 360 J, depending on the device in use. If a shockable rhythm recurs after successful defibrillation (with or without ROSC), give the next shock with the energy level that had previously been successful or higher.

Monophasic defibrillators

The monophasic waveform does not defibrillate as effectively as the biphasic waveform. Therefore, when using a monophasic defibrillator use 360 J for the first and all subsequent shocks.

Importance of uninterrupted chest compressions

The importance of early, uninterrupted chest compression is emphasised throughout this manual; they should be interrupted only for rhythm checking and shock delivery, and resumed as soon as a shock has been delivered. When two rescuers are present, the rescuer operating the defibrillator applies the electrodes whilst CPR is in progress. With manual defibrillation, it is possible to perform CPR during charging thereby reducing the pre-shock pause (interval from stopping compressions to shock delivery) to < 5 s. When using manual defibrillation, the entire process of pausing chest compressions, standing clear, delivering the shock and immediately resuming chest compressions should be achievable in < 5 s.

Safety

Attempted defibrillation should be undertaken without risk to members of the resuscitation team. This is achieved best by using self-adhesive pad electrodes as this eliminates the possibility of anyone touching any part of the electrode. Be wary of wet surroundings or clothing - wipe any water from the patient's chest before attempted defibrillation. No part of any person should make direct or indirect contact with the patient. Do not hold intravenous infusion equipment or the patient's trolley during shock delivery. The operator must ensure that everyone is clear of the patient before delivering a shock.

Gloves may provide limited protection from the electric current; therefore it is strongly recommended that all members of the resuscitation team wear gloves.

Safe use of oxygen during defibrillation

There are several reports of fires being caused in an oxygen-enriched atmosphere by sparking from poorly applied defibrillator paddles and most have resulted in significant burns to the patient. The use of self-adhesive pads is far less likely to cause sparks than manual paddles - no fires have been reported in association with the use of self-adhesive pads. The following are recommended as good practice:

- Take off any oxygen mask or nasal cannulae and place them at least 1 m away from the patient's chest.

- Leave the ventilation bag connected to the tracheal tube or supraglottic airway device, no increase in oxygen concentration occurs in the zone of defibrillation, even with an oxygen flow of 15 l min⁻¹. Alternatively, disconnect the ventilation bag from the tracheal tube or supraglottic airway device and remove it at least 1 m from the patient's chest during defibrillation.

- If the patient is connected to a ventilator, for example in the operating room or critical care unit, leave the ventilator tubing (breathing circuit) connected to the tracheal tube unless chest compressions prevent the ventilator from delivering adequate tidal volumes. In this case, the ventilator is usually substituted by a ventilation bag, which can be left connected or detached and removed to a distance of at least 1 m. If the ventilator tubing is disconnected, ensure that it is kept at least 1 m from the patient or, better still, switch the ventilator off; modern ventilators generate high oxygen flows when disconnected. During normal use, when connected to a tracheal tube, oxygen from a ventilator in the critical care unit will be vented from the main ventilator housing well away from the defibrillation zone. Patients in the critical care unit may be dependent on positive end expiratory pressure (PEEP) to maintain adequate oxygenation; during cardioversion, when the spontaneous circulation potentially enables blood to remain well oxygenated, it is particularly appropriate to leave the critically ill patient connected to the ventilator during shock delivery.

Automated external defibrillators

Automated external defibrillators are sophisticated, reliable, computerised devices that use voice and visual prompts to guide lay rescuers and healthcare professionals to attempt defibrillation safely in cardiac arrest victims (Figure 9.4). Advances in technology, particularly with respect to battery capacity, and software arrhythmia analysis have enabled the mass production of relatively cheap, reliable and easily operated portable defibrillators. Shock-advisory defibrillators have ECG-analysis capability but can usually be manually over-ridden by healthcare providers capable of rhythm recognition.

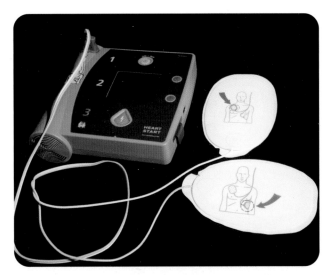

Figure 9.4 Automated external defibrillator (AED)

Automated rhythm analysis

Automated external defibrillators have microprocessors that analyse several features of the ECG, including frequency and amplitude. Some AEDs are programmed to detect spontaneous movement by the patient or others. Developing technology should soon enable AEDs to provide information about frequency and depth of chest compressions during CPR that may improve resuscitation performance by all rescuers.

Automated external defibrillators have been tested extensively against libraries of recorded cardiac rhythms and in many trials in adults and children. They are extremely accurate in rhythm analysis. Although AEDs are not designed to deliver synchronised shocks, all AEDs will recommend shocks for VT if the rate and R-wave morphology exceed preset values.

In-hospital use of AEDs

Delayed defibrillation may occur when patients sustain cardiac arrest in unmonitored hospital beds and in outpatient departments. In these areas several minutes may elapse before resuscitation teams arrive with a defibrillator and deliver shocks. Two non-randomised studies of adults with in-hospital cardiac arrest from shockable rhythms showed higher survival-to-hospital discharge rates when defibrillation was provided through an AED program than with manual defibrillation alone. Despite limited evidence, AEDs should be considered for the hospital setting as a way to facilitate defibrillation as soon as possible (within 3 min of collapse at the most) especially in areas where staff have no rhythm recognition skills or where they use defibrillators infrequently. An effective system for training and retraining should be in place. Adequate numbers of staff should be trained to enable achievement of the goal of providing the first shock within 3 min of collapse anywhere in the hospital.

Training in the use of AEDs can be achieved much more rapidly and easily than for manual defibrillators. Automated equipment has made attempted defibrillation available to a much wider range of medical, nursing, paramedical, and lay workers (e.g. police and first-aiders - 'first-responder defibrillation'). Healthcare providers with a duty to perform CPR should be trained, equipped, and authorised to perform defibrillation. First-responder attempted defibrillation is vital, as the delay to delivery of the first shock is the main determinant of survival in cardiac arrest.

Public access defibrillation (PAD) programmes

Public access defibrillation (PAD) and first responder AED programmes may increase the number of victims who receive bystander CPR and early defibrillation, thus improving survival from out-of-hospital cardiac arrest. These programmes require an organised and practised response with rescuers trained and equipped to recognise emergencies, activate the EMS system, provide CPR, and use the AED. Lay rescuer AED programmes with very rapid response times in airports, on aircraft, or in casinos, and uncontrolled studies using police officers as first responders have achieved reported survival rates as high as 49 - 74%.

Recommended elements for PAD programmes include:

- a planned and practised response;

- training of anticipated rescuers in CPR and use of the AED;

- link with the local EMS system;

- programme of continuous audit (quality improvement).

Public access defibrillation programmes are most likely to improve survival from cardiac arrest if they are established in locations where witnessed cardiac arrest is likely to occur. Suitable sites might include airports, casinos and sports facilities. Approximately 80% of out-of-hospital cardiac arrests occur in private or residential settings; this fact inevitably limits the overall impact that PAD programmes can have on survival rates.

AED Algorithm

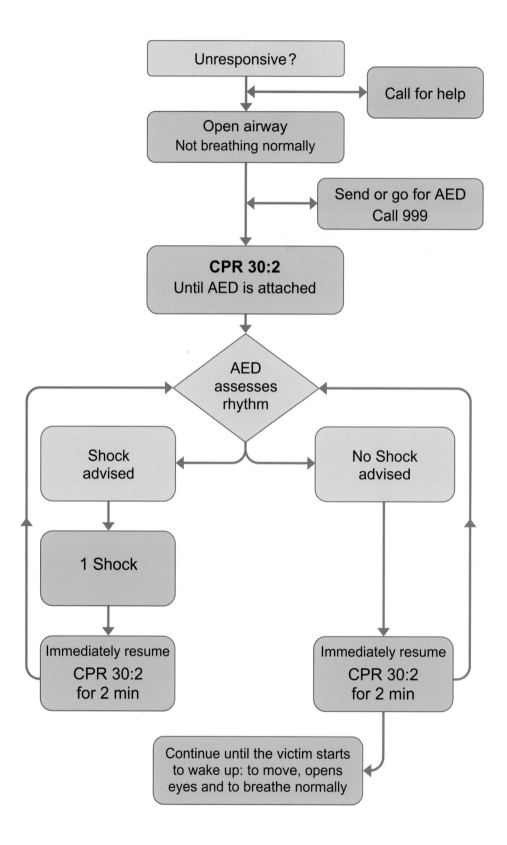

Figure 9.5 AED Algorithm

Sequence for use of an AED or shock-advisory defibrillator

1   Make sure the victim, any bystanders, and you are safe

2   If the victim is unresponsive and not breathing normally:

-   Send someone for the AED and call for an ambulance or resuscitation team. If you are on your own, do this yourself.

3   Start CPR according to the guidelines (Chapter 5).

4   As soon as the AED arrives:

-   Switch on the AED and attach the electrode pads. If more than one rescuer is present, continue CPR while this is done.

-   Follow the voice/visual directions.

-   Ensure that nobody touches the victim whilst the AED is analysing the rhythm.

5A   If a shock **IS** indicated:

-   Ensure that nobody touches the victim (Figure 9.6a).

-   Push the shock button (Figure 9.6b) as directed.

-   Continue as directed by the voice/visual prompts.

5B   If **NO** shock is indicated:

-   Immediately resume CPR using a ratio of 30 compressions to 2 rescue breaths (Figure 9.6c).

-   Continue as directed by the voice/visual prompts.

6   Continue to follow the AED prompts until:

-   Qualified help (e.g. ambulance or resuscitation team) arrives and takes over.

-   The victim starts to breathe normally, or

-   You become exhausted.

Notes

●   The carrying case with the AED must contain some strong scissors for cutting through clothing and a disposable razor for shaving excessive chest hair in order to obtain good electrode contact.

●   If ALS providers are using the AED, they should implement other ALS interventions (advanced airway, ventilation, IV access, drug delivery, etc.) according to local protocols.

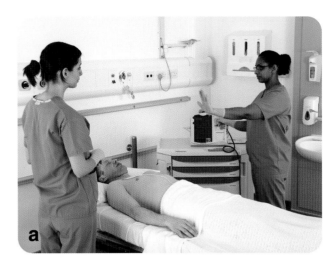

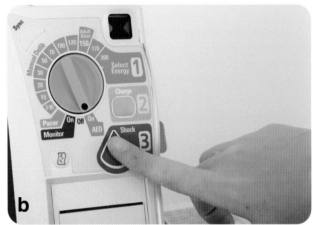

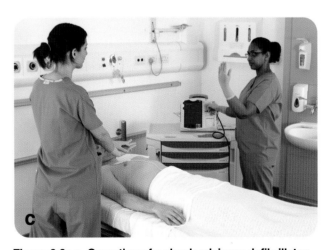

Figure 9.6a-c Operation of a shock-advisory defibrillator and efficient CPR

Manual defibrillation

Manual defibrillators have several advantages over AEDs. They enable the operator to diagnose the rhythm and deliver a shock rapidly without having to wait for rhythm analysis. This minimises the interruption in chest compressions. Manual defibrillators often have additional functions, such as the ability to deliver synchronised shocks, and external pacing facilities. The main disadvantage of these devices is that the operator has to

ALS

be skilled in ECG rhythm recognition; therefore, in comparison with AEDs, extra training is required.

Sequence for use of a manual defibrillator

This sequence is an integral part of the advanced life support treatment algorithm in Chapter 6.

1. Confirm cardiac arrest - check for signs of life or if trained to do so, breathing and pulse simultaneously.

2. Call resuscitation team.

3. Perform uninterrupted chest compressions while applying self-adhesive defibrillation/monitoring pads (Figure 9.7) - one below the right clavicle and the other in the V6 position in the midaxillary line.

4. Plan actions before pausing CPR for rhythm analysis and communicate these to the team.

5. Stop chest compressions; confirm VF from the ECG.

6. Resume chest compressions immediately; simultaneously, the designated person selects the appropriate energy on the defibrillator (150 - 200 J biphasic for the first shock and 150 - 360 J biphasic for subsequent shocks) and presses the charge button (Figure 9.8).

7. While the defibrillator is charging, warn all rescuers other than the individual performing the chest compressions to "stand clear" and remove any oxygen delivery device as appropriate. Ensure that the rescuer giving the compressions is the only person touching the patient.

8. Once the defibrillator is charged, tell the rescuer doing the chest compressions to "stand clear"; when clear, give the shock.

9. Without reassessing the rhythm or feeling for a pulse, restart CPR using a ratio of 30:2, starting with chest compressions.

10. Continue CPR for 2 min; the team leader prepares the team for the next pause in CPR.

11. Pause briefly to check the monitor.

12. If VF/VT, repeat steps 6 - 11 above and deliver a second shock.

13. If VF/VT persists repeat steps 6 - 8 above and deliver a third shock. Resume chest compressions immediately and then give adrenaline 1 mg IV and amiodarone 300 mg IV while performing a further 2 min CPR.

14. Repeat this 2 min CPR - rhythm/pulse check - defibrillation sequence if VF/VT persists.

15. Give further adrenaline 1 mg IV after alternate shocks (i.e. approximately every 3 - 5 min).

16. If organised electrical activity is seen during the pause to check the monitor, feel for a pulse:

     a. If a pulse is present, start post-resuscitation care.
     b. If no pulse is present, continue CPR and switch to the non-shockable algorithm.

17. If asystole is seen, continue CPR and switch to the non-shockable algorithm.

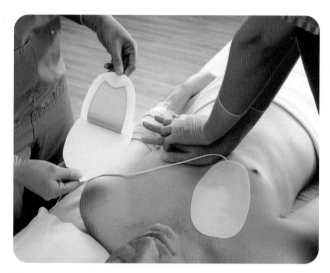

Figure 9.7 Applying defibrillator pads

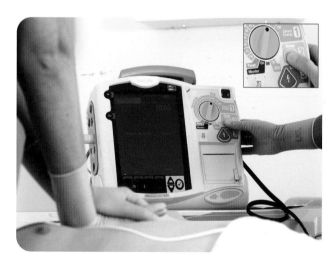

Figure 9.8 Charging during chest compressions

Prehospital defibrillation

Although previous guidelines have recommended that a period of CPR before defibrillation may be beneficial after prolonged collapse, recent studies have failed to confirm the value of this. Furthermore, the duration of collapse before the arrival of the EMS is often difficult to assess accurately. However, there is evidence that performing chest compressions while retrieving, applying and charging the defibrillator improves the probability of survival. For these reasons, when attending any cardiac arrest not witnessed by EMS personnel, one member of the EMS team should provide good-quality CPR until the other is ready to deliver a shock. Do not give a specified period of CPR before rhythm analysis and shock delivery (see Chapter 14).

Laypeople and first responders using AEDs should attach the device as soon as possible and follow the prompts.

Defibrillation with an AED in children

A standard AED using the energy settings already described is suitable for defibrillation of children above the age of 8 years. For defibrillation of children between 1 and 8 years, special paediatric electrodes with integral energy attenuators are recommended; these reduce the delivered energy to that recommended for manual defibrillation. If these electrodes are not available, use standard adult electrodes, ensuring that they do not overlap, and adult AED settings. For children below 1 year of age, based on some case reports documenting successful use in this group, it is acceptable to use an AED if no other option is available.

Synchronised cardioversion

If electrical cardioversion is used to convert atrial or ventricular tachyarrhythmias, the shock must be synchronised to occur with the R wave (not the T wave) of the electrocardiogram. By avoiding the relative refractory period, the risk of inducing VF is minimised. Most manual defibrillators incorporate a switch that enables the shock to be triggered by the R wave on the electrocardiogram. Electrodes are applied to the chest wall and cardioversion is achieved in the same way as attempted defibrillation but the operator must anticipate the slight delay between pressing the buttons and the discharge of the shock when the next R wave occurs. Do not move the defibrillator electrodes during this interval; otherwise the QRS complex will not be detected.

Synchronisation can be difficult in VT because of the wide-complex and variable forms of ventricular arrhythmia. If synchronisation fails, give unsynchronised shocks to the unstable patient in VT to avoid prolonged delay in restoring sinus rhythm. Ventricular fibrillation or pulseless VT requires unsynchronised shocks. Conscious patients must be anaesthetised or sedated before attempting synchronised cardioversion.

With some defibrillators, the synchronised mode has to be reset if a second shock is required. Other machines remain in the synchronised mode; be careful not to leave the synchronisation switch in the 'on' position following use as this will inhibit discharge of the defibrillator when it is next used for treating VF/VT.

Energy doses for cardioversion are discussed in Chapter 11.

Cardiac pacemakers and implantable cardioverter-defibrillators

If the patient has a cardiac pacemaker or implantable cardioverter-defibrillator (ICD), be careful when placing the electrodes. Although modern pacemakers are fitted with protection circuits, the current may travel along the pacemaker wire or ICD lead causing burns where the electrode tip makes contact with the myocardium. This may increase resistance at the contact point and gradually increase the threshold for pacing. Place the defibrillator electrodes at least 8 cm from the pacemaker unit to minimise the risk. Alternatively place the pads in the antero-posterior or postero-lateral position as described above. If resuscitation is successful following defibrillation, check the pacemaker threshold regularly over the next two months. Recent case reports have documented rescuers receiving shocks from ICDs when in contact with the patient during CPR. It is particularly important to wear gloves and avoid skin-to-skin contact with the patient while performing CPR as there is no warning before the ICD discharges.

Internal defibrillation

Internal defibrillation using paddles applied directly across the ventricles requires considerably less energy than that used for external defibrillation. Biphasic shocks are substantially more effective than monophasic shocks for direct defibrillation. For biphasic shocks, use 10 - 20 J, delivered directly to the myocardium through internal paddles. Monophasic shocks require approximately double these energy levels. Do not exceed 50 J when using internal defibrillation - failure to defibrillate at these energy levels requires myocardial optimisation before defibrillation is attempted again.

Key learning points

- For the patient in VF, early defibrillation is the only effective means of restoring a spontaneous circulation.

- When using a defibrillator, minimise interruptions in chest compressions.

Further reading

Deakin CD, Morrison LJ, Morley PT, et al. Part 8: Advanced Life Support. 2010 International Consensus on Cardiopulmonary Resuscitation and Emergency Cardiovascular Care Science with Treatment Recommendations. Resuscitation 2010; 81: e93-e169.

Deakin CD, Nolan JP, Soar J, Sunde K, Koster R, Smith GB, Perkins GD. European Resuscitation Council Guidelines for Resuscitation 2010. Section 4: Adult advanced life support. Resuscitation 2010;81:1305-52.

Deakin CD, Nolan JP, Sunde K, Koster R. European Resuscitation Council Guidelines for Resuscitation 2005. Section 3: Electrical therapies: automated external defibrillators, defibrillation, cardioversion and pacing. Resuscitation 2010;81:1293-1304.

Sunde K, Jacobs I, Deakin CD, et al. Part 6: Defibrillation. 2010 International Consensus on Cardiopulmonary Resuscitation and Emergency Cardiovascular Care Science with Treatment Recommendations. Resuscitation 2010;81: e71-e85.

Cardiac Pacing

Introduction

In some cardiac arrest or peri-arrest settings, appropriate use of cardiac pacing can be life-saving. Non-invasive pacing may be used to maintain cardiac output temporarily while expert help to deliver longer-term treatment is obtained. Non-invasive pacing can be established rapidly and is well within the capabilities of an ALS provider.

The ALS provider does not need to have a detailed technical knowledge of permanent cardiac pacemakers and implanted cardioverter defibrillators (ICDs) but needs to be able to recognise when one of these devices is present, when they are failing, and how the presence of an implanted device may influence the management of a cardiac arrest.

The cardiac impulse – its formation and its failure

The electrical activity that stimulates each normal heartbeat arises in the sino-atrial (SA) node. This depolarises spontaneously and regularly without any external stimulus. Such behaviour is termed automaticity, and any cardiac tissue that possesses it is capable of initiating a heartbeat and behaving as the heart's natural pacemaker. Different parts of the conducting system depolarise spontaneously at different rates (Figure 10.1). The fastest pacemaker will provide the cardiac rhythm and slower natural pacemakers will only take over if the faster ones fail. Examples may be seen in sinus arrest or extreme sinus bradycardia when the atrioventricular (AV) node may

take over and provide a junctional escape rhythm, and in complete atrioventricular block (complete heart block - CHB) when the escape rhythm arises from the ventricular myocardium or from conducting tissue below the atrioventricular node.

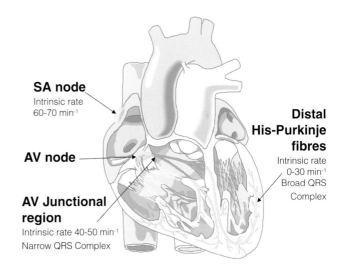

SA node
Intrinsic rate
60-70 min⁻¹

AV node

AV Junctional region
Intrinsic rate 40-50 min⁻¹
Narrow QRS Complex

Distal His-Purkinje fibres
Intrinsic rate
0-30 min⁻¹
Broad QRS
Complex

Figure 10.1 Cardiac conducting system

When CHB occurs at the level of the AV node, the most rapid automatic activity arises from cells immediately below the block and these become the new pacemaker. The intrinsic rate of these cells is relatively fast (often about 50 min⁻¹). The resulting escape rhythm is usually relatively stable and unlikely to fail and cause asystole.

The QRS complexes resulting from this type of block are narrow because the impulse is transmitted to the ventricles rapidly through an intact His-Purkinje system. This situation may be seen complicating acute inferior myocardial infarction. In this setting, narrow-complex CHB may not require pacing because the heart rate is often not especially slow and the risk of asystole is usually low.

Complete heart block can occur lower in the conducting system, for example, when all the fibres of the bundle branches are involved following anteroseptal myocardial infarction, or as a result of other disease including degenerative fibrosis and valve disease. Any automatic activity arising below this block in the distal Purkinje fibres is likely to be slow and unreliable. In this situation, the resulting QRS complexes will be broad, since the impulse passes slowly through ventricular muscle rather then rapidly through the His-Purkinje system. The unreliable escape rhythm may fail briefly, leading to syncope (Stokes-Adams attack), or completely, causing ventricular standstill and cardiac arrest. Broad-complex CHB requires

? temporary pacing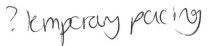

cardiac pacing, and the occurrence of significant ventricular pauses makes this urgent, as this implies a risk of asystole. The possible risk of more severe AV block and asystole should always be considered in a patient who has presented with syncope and has any ECG evidence of conduction delay (e.g. long PR interval or bundle branch block). Such patients require at least cardiac monitoring and expert assessment.

In the peri-arrest setting, artificial pacemakers are used when the cardiac rhythm is unduly slow or unreliable and not responding to the treatment described in the peri-arrest algorithm for bradycardia (Chapter 11). However, pacing will be successful only if the heart is able to respond to the pacing stimulus. In the setting of cardiac arrest the continued presence of P waves makes this more likely.

Pacing is rarely successful in asystole in the absence of P waves and should not be attempted routinely in this situation.

The stimulus to the myocardium may be either mechanical, as in percussion pacing, or electrical as in transcutaneous and transvenous pacing.

If a pacing stimulus induces an immediate QRS complex this is referred to as 'capture'. Always check that electrical activity seen on the ECG is accompanied by mechanical activity producing a palpable pulse.

Methods of pacing

Methods of pacing are classified as:

Non-invasive

- Percussion pacing ('fist pacing')
- Transcutaneous pacing

Invasive

- Temporary transvenous pacing
- Permanent pacing with an implanted pacemaker

Implanted devices that deliver pacing include pacemakers implanted for the treatment of bradycardia, biventricular pacemakers implanted for the treatment of heart failure (cardiac resynchronisation therapy) and implanted cardioverter defibrillators (ICDs) that also have a pacemaker function.

Non-invasive pacing

Percussion pacing

When bradycardia is so profound that it causes clinical cardiac arrest, percussion pacing can be used in

preference to CPR because it is capable of producing an adequate cardiac output with minimal trauma to the patient. It is more likely to be successful when ventricular standstill is accompanied by continuing P wave activity (Chapter 8).

How to perform percussion pacing

- With the side of a closed fist deliver repeated firm blows to the precordium lateral to the lower left sternal edge.

- Raise the hand about 10 cm above the chest for each blow.

- If initial blows do not produce a QRS complex try using slightly harder blows and try moving the point of contact around the precordium until a site is found that produces repeated ventricular stimulation.

Percussion pacing is not as reliable as electrical pacing in stimulating QRS complexes. If percussion does not produce a pulsed rhythm promptly, regardless of whether or not it stimulates QRS complexes, start CPR immediately.

Like CPR, percussion pacing is an emergency measure that is used to try to maintain circulation to vital organs and enable either recovery of a spontaneous cardiac rhythm or transcutaneous or transvenous pacing.

Transcutaneous pacing

Compared with transvenous pacing, non-invasive transcutaneous pacing has the following advantages:

- it can be established very quickly;

- it is easy to perform and requires a minimum of training;

- it can be initiated by nurses, paramedics and doctors, while waiting for expert help to establish transvenous pacing.

The major disadvantage of transcutaneous pacing in the conscious patient is discomfort. The pacing impulse stimulates painful contraction of chest wall muscles as well as causing some direct discomfort. Many defibrillators incorporate a facility for transcutaneous pacing and the availability of multifunction, adhesive electrode pads capable of ECG monitoring, pacing, cardioversion, and defibrillation have made these units particularly versatile. Stand-alone non-invasive pacing devices may also be available in some hospital departments.

Most modern transcutaneous pacing systems are capable of demand pacing: intrinsic QRS complexes are sensed and pacing stimuli delivered only when needed.

How to perform transcutaneous pacing

- Avoid any unnecessary delay in starting pacing, but pay careful attention to technique to increase the chance of success.

- Using scissors or a razor, quickly remove excess chest hair from the skin where the electrode pad is to be applied.

- Make sure that the skin is dry.

- Attach ECG monitoring electrodes and leads if necessary - these are needed with some transcutaneous pacing devices.

- Position the electrode pads in the conventional right pectoral-apical positions if possible (Figure 10.2a). If this is prevented (e.g. by chest trauma) anterior-posterior (A-P) positions can be used (Figure 10.2b-d).

- If you are using a pacing device that is not capable of defibrillation, use A-P positions for the pacing electrodes so that defibrillator pads can still be used in the 'conventional' right pectoral and apical positions if cardiac arrest occurs.

- For right pectoral-apical positions place one electrode over the right pectoral muscle, just below the clavicle. Place the apical pad in the mid-axillary line, overlying the V6 ECG electrode position. It is important that this electrode is placed sufficiently laterally. Apply this pad to the chest wall, not over any breast tissue.

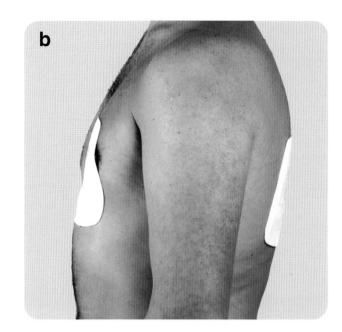

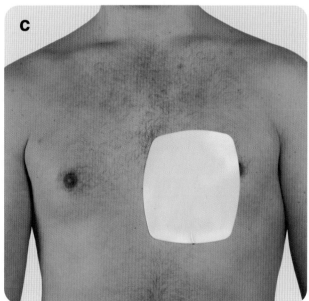

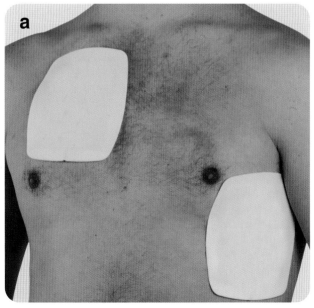

Figure 10.2a Pectoral-apical pad positions for external pacing

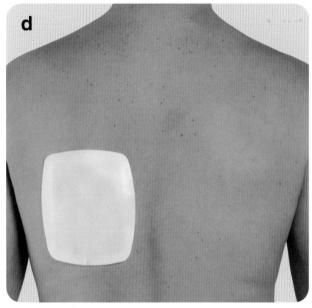

Figure 10.2b - d. Anterior-posterior (AP) pad positions for external pacing.

ALS

- For A-P positions place the anterior electrode on the left anterior chest wall, beside the sternum, overlying the V2 and V3 ECG electrode positions. Place the posterior electrode between the lower part of the left scapula and the spine, at the same horizontal level on the trunk as the anterior electrode.

- Different transcutaneous pacing devices have different properties. For example some require the operator to increase the current delivered with each pacing stimulus until electrical capture is achieved, whilst others use a constant current that cannot be adjusted and longer pulse duration (duration of the pacing stimulus) than other devices. Make sure that you are familiar with the operation of the device that you are using.

- Most transcutaneous pacing devices offer pacing in demand mode; the pacemaker will be inhibited if it detects a spontaneous QRS complex. However, if there is a lot of movement artefact on the ECG this may inhibit the pacemaker. Avoid movement artefact as far as possible. If artefact still appears to be inhibiting the pacemaker, switch to fixed-rate pacing mode.

- Select an appropriate pacing rate. This will usually be in the range of 60 - 90 min⁻¹ for adults, but in some circumstances (for example complete AV block with an idioventricular rhythm at 50 min⁻¹) a slower pacing rate of 40 or even 30 min⁻¹ may be appropriate to deliver pacing only during sudden ventricular standstill or more extreme bradycardia.

- If the pacing device has an adjustable energy output set this at its lowest value and turn on the pacemaker. Gradually increase the output while observing the patient and the ECG. As the current is increased the muscles of the chest wall will contract with each impulse and a pacing spike will appear on the ECG (Figure 10.3a). Increase the current until each pacing spike is followed immediately by a QRS complex, indicating electrical capture (typically with a current of 50 - 100 mA using a device with adjustable output). This means that the pacing stimuli are causing depolarisation of the ventricles (Figure 10.3b).

- Check that the apparent QRS complex is followed by a T wave. Occasionally, artefact generated by the pacing current travelling through the chest may be mistaken for a QRS complex, but such artefact will not be followed by a T wave (Figure 10.3a).

- If the highest current setting is reached and electrical capture has not occurred, try changing the electrode positions. Continued failure to achieve electrical capture may indicate non-viable myocardium, but other conditions (e.g. hyperkalaemia) may prevent successful pacing.

Having achieved electrical capture with the pacemaker, check for a pulse. A palpable pulse confirms the presence

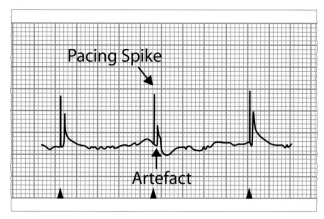

Figure 10.3a Transcutaneous pacing. Appearance of pacing spikes on ECG

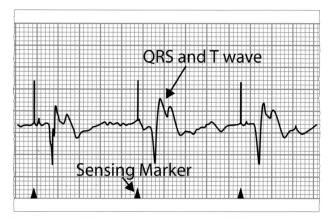

Figure 10.3b. Transcutaneous pacing. ECG shows ventricular capture after each pacing spike

of a mechanical response of the heart to the paced QRS complex (i.e. contraction of the myocardium). Absence of a pulse in the presence of good electrical capture constitutes pulseless electrical activity (PEA). The most likely cause is severe myocardial failure but consider other possible causes of PEA in these circumstances.

Conscious patients usually experience considerable discomfort during transcutaneous pacing. Warn patients in advance that this may happen. They will often require intravenous analgesia and/or sedation if prolonged transcutaneous pacing is necessary. If sedation is used, reassess the patient frequently (ABCDE) because sedative drugs may suppress respiratory effort.

When defibrillating a patient who has pacing-only electrode pads in place, apply the defibrillator paddles at least 2 - 3 cm from the pacing electrodes to prevent arcing of the defibrillation current.

Chest compressions can be given and other manual contact with the patient maintained as necessary with transcutaneous electrodes in place. There is no hazard from transcutaneous pacing to other people who are in contact with the patient. However, there is no benefit in trying to deliver transcutaneous pacing during chest compressions, so it is best to turn off the pacemaker whilst CPR is in progress.

When transcutaneous pacing produces an adequate cardiac output seek expert help immediately to insert a transvenous pacing lead.

Invasive pacing

Temporary transvenous pacing

It is rare to have to attempt to insert a transvenous pacing wire during a cardiac arrest. In this setting, use non-invasive pacing to attempt to establish a cardiac output, and then seek expert help to establish transvenous pacing.

Failure of an existing temporary transvenous pacing system may cause cardiac arrest, particularly when the patient is pacing-dependent. Temporary transvenous pacing systems can fail in three ways:

1. High threshold

When a temporary pacing lead is inserted the usual aim is to position its tip in the apex of the right ventricle, where it is least likely to be displaced. After positioning the lead, it is used to pace the heart and the voltage delivered by the pacemaker is decreased and increased to determine the minimum voltage needed to stimulate the ventricle. This is termed the pacing threshold and the usual aim is to achieve a threshold of < 1 V at the time of lead insertion. Higher thresholds suggest that the electrode is not making satisfactory contact with the myocardium, and the lead may need to be repositioned.

It is usual to pace the heart with a 3 - 4 V stimulus, well above the initial pacing threshold. Over the first days and weeks after insertion of a pacing lead (temporary or permanent) a rise in the threshold can be expected.

Check the threshold on temporary pacing leads at least daily to make sure that the output of the pacemaker is well above the threshold. If not, loss of capture may occur. This is seen on the ECG as a pacing spike without a subsequent QRS complex. Loss of capture may be intermittent, so any apparent 'missed beat' of this nature should prompt a repeat check of the pacing threshold.

If loss of capture occurs because of a high threshold, increase the output of the pacemaker immediately to well above the threshold. A sudden increase in pacing threshold may be caused by lead displacement, so obtain prompt expert help, as repositioning of the lead may be required.

2. Loss of electrical continuity

Modern temporary transvenous pacing leads are bipolar. One electrode is at the tip of the lead and the second is about 1 cm proximal to the tip. Each electrode is connected by the lead to separate connectors at the other end, outside the patient. These are usually inserted into sockets at one end of a connecting cable that in turn is connected to the terminals of the pacemaker.

Make sure that all connections between the lead and the pacemaker are making good secure contact that is unlikely to be lost easily, for example by minor movement of the lead or cable.

Loss of contact at any point will stop delivery of the pacing stimulus to the heart, seen on the ECG as absence of a pacing spike. This may be intermittent and symptomless, or may be sudden and total and may cause syncope or cardiac arrest in asystole. When pacing failure is accompanied by loss of the pacing spike on the ECG, check all connections immediately; check that the pacemaker has not been turned off inadvertently and check that its batteries are not depleted. If no such cause is present another possible explanation is a fracture of a wire within its insulation. This usually causes intermittent pacing failure and the fracture is more likely to be in the connecting cable than in the pacing lead. If this is suspected change the connecting cable immediately.

3. Electrode displacement

The tip of an endocardial transvenous pacing lead is usually positioned in the apex of the right ventricle. There should be enough slack in the lead as it passes through the right atrium to allow for changes in posture and deep inspiration, but not so much as to encourage displacement of the lead tip.

The tip of a pacing lead may also perforate the wall of the right ventricle and enter the pericardium with little or no apparent change in position on chest X-ray. Very rarely, this may cause pericardial tamponade, so consider this possibility if a patient with a recently implanted pacing lead suffers cardiac arrest with pulseless electrical activity.

When displacement or perforation occurs, the ECG will still show a pacing spike, but there is likely to be intermittent or complete loss of capture of the pacing stimulus, so the pacing spikes are not followed consistently by QRS complexes. When a pacing lead displaces but remains in the right ventricle it may trigger ventricular extrasystoles or more serious ventricular arrhythmia, including VT and VF. When transvenous pacing fails, there is a risk of ventricular standstill. This may be relatively short-lived and cause syncope, or prolonged and cause cardiac arrest in asystole. In this situation use non-invasive pacing until effective transvenous pacing has been re-established.

Implanted permanent pacing systems

Problems with permanent pacing systems are rare, because the connections between pacing electrodes and the pacemaker are much more secure. Occasional fracture of a permanent pacing lead may occur, usually following trauma such as a fall on to an outstretched arm on the side of the pacemaker. This may cause permanent or intermittent loss of the pacing spike.

When assessing a patient using the ABCDE approach check (during 'E') for the presence of an implanted device. These devices are usually implanted below the clavicle, often but not always on the left side. If a device is identified consider whether it is a pacemaker or an ICD and in the case of a pacemaker try to establish whether it was implanted as treatment for bradyarrhythmia or as treatment for heart failure.

If a patient with an implanted pacemaker or ICD has a cardiac arrest or requires cardioversion, place defibrillation pads at least 8 cm from the device. Devices that are implanted below the left clavicle usually present no problem with the use of standard defibrillator paddle positions. If a device has been implanted below the right clavicle, use A-P positions for defibrillation or cardioversion if possible. This is most easily and safely achieved using self-adhesive electrode pads rather than hand-held defibrillator paddles.

Biventricular pacing systems

Until relatively recently, the usual reason for implantation of a permanent pacemaker has been the treatment of bradycardia, caused mostly by malfunction of the sino-atrial node or atrioventricular conduction. In recent years there has been increasing use of biventricular pacemakers as 'cardiac resynchronisation therapy' in patients with heart failure. Most of these patients do not require pacing for bradycardia. Pacing the apex of the right ventricle and the lateral wall of the left ventricle simultaneously improves the co-ordination of left ventricular contraction. These pacemakers require the same precautions during defibrillation and cardioversion as any other pacemaker, but failure of a pacemaker that has been inserted for this purpose will not usually cause any major change in heart rate or any dangerous rhythm abnormality.

Implantable cardioverter-defibrillators

These devices resemble large implanted pacemakers. Many of them can function as demand pacemakers in the event of bradycardia and some will also deliver biventricular pacing for heart failure, as well as delivering defibrillation if required. National and international guidelines define indications for the implantation of an ICD, but accumulating evidence for improved survival after major myocardial infarction and in patients with heart failure has increased the use of these devices. Unlike a simple pacemaker, the primary function of an ICD is to terminate a life-threatening tachyarrhythmia. A 'simple' ICD can deliver a defibrillatory shock when it detects VF or very fast VT. More sophisticated devices can be programmed also to deliver critically timed pacing stimuli to attempt to terminate VT that is not especially fast and is unlikely to cause cardiac arrest, resorting to defibrillation only if the VT accelerates or degenerates into VF.

ICDs are implanted usually in the pectoral region in a similar position to pacemakers. Though these devices may seem complex, the means by which they sense changes in cardiac rhythm is relatively simple, depending mainly upon detection of rapid heart rates. Consequently, ICDs will occasionally misdiagnose an arrhythmia, or misinterpret other electrical signals, and deliver inappropriate shocks, which are very unpleasant for a conscious patient. Implantable cardioverter defibrillators can be disabled temporarily by holding or taping a magnet on the skin over the device. Seek expert help if ICD malfunction is suspected, as it may require reprogramming.

If a patient with an ICD has a cardiac arrest that is not terminated by the ICD, deliver CPR in the usual way. Until recently, it was thought that chest compressions could be undertaken without risk to the rescuer, even if the ICD delivers an internal shock to the patient during chest compression. However, there have been rare reports of rescuers receiving shocks from an ICD. This risk is minimised by wearing gloves. If a shockable cardiac arrest rhythm is present and is not terminated by the ICD, use external defibrillation in a standard fashion, taking the same precautions with choice of defibrillator paddle positions as in a patient with an implanted pacemaker.

Consider the possible requirement for ICD implantation in any patient who has been resuscitated from cardiac arrest in a shockable rhythm outside the context of proven acute ST segment elevation myocardial infarction. All such patients should be referred before discharge from hospital for assessment by a cardiologist with expertise in heart rhythm disorders.

Key learning points

- Non-invasive pacing can be delivered by any ALS provider and is the immediate treatment for bradyarrhythmia that is a potential risk to the patient who does not respond to initial drug treatment.

- Non-invasive pacing is a temporary measure to be used until either a stable and effective spontaneous rhythm returns, or a competent person establishes transvenous pacing.

- Special precautions are necessary during resuscitation attempts in patients with implanted pacemakers and ICDs.

- The possible need for an ICD should be considered in patients resuscitated from cardiac arrest in VT or VF, in whom there is a possible risk of recurrence.

Further reading

Deakin CD, Nolan JP, Sunde K, Koster RW. European Resuscitation Council Guidelines for Resuscitation 2010. Section 3. Electrical Therapies: Automated External Defibrillators, Defibrillation, Cardioversion and Pacing. Resuscitation 2010;81:e32-40.

National Institute for Clinical Health & Excellence 2006. Technology Appraisal 95. Implantable cardioverter defibrillators for arrhythmias. Review of Technology Appraisal 11. www.nice.org.uk

Peri-arrest Arrhythmias

CHAPTER 11

Learning outcomes

To understand:

▶ **The importance of arrhythmias that may precede or follow a cardiac arrest**

▶ **How to assess peri-arrest arrhythmias**

▶ **The principles of treatment of peri-arrest arrhythmias**

Introduction

Rhythm abnormalities that occur in the peri-arrest period may be considered in two main categories:

- **Arrhythmias that may lead to cardiac arrest** - many rhythm abnormalities occur without causing cardiac arrest: they are a relatively common complication of acute myocardial infarction (AMI) but are also common in patients with other cardiac abnormalities and in people who do not have coronary disease or structural heart disease. Untreated, some of these arrhythmias may lead to cardiac arrest or to avoidable deterioration in the patient's condition. Others may require no immediate treatment.

- **Arrhythmias that occur after initial resuscitation from cardiac arrest** - these often indicate that the patient's condition is still unstable and that there is a risk of deterioration or further cardiac arrest.

You should be able to recognise common arrhythmias and to know how to assess whether or not they require immediate treatment. The treatment algorithms described in this section have been designed to enable the non-specialist advanced life support (ALS) provider to treat a patient effectively and safely in an emergency; for this reason they have been kept as simple as possible. If patients are not acutely ill there may be treatment options, including the use of drugs (oral or parenteral) that will be less familiar to the non-expert. In this situation you should, whenever possible, seek advice from cardiologists or other senior doctors with the appropriate expertise.

Sequence of actions

When an arrhythmia is present or suspected, start by assessing the patient using the ABCDE approach, including early establishment of cardiac monitoring (see Chapter 8). Assess the patient specifically for adverse features (see below). Insert an intravenous cannula and, if appropriate, give oxygen. Whenever possible, record a 12-lead ECG at the earliest opportunity. This will help to identify the precise rhythm, either before treatment or retrospectively, if necessary with the help of an expert. Clinical assessment is of limited value in identifying the precise rhythm abnormality.

When you assess any patient with an arrhythmia address two factors:

1. the condition of the patient (presence or absence of adverse features)

2. the nature of the arrhythmia.

Adverse features

The presence or absence of adverse signs or symptoms will dictate the urgency and choice of treatment for most arrhythmias. The following adverse features indicate that a patient is unstable and at risk of deterioration, wholly or partly because of the arrhythmia:

- Shock - hypotension (systolic blood pressure < 90 mmHg), pallor, sweating, cold extremities, confusion or impaired consciousness.

- Syncope - transient loss of consciousness because of global reduction in blood flow to the brain.

- Heart failure - pulmonary oedema and/or raised jugular venous pressure (with or without peripheral oedema and liver enlargement).

- Myocardial ischaemia - typical ischaemic chest pain and/or evidence of myocardial ischaemia on a 12-lead ECG.

- Extremes of heart rate - in addition to the above adverse features it may be appropriate to consider extremes of heart rate as adverse signs in themselves, requiring more urgent assessment and treatment than less extreme tachycardia or bradycardia with no adverse signs.

  (a) Extreme tachycardia: when heart rate increases, diastole is shortened to a greater degree than systole. Rhythm abnormalities that cause very fast heart rates (e.g. > 150 min^{-1}) reduce cardiac output dramatically (because diastole is very short and the heart does not have time to fill properly) and reduce coronary blood flow (because this mostly occurs during diastole), potentially causing myocardial ischaemia. The faster the heart rate, the less well it will be tolerated.

(b) Extreme bradycardia: in general, the slower the bradycardia the less well it will be tolerated and heart rates below 40 min^{-1} are often tolerated poorly. This is especially so when people have severe heart disease and cannot compensate for the bradycardia by increasing stroke volume. Some people with very severe heart disease require faster than normal heart rates to maintain cardiac output, and even a 'normal' heart rate may be inappropriately slow for them.

Treatment options

Depending on the clinical status of the patient (i.e. the presence or absence of adverse features) and the nature of the arrhythmia, immediate treatments can be categorised under four headings:

1) Electrical (cardioversion for tachyarrhythmia or pacing for bradyarrhythmia)

2) Simple clinical intervention (e.g. vagal manoeuvres, percussion pacing)

3) Pharmacological (drug treatment)

4) No treatment needed

Most drugs act more slowly and less reliably than electrical treatments, so electrical treatment is usually the preferred treatment for an unstable patient with adverse features.

If a patient develops an arrhythmia as a complication of some other condition (e.g. infection, AMI, heart failure), make sure that the underlying condition is assessed and treated appropriately, involving relevant experts if necessary.

Subsequent monitoring and treatment

After successful treatment of an arrhythmia continue to monitor the patient until you are confident that the risk of further arrhythmia is low. Remember always to record a 12-lead ECG **after** successful treatment of an arrhythmia because this may show abnormalities (or absence of abnormalities) that will be important in planning future management. Correct all reversible factors that may predispose to further arrhythmia. Ensure that appropriate further expert help and advice is obtained at the most appropriate time for the patient.

Tachyarrhythmia

If the patient has adverse features

These imply that the patient's condition is unstable and at risk of deterioration; if this appears to be because of the presence of tachyarrhythmia, attempt to correct this using synchronised cardioversion (Figure 11.1). In people with otherwise normal hearts, adverse signs and symptoms are uncommon if the heart rate is < 150 min^{-1}. Patients with impaired cardiac function, structural heart disease or other serious medical conditions (e.g. severe lung disease) may be symptomatic and unstable during arrhythmias with heart rates between 100 and 150 min^{-1}.

If cardioversion fails to terminate the arrhythmia, and adverse features persist, give amiodarone 300 mg IV over 10 - 20 min and attempt further synchronised cardioversion. The loading dose of amiodarone can be followed by an infusion of 900 mg over 24 h, given into a large vein (preferably via central venous cannula).

Synchronised cardioversion

Carry out cardioversion under general anaesthesia or conscious sedation, administered by a healthcare professional competent in the technique being used. Ensure that the defibrillator is set to deliver a synchronised shock. This delivers the shock to coincide with the R wave. An unsynchronised shock could coincide with a T wave and cause ventricular fibrillation (VF).

For a broad-complex tachycardia or atrial fibrillation, start with 120 - 150 J biphasic shock (200 J monophasic) and increase in increments if this fails. Atrial flutter and regular narrow-complex tachycardia will often be terminated by lower-energy shocks: start with 70 - 120 J biphasic (100 J monophasic). For atrial fibrillation and flutter use anteroposterior defibrillator pad positions when it is practicable to do so.

When delivering the shock, press the shock button and keep it pressed until after the shock has occurred - there may be a slight delay before the shock is delivered.

If a second shock is needed, reactivate the synchronisation switch if necessary.

If the patient has no adverse features

If there are no adverse features consider using drug treatment in the first instance. Assess the ECG and measure the QRS duration. If the QRS duration is 0.12 s (3 small squares at ECG paper speed 25 mm s^{-1}) or more this is a broad complex tachycardia. If the QRS duration is < 0.12 s it is a narrow complex tachycardia. Following any drug therapy, continue to reassess the patient (ABCDE)

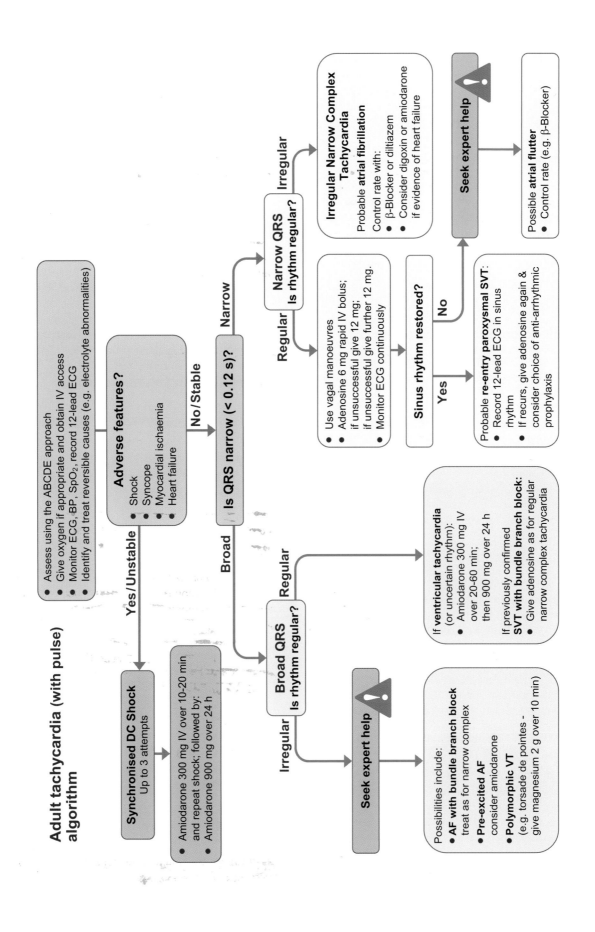

Figure 11.1 Tachycardia algorithm

Adult tachycardia (with pulse) algorithm

- Assess using the ABCDE approach
- Give oxygen if appropriate and obtain IV access
- Monitor ECG, BP, SpO₂, record 12-lead ECG
- Identify and treat reversible causes (e.g. electrolyte abnormalities)

Adverse features?
- Shock
- Syncope
- Myocardial ischaemia
- Heart failure

Yes/Unstable

Synchronised DC Shock
Up to 3 attempts

- Amiodarone 300 mg IV over 10-20 min and repeat shock; followed by:
- Amiodarone 900 mg over 24 h

No/Stable

Is QRS narrow (< 0.12 s)?

Broad

Broad QRS
Is rhythm regular?

Regular

If **ventricular tachycardia** (or uncertain rhythm):
- Amiodarone 300 mg IV over 20-60 min; then 900 mg over 24 h

If previously confirmed **SVT with bundle branch block:**
- Give adenosine as for regular narrow complex tachycardia

Irregular

Seek expert help

Possibilities include:
- **AF with bundle branch block** treat as for narrow complex
- **Pre-excited AF** consider amiodarone
- **Polymorphic VT** (e.g. torsade de pointes - give magnesium 2 g over 10 min)

Narrow

Narrow QRS
Is rhythm regular?

Regular

- Use vagal manoeuvres
- Adenosine 6 mg rapid IV bolus; if unsuccessful give 12 mg; if unsuccessful give further 12 mg.
- Monitor ECG continuously

Sinus rhythm restored?

Yes

Probable **re-entry paroxysmal SVT**:
- Record 12-lead ECG in sinus rhythm
- If recurs, give adenosine again & consider choice of anti-arrhythmic prophylaxis

No

Seek expert help

Possible **atrial flutter**
- Control rate (e.g. β-Blocker)

Irregular

Irregular Narrow Complex Tachycardia
Probable **atrial fibrillation**
Control rate with:
- β-Blocker or diltiazem
- Consider digoxin or amiodarone if evidence of heart failure

and monitor heart rate and rhythm to assess the response to treatment. Some anti-arrhythmic drugs cause myocardial depression, which may cause or worsen heart failure or hypotension, and in some cases an anti-arrhythmic drug may cause other tachyarrhythmia or provoke severe bradycardia.

Broad-complex tachycardia

Broad-complex tachycardia (QRS ≥ 0.12 s) may be ventricular in origin or may be a supraventricular rhythm with aberrant conduction (i.e. bundle branch block). In the patient with adverse features the distinction is irrelevant. Attempt synchronised cardioversion as described above. If a patient has a broad-complex tachycardia but no adverse features, next determine whether the rhythm is regular or irregular.

Regular broad-complex tachycardia

A regular broad-complex tachycardia may be ventricular tachycardia (VT) or a supraventricular rhythm with bundle branch block.

If the broad complex tachycardia is considered to be VT, treat with amiodarone 300 mg intravenously over 20 - 60 minutes, followed by an infusion of 900 mg over 24 h. If a regular broad-complex tachycardia is known to be a supraventricular arrhythmia with bundle branch block, and the patient is stable, use the treatment strategy indicated for narrow-complex tachycardia (below).

Irregular broad-complex tachycardia

This is most likely to be atrial fibrillation (AF) with bundle branch block, but careful examination of a 12-lead ECG (if necessary by an expert) may provide confident identification of the rhythm. Other possible causes are AF with ventricular pre-excitation (in patients with Wolff-Parkinson-White [WPW] syndrome), or polymorphic VT (e.g. torsade de pointes), but polymorphic VT is unlikely to be present without adverse features. Seek expert help with the assessment and treatment of irregular broad-complex tachyarrhythmia.

Treat torsade de pointes VT by stopping immediately all drugs known to prolong the QT interval. Correct electrolyte abnormalities, especially hypokalaemia. Give magnesium sulphate 2 g IV over 10 min. Obtain expert help, as other treatment (e.g. overdrive pacing) may be indicated to prevent relapse once the arrhythmia has been corrected. If adverse features develop, which is common, arrange immediate synchronised cardioversion. If the patient becomes pulseless, attempt defibrillation immediately (ALS algorithm).

Narrow-complex tachycardia

Examine the ECG to determine if the rhythm is regular or irregular. Regular narrow-complex tachycardias include sinus tachycardia, atrioventricular nodal re-entry tachycardia (AVNRT) - the commonest type of regular narrow-complex tachyarrhythmia, atrioventricular re-entry tachycardia (AVRT) - due to WPW syndrome, and atrial flutter with regular AV conduction (usually 2:1).

An irregular narrow-complex tachycardia is most likely to be AF, or sometimes atrial flutter with variable AV conduction ('variable block').

Regular narrow-complex tachycardia

Sinus tachycardia

Sinus tachycardia is not an arrhythmia. This is a common physiological response to stimuli such as exercise or anxiety. In a sick patient it may occur in response to many conditions including pain, infection, anaemia, blood loss, and heart failure. Treatment is directed at the underlying cause; trying to slow sinus tachycardia that has occurred in response to most of these situations will make the situation worse. Do not attempt to treat sinus tachycardia with cardioversion or anti-arrhythmic drugs.

AVNRT and AVRT (paroxysmal supraventricular tachycardia)

Atrioventricular nodal re-entry tachycardia is the commonest type of paroxysmal supraventricular tachycardia (SVT), often seen in people without any other form of heart disease. It is uncommon in the peri-arrest setting. It causes a regular, narrow-complex tachycardia, often with no clearly visible atrial activity on the ECG. The heart rate is usually well above the upper limit of sinus rate at rest (100 min⁻¹). It is usually benign, unless there is additional, co-incidental, structural heart disease or coronary disease, but it may cause symptoms that the patient finds frightening.

Atrioventricular re-entry tachycardia occurs in patients with the WPW syndrome, and is also usually benign, unless there is additional structural heart disease. The common type of AVRT is a regular narrow-complex tachycardia, usually with no visible atrial activity on the ECG. Like AVNRT, it may cause frightening symptoms.

Atrial flutter with regular AV conduction (often 2:1 block)

This produces a regular narrow-complex tachycardia. It may be difficult to see atrial activity and identify flutter waves on the ECG with confidence, so the rhythm may be indistinguishable, at least initially, from AVNRT or AVRT.

Typical atrial flutter has an atrial rate of about 300 min⁻¹, so atrial flutter with 2:1 conduction produces a tachycardia of about 150 min⁻¹. Much faster rates (160 min⁻¹ or more) are unlikely to be caused by atrial flutter with 2:1 conduction. Regular tachycardia with slower rates (125 - 150 min⁻¹) may be caused by atrial flutter with 2:1 conduction, usually when the rate of the atrial flutter has been slowed by drug therapy.

Treatment of regular narrow-complex tachyarrhythmia

If the patient has adverse features and is at risk of deterioration because of the tachyarrhythmia, perform synchronised cardioversion. In this situation it is reasonable to attempt vagal manoeuvres (see below) or to give intravenous adenosine (see below) to a patient with a regular narrow-complex tachyarrhythmia while preparations are being made for synchronised cardioversion. However, do not delay electrical cardioversion if these treatments fail to terminate the arrhythmia.

In the absence of adverse features:

1. Start with vagal manoeuvres. Carotid sinus massage or the Valsalva manoeuvre will terminate up to a quarter of episodes of paroxysmal SVT. Record an ECG (preferably 12-lead) during each manoeuvre. If the rhythm is atrial flutter with 2:1 conduction, slowing of the ventricular response will often occur and reveal flutter waves.

2. If the arrhythmia persists and is not atrial flutter, give adenosine 6 mg as a very rapid intravenous bolus. Use a relatively large cannula and large (e.g. antecubital) vein. Warn the patient that they will feel unwell and probably experience chest discomfort for a few seconds after the injection. Record an ECG (preferably 12-lead) during the injection. If the ventricular rate slows transiently, but then speeds up again, look for atrial activity, such as atrial flutter or other atrial tachycardia, and treat accordingly. If there is no response to adenosine 6 mg, give a 12 mg bolus. If there is no response give one further 12 mg bolus. Apparent lack of response to adenosine will occur if the bolus is given too slowly or into a peripheral vein.

3. Vagal manoeuvres or adenosine will terminate almost all AVNRT or AVRT within seconds. Failure to terminate a regular narrow-complex tachycardia with adenosine suggests an atrial tachycardia such as atrial flutter (unless the adenosine has been injected too slowly or into a small peripheral vein).

4. If adenosine is contra-indicated, or fails to terminate a regular narrow complex tachycardia without demonstrating that it is atrial flutter, consider giving a calcium-channel blocker, for example verapamil 2.5 - 5 mg intravenously over 2 min.

Rapid narrow-complex tachycardia with no pulse

Rarely, a very rapid (usually > 250 min^{-1}) narrow-complex tachycardia can impair cardiac output to such an extent that the pulse may be impalpable and consciousness impaired. If the patient is pulseless and unconscious this situation is pulseless electrical activity (PEA) and you should start CPR. As the arrhythmia is potentially treatable by DC shock the most appropriate treatment then is immediate synchronised cardioversion, so this is an exception to the non-shockable limb of the ALS algorithm (Chapter 6).

Irregular narrow-complex tachycardia

An irregular narrow-complex tachycardia is most likely to be AF with a rapid ventricular response or, less commonly, atrial flutter with variable AV conduction. Record a 12-lead ECG to identify the rhythm.

If the patient has adverse features and is at risk of deterioration because of the tachyarrhythmia, perform synchronised cardioversion. In the absence of contraindications, start anticoagulation, initially with low-molecular-weight heparin or unfractionated heparin (see below), at the earliest opportunity. Do not allow this treatment to delay cardioversion.

If there are no adverse features, immediate treatment options include:

*   rate control by drug therapy;

*   rhythm control using drugs to achieve chemical cardioversion;

*   rhythm control by synchronised cardioversion;

*   treatment to prevent complications (e.g. anticoagulation).

Obtain expert help to determine the most appropriate treatment for the individual patient. The longer a patient remains in AF the greater is the likelihood of atrial thrombus developing. In general, patients who have been in AF for > 48 h should not be treated by cardioversion (electrical or chemical) until they have been fully anticoagulated for at least 3 weeks, or unless trans-oesophageal echocardiography has detected no evidence of atrial thrombus. If the clinical situation dictates that cardioversion is needed more urgently, give either regular low-molecular-weight heparin in therapeutic dose or an intravenous bolus injection of unfractionated heparin followed by a continuous infusion to maintain the activated partial thromboplastin time (APTT) at 1.5 - 2 times the reference control value. Continue heparin therapy and commence oral anticoagulation after successful cardioversion. Seek expert advice on the duration of anticoagulation, which should be a minimum of 4 weeks, often substantially longer.

If the aim is to control heart rate, the usual drug of choice is a beta-blocker. Diltiazem may be used in patients in whom beta blockade is contraindicated or not tolerated. Digoxin may be used in patients with heart failure.

Amiodarone may be used to assist with rate control but is most useful in maintaining rhythm control. Magnesium is also used but the data supporting this are limited. When possible seek expert help in selecting the best choice of treatment for rate control in each individual patient.

If the duration of AF is < 48 h and rhythm control is considered the appropriate strategy, chemical cardioversion may be appropriate. Seek expert help with the use of drugs such as flecainide. Do not use flecainide in the presence of heart failure, known left ventricular impairment or ischaemic heart disease, or a prolonged QT interval. Amiodarone (300 mg intravenously over 20 - 60 min followed by 900 mg over 24 h) may be used to attempt chemical cardioversion but is less often effective and takes longer. Electrical cardioversion remains an option in this setting and will restore sinus rhythm in more patients than chemical cardioversion.

Seek expert help if a patient with AF is known or found to have ventricular pre-excitation (WPW syndrome). Avoid using adenosine, diltiazem, verapamil, or digoxin in patients with pre-excited AF or atrial flutter as these drugs block the AV node and may cause a relative increase in pre-excitation.

Bradyarrhythmia

Bradycardia is defined as a resting heart rate of < 60 min^{-1}. It may be

- physiological (e.g. in athletes);

- cardiac in origin (e.g. atrioventricular block or sinus node disease);

- non-cardiac in origin (e.g. vasovagal, hypothermia, hypothyroidism, hyperkalaemia);

- drug-induced (e.g. beta blockade, diltiazem, digoxin, amiodarone).

Assess the patient with bradycardia using the ABCDE approach. Consider the potential cause of the bradycardia and look for adverse signs (Figure 11.2). Treat any reversible causes of bradycardia identified in the initial assessment.

If the patient has adverse features

If adverse features are present start to treat the bradycardia. Initial treatment is usually pharmacological; pacing is used for patients in whom initial pharmacological treatment is ineffective or inadequate and those with risk factors for asystole.

Pharmacological treatment for bradycardia

If adverse features are present, give atropine, 500 mcg, intravenously and, if necessary, repeat every 3 - 5 min to a total of 3 mg. Doses of atropine of < 500 mcg can cause paradoxical slowing of the heart rate. In healthy volunteers a dose of 3 mg produces the maximum achievable increase in resting heart rate. Use atropine cautiously in the presence of acute myocardial ischaemia or myocardial infarction; the resulting increase in heart rate may worsen ischaemia or increase the size of the infarct.

If bradycardia with adverse signs persists despite atropine, cardiac pacing should be considered. If pacing cannot be achieved promptly, consider the use of second-line drugs. Seek expert help to select the most appropriate choice.

In some clinical settings second-line drugs may be appropriate before the use of cardiac pacing. For example, consider giving intravenous glucagon if a beta-blocker or calcium channel blocker is a likely cause of the bradycardia. Consider using digoxin-specific antibody fragments for bradycardia caused by digoxin toxicity. Consider using theophylline (100 - 200 mg by slow intravenous injection) for bradycardia complicating acute inferior wall myocardial infarction, spinal cord injury or cardiac transplantation. Do not give atropine to patients with cardiac transplants. Their hearts are denervated and will not respond to vagal blockade by atropine, which may cause paradoxical sinus arrest or high-grade AV block. Other options for second-line drug therapy include infusion of isoprenaline (5 mcg min^{-1} starting dose), adrenaline (2 - 10 mcg min^{-1}), or dopamine (2.5 - 10 mcg kg^{-1} min^{-1}).

Cardiac pacing for bradycardia

In a patient with bradycardia and adverse features, if there is no response to atropine or if atropine is unlikely to be effective, initiate transcutaneous pacing immediately (see chapter 10). In the presence of severe bradycardia, use percussion pacing as an interim measure until transcutaneous pacing is achieved. Give serial rhythmic blows with the closed fist over the left lower edge of the sternum to stimulate the heart at a rate of 50 - 70 beats min^{-1}.

Transcutaneous pacing can be painful and may fail to achieve effective electrical 'capture' (i.e. a QRS complex after the pacing stimulus) or fail to achieve a mechanical response (i.e. palpable pulse). Verify electrical capture on the monitor or ECG and check that it is producing a pulse. Reassess the patient's condition (ABCDE). Use analgesia and sedation as necessary to control pain; remember that sedation may compromise respiratory effort so continue to reassess the patient at frequent intervals. Attempt to identify the cause of the bradyarrhythmia.

Seek expert help to assess the need for temporary transvenous pacing and to initiate this when appropriate. Consider temporary transvenous pacing if there is documented recent asystole (ventricular standstill of > 3 s), Mobitz type II AV block, or complete (third-degree) AV block (especially with broad QRS or initial heart rate < 40 min^{-1}).

Adult bradycardia algorithm

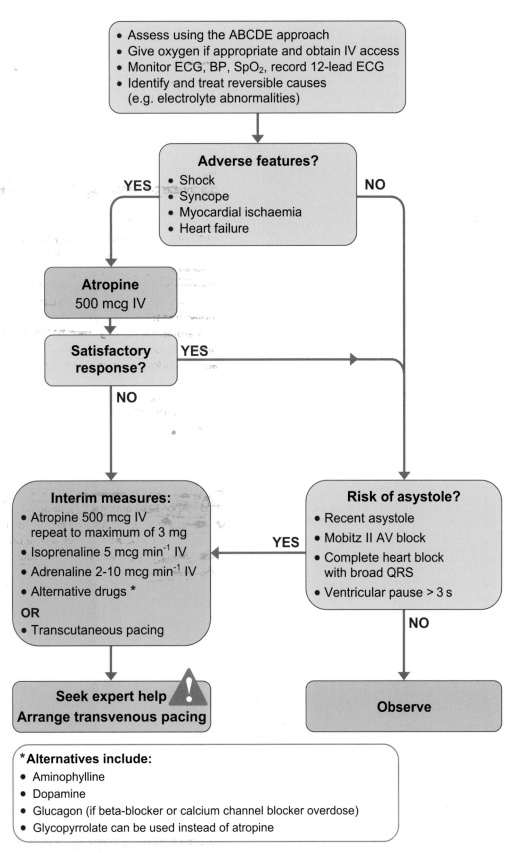

- Assess using the ABCDE approach
- Give oxygen if appropriate and obtain IV access
- Monitor ECG, BP, SpO₂, record 12-lead ECG
- Identify and treat reversible causes
  (e.g. electrolyte abnormalities)

Adverse features?
- Shock
- Syncope
- Myocardial ischaemia
- Heart failure

YES   NO

Atropine
500 mcg IV

Satisfactory response?   YES

NO

Interim measures:
- Atropine 500 mcg IV
  repeat to maximum of 3 mg
- Isoprenaline 5 mcg min⁻¹ IV
- Adrenaline 2-10 mcg min⁻¹ IV
- Alternative drugs *

OR
- Transcutaneous pacing

YES

Risk of asystole?
- Recent asystole
- Mobitz II AV block
- Complete heart block
  with broad QRS
- Ventricular pause > 3 s

NO

Seek expert help
Arrange transvenous pacing

Observe

*Alternatives include:**
- Aminophylline
- Dopamine
- Glucagon (if beta-blocker or calcium channel blocker overdose)
- Glycopyrrolate can be used instead of atropine

Figure 11.2 Bradycardia algorithm

If the patient has no adverse features

In a patient with bradycardia and no adverse features or high risk of progression to asystole, do not initiate immediate treatment. Continue to monitor the patient. Assess the patient to identify the cause of the bradycardia. If the cause is physiological or reversible (e.g. by stopping suppressant drug therapy) no further treatment may be needed. Seek expert help to arrange appropriate further assessment and treatment for those with other causes of bradycardia.

Key learning points

- Arrhythmias occurring after resuscitation from cardiac arrest and ROSC may need treatment to stabilise the patient and prevent recurrence of cardiac arrest.

- In other settings some arrhythmias may require prompt treatment to prevent deterioration, including progression to cardiac arrest, and others do not require immediate treatment.

- The urgency for treatment and the best choice of treatment is determined by the condition of the patient (presence or absence of adverse features) and by the nature and cause of the arrhythmia.

- Assessment of a patient with an arrhythmia should follow the ABCDE approach.

- Whenever possible the arrhythmia should be documented on a 12-lead ECG.

Further reading

Blomstrom-Lundqvist C, Scheinmann M M (Co-chairs). American College of Cardiology/American Heart Association Task Force and the European Society of Cardiology Committee for Practice Guidelines. ACC/AHA/ESC Guidelines for the Management of Patients With Supraventricular Arrhythmias. www.escardio.org

Moya A, Sutton R (Co-chairs). The Task Force for the Diagnosis and Management of Syncope of the European Society of Cardiology (ESC). Guidelines for the diagnosis and management of syncope (version 2009). www.escardio.org

Ryden L, Fuster F (Co-chairs). American College of Cardiology/American Heart Association Task Force and the European Society of Cardiology Committee for Practice Guidelines and Policy Conferences. ACC/AHA/ESC guidelines for the management of patients with atrial fibrillation. www.escardio.org

Vardas P E (Chairperson). The Task Force for Cardiac Pacing and Cardiac Resynchronization Therapy of the European Society of Cardiology. Guidelines for cardiac pacing and cardiac resynchronization therapy. www.escardio.org

Zipes D P, Camm J A (Co-chairs). A report of the American College of Cardiology/American Heart Association Task Force and the European Society of Cardiology Committee for Practice Guidelines. ACC/AHA/ESC 2006 guidelines for management of patients with ventricular arrhythmias and the prevention of sudden death. www.escardio.org

Cardiac Arrest in Special Circumstances

Learning outcomes

To understand how resuscitation techniques are modified in the special circumstances of:

▶ **Life-threatening electrolyte disorders**

▶ **Poisoning**

▶ **Accidental hypothermia**

▶ **Hyperthermia**

▶ **Drowning**

▶ **Asthma**

▶ **Anaphylaxis**

▶ **Cardiac arrest following cardiac surgery**

▶ **Trauma**

▶ **Pregnancy**

▶ **Electrocution**

Introduction

Resuscitation needs to be modified in specific circumstances. Early recognition of signs and symptoms and effective treatment will often prevent cardiac arrest. These conditions account for a large proportion of cardiac arrests in younger patients with no co-existing disease. It is essential to ask for appropriate expert help early for most of these conditions as they will require specialist interventions.

Survival in all these conditions still relies on using the ABCDE approach to help prevent cardiac arrest. If cardiac arrest does occur, high quality CPR with minimal interruption and treatment of reversible causes are still the most important interventions.

Life-threatening electrolyte disorders

Electrolyte abnormalities can cause cardiac arrhythmias or cardiorespiratory arrest. Potassium disorders pose the greatest risk. Consider starting treatment in life-threatening electrolyte disorders before laboratory results are available. Electrolyte values for definitions are quoted as a guide to clinical decision-making. The precise values that trigger treatment decisions will depend on the patient's clinical condition and rate of change of electrolyte values.

Prevention of electrolyte disorders

- Treat life-threatening electrolyte abnormalities before cardiac arrest occurs.

- Remove precipitating factors (e.g. drugs) and monitor electrolyte concentrations to prevent recurrence of the abnormality.

- Monitor renal function in patients at risk of electrolyte disorders (e.g. patients with chronic kidney disease, heart failure).

- Review renal replacement therapy (e.g. haemodialysis) regularly to avoid inappropriate electrolyte shifts during treatment.

Potassium disorders

Potassium homeostasis

Extracellular potassium concentration is regulated tightly between 3.5 - 5.0 mmol l^{-1}. A large concentration gradient normally exists between intracellular and extracellular fluid compartments. Evaluation of serum potassium must take into consideration the effects of changes in serum pH. When serum pH decreases (acidaemia), serum potassium concentration increases, because potassium shifts from the cellular to the vascular space. When serum pH increases (alkalaemia), serum potassium concentration decreases because potassium shifts into cells. Anticipate the effects of pH changes on serum potassium during therapy for hyperkalaemia or hypokalaemia.

Hyperkalaemia

Hyperkalaemia is usually caused by increased potassium release from cells or impaired excretion by the kidneys.

Definition

There is no universal definition. We have defined hyperkalaemia as a serum potassium concentration > 5.5 mmol l^{-1}; in practice, hyperkalaemia is a continuum. As the potassium concentration increases, the risk of adverse events increases and the need for urgent treatment increases. Severe hyperkalaemia has been defined as a serum potassium concentration > 6.5 mmol l^{-1}.

Causes

The causes of hyperkalaemia include:

- renal failure;

- drugs - angiotensin converting enzyme inhibitors (ACEI), angiotensin II receptor blockers (ARB), potassium sparing diuretics, non-steroidal anti-inflammatory drugs (NSAIDs), beta-blockers, trimethoprim;

- tissue breakdown (skeletal muscle (rhabdomyolysis), tumour lysis, haemolysis);

- metabolic acidosis;

- endocrine disorders (Addison's disease);

- hyperkalaemic periodic paralysis;

- diet (may be the principal cause in patients receiving chronic renal replacement therapy).

Abnormal erythrocytes or thrombocytosis may cause a spuriously high potassium concentration. The risk of hyperkalaemia increases when there is a combination of causative factors such as the concomitant use of ACEI and NSAIDs or potassium sparing diuretics.

Recognition of hyperkalaemia

Exclude hyperkalaemia in all patients with an arrhythmia or cardiac arrest. Patients can present with weakness progressing to flaccid paralysis, paraesthesia, or depressed deep tendon reflexes. The effect of hyperkalaemia on the ECG depends on the absolute serum potassium concentration as well as the rate of increase (Figure 12.1).

ECG changes with hyperkalaemia are usually progressive and include:

- first degree heart block (prolonged PR interval) (> 0.2 s);

- flattened or absent P waves;

- tall, peaked (tented) T waves (T wave larger than R wave in more than one lead);

- ST-segment depression;

- S and T wave merging (sine wave pattern);

- widened QRS (> 0.12 s);

- bradycardia (sinus bradycardia or AV block);

- ventricular tachycardia;

- cardiac arrest (PEA, VF/VT, asystole).

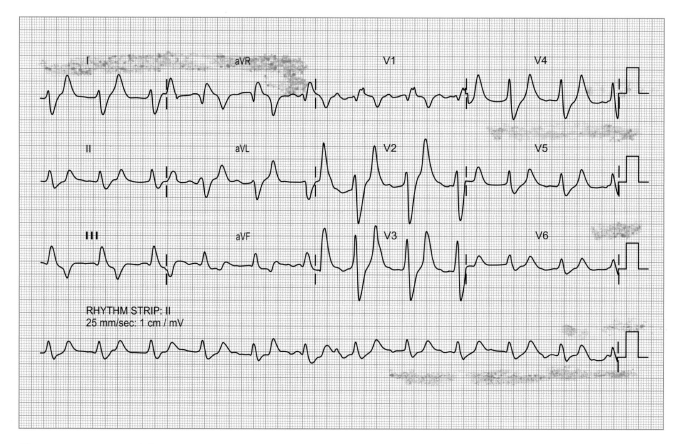

Figure 12.1 12-lead ECG showing features of hyperkalaemia

Most patients will have ECG abnormalities at a serum potassium concentration > 6.7 mmol l^{-1}. The use of a blood gas analyser that measures potassium helps reduce delays in recognition.

Treatment of hyperkalaemia

The five key steps in treating hyperkalaemia are:

1. Cardiac protection by antagonising the effects of hyperkalaemia.

2. Shifting potassium into cells.

3. Removing potassium from the body.

4. Monitoring serum potassium concentration for rebound hyperkalaemia.

5. Prevention of recurrence of hyperkalaemia.

When hyperkalaemia is strongly suspected, e.g. in the presence of ECG changes, start life-saving treatment even before laboratory results are available. Involve expert help from renal or intensive care teams at an early stage especially for those patients who might require renal replacement therapies (e.g. haemodialysis).

Patient not in cardiac arrest

Assess ABCDE (Airway, Breathing, Circulation, Disability, Exposure) and correct any abnormalities. If hypovolaemic, give fluid to enhance urinary potassium excretion. Obtain intravenous access, check serum potassium and record an ECG. Treatment is determined according to severity of hyperkalaemia. Approximate values are provided to guide treatment.

Mild elevation (5.5 - 5.9 mmol l^{-1}): remove potassium from the body with:

- Potassium exchange resins - calcium resonium 15 - 30 g OR sodium polystyrene sulfonate (Kayexalate) 15 - 30 g in 50 - 100 ml of 20 % sorbitol, given either orally or by retention enema (onset in 1 - 3 h; maximal effect at 6 h), or

- Diuretics: furosemide 1 mg kg^{-1} IV slowly (onset with the diuresis).

Address the cause of hyperkalaemia to correct and avoid further rise in serum potassium (e.g. drugs, diet)

Moderate elevation (6 - 6.4 mmol l^{-1}) without ECG changes: use strategies above plus:

- Shift potassium into cells with glucose/insulin: 10 units short-acting Insulin and 25 g glucose IV over 15 - 30 min (onset in 15 - 30 min; maximal effect at 30 - 60 min; monitor blood glucose).

- Consider renal replacement therapy (e.g. haemodialysis) to remove potassium from the body if patient is oliguric or potassium level increasing or not improving. Haemodialysis is more efficient than peritoneal dialysis at removing potassium (immediate onset; 25 - 30 mmol potassium h^{-1} removed with haemodialysis). Seek expert help.

Severe elevation (≥ 6.5 mmol l^{-1}) without ECG changes: seek expert help and shift potassium into cells with:

- Glucose/insulin (see above)

- Salbutamol 5 mg nebulised. Several doses (10 - 20 mg) may be required (onset in 15 - 30 min).

- Sodium bicarbonate: 50 mmol IV over 5 to 15 min if metabolic acidosis present (onset in 15 - 30 min). Bicarbonate alone is less effective than glucose plus insulin or nebulised salbutamol; it is best used in conjunction with these medications.

Remove potassium from the body with multiple strategies above.

Severe elevation (≥ 6.5 mmol l^{-1}) WITH toxic ECG changes (Figure 12.1): SEEK EXPERT HELP and protect the heart first with:

- Calcium chloride: 10 ml 10% calcium chloride IV over 2 - 5 min to antagonise the toxic effects of hyperkalaemia at the myocardial cell membrane. This protects the heart by reducing the risk of VF, but does not lower serum potassium (onset in 1 - 3 min).

- Use potassium removal and shifting strategies stated above.

- Prompt specialist referral is essential. In hospitals without a dedicated renal unit, intensive care units can often provide emergency renal replacement therapies.

Patient in cardiac arrest

Modifications to BLS
There are no modifications to basic life support in the presence of electrolyte abnormalities.

Modifications to ALS
Follow the ALS algorithm. Hyperkalaemia can be confirmed rapidly using a blood gas analyser if available.

Cardiac arrest: protect the heart first; then use shifting and removal strategies

- Calcium chloride: 10 ml 10% calcium chloride IV by rapid bolus injection to antagonise the toxic effects of hyperkalaemia at the myocardial cell membrane.

- Sodium bicarbonate: 50 mmol IV by rapid injection (if severe acidosis or renal failure).

- Glucose/insulin: 10 units short-acting insulin and 25 g glucose IV by rapid injection.

- Haemodialysis: consider this for cardiac arrest induced by hyperkalaemia which is resistant to medical treatment. Several dialysis modes have been used safely and effectively in cardiac arrest, but this may only be available in specialist centres that offer acute renal replacement therapy in critically ill patients.

Indications for haemodialysis

Haemodialysis is the most effective method for removal of potassium from the body. The principle mechanism of action is the diffusion of potassium ions across the membrane down the potassium ion gradient. The typical decline in serum potassium is 1 mmol l^{-1} in the first 60 min, followed by 1 mmol l^{-1} over the next 2 h.

Consider haemodialysis early for hyperkalaemia associated with established renal failure, oliguric acute kidney injury (< 400 ml day^{-1} urine output) or when there is marked tissue breakdown. Dialysis is also indicated when hyperkalaemia is resistant to medical treatment. Serum potassium frequently rebounds after initial treatment. In unstable patients continuous renal replacement therapy (e.g. continuous veno-veno haemodiafiltration) is less likely to compromise cardiac output than intermittent haemodialysis. This is now widely available in many intensive care units.

Cardiac arrest during haemodialysis

- Primary cardiac arrest is common in patients on long-term haemodialysis

- Call the resuscitation team and seek expert help immediately.

- Start resuscitation according to standard protocols ensuring high quality CPR and minimising interruptions.

- A trained dialysis nurse should be assigned to the dialysis machine.

- VF/ VT is more common in patients undergoing haemodialysis than in the general population.

- All of the standard reversible causes (4 Hs and 4 Ts) apply to dialysis patients. Electrolyte disorders, particularly hyperkalaemia, and fluid overload (e.g. pulmonary oedema) are most common causes.

- Some haemodialysis machine manufacturers

recommend disconnection from dialysis equipment for defibrillation. Renal units should have a protocol based on their equipment for disconnection for defibrillation and a number of methods have been described. In clinical practice, following standard safety protocols for defibrillation will be safe for the patient and resuscitation team.

- In life-threatening circumstances and cardiac arrest, vascular access used for dialysis can be used to give drugs.

Hypokalaemia

Hypokalaemia is common in hospital patients. Hypokalaemia increases the incidence of arrhythmias, particularly in patients with pre-existing heart disease and in those treated with digoxin.

Definition

Hypokalaemia is defined as serum potassium < 3.5 mmol l^{-1}. Severe hypokalaemia is defined as potassium < 2.5 mmol l^{-1} and may be associated with symptoms.

Causes

Causes of hypokalaemia include:

- gastrointestinal losses (diarrhoea);

- drugs (diuretics, laxatives, steroids, adrenaline, isoprenaline, etc);

- renal losses (renal tubular disorders, diabetes insipidus, dialysis);

- endocrine disorders (Cushing's Syndrome, hyperaldosteronism);

- metabolic alkalosis;

- magnesium depletion;

- poor dietary intake.

Treatment for hyperkalaemia can also induce hypokalaemia.

Recognition of hypokalaemia

Exclude hypokalaemia in every patient with an arrhythmia or cardiac arrest. In dialysis patients, hypokalaemia occurs commonly at the end of a haemodialysis session or during treatment with continuous ambulatory peritoneal dialysis (CAPD).

As serum potassium concentration decreases, the nerves and muscles are predominantly affected, causing fatigue, weakness, leg cramps or constipation. In severe cases (K$^+$< 2.5 mmol l^{-1}), rhabdomyolysis, ascending paralysis and respiratory difficulties may occur.

ECG features of hypokalaemia are:

- U waves;

- T wave flattening;

- ST segment changes;

- arrhythmias (especially if patient is taking digoxin);

- cardiorespiratory arrest (PEA, VF/VT, asystole).

Treatment of hypokalaemia

This depends on the severity of hypokalaemia and the presence of symptoms and ECG abnormalities. Gradual replacement of potassium is preferable, but in an emergency intravenous potassium is required. Seek expert help. The maximum recommended IV infusion rate of potassium is 20 mmol h^{-1}, but more rapid infusion (e.g. 2 mmol min^{-1} for 10 min, followed by 10 mmol over 5 - 10 min) is indicated for unstable arrhythmias when cardiac arrest is imminent or has occurred. Continuous ECG monitoring is essential during IV infusion. Adjust the dose after repeated sampling of serum potassium levels.

Patients who are potassium deficient can also be deficient in magnesium. Repletion of magnesium stores will facilitate more rapid correction of hypokalaemia and is recommended in severe cases of hypokalaemia.

Calcium and magnesium disorders

The recognition and management of calcium and magnesium disorders is summarised in Table 12.1.

Disorder	Causes	Presentation	ECG	Treatment
Hypercalcaemia Total Calcium* > 2.6 mmol l^{-1}	Primary or tertiary hyperparathyroidism Malignancy Sarcoidosis Drugs	Confusion Weakness Abdominal pain Hypotension Arrhythmias Cardiac arrest	Short QT interval Prolonged QRS Interval Flat T waves AV block Cardiac arrest	Fluid replacement IV Furosemide 1mg kg^{-1} IV Hydrocortisone 200 - 300mg IV Pamidronate 30 - 90mg IV Treat underlying cause
Hypocalcaemia Total Calcium* < 2.1 mmol l^{-1}	Chronic renal failure Acute pancreatitis Calcium channel blocker overdose Toxic shock syndrome Rhabdomyolysis Tumour lysis syndrome	Paraesthesia Tetany Seizures AV - block Cardiac arrest	Prolonged QT interval T wave inversion Heart block Cardiac arrest	Calcium chloride 10% 10 - 40ml IV Magnesium sulphate 50% 4 - 8 mmol (if necessary) IV
Hypermagnesaemia [Magnesium] > 1.1 mmol l^{-1}	Renal failure Iatrogenic	Confusion Weakness Respiratory depression AV - block Cardiac arrest	Prolonged PR and QT intervals T wave peaking AV - block Cardiac arrest	Consider treatment when [Magnesium] > 1.75 mmol l^{-1} Calcium chloride 10% 5-10ml IV repeated if necessary Ventilatory support if necessary Saline diuresis - 0.9% saline
Hypomagnesaemia [Magnesium] < 0.6 mmol l^{-1}	GI loss Polyuria Starvation Alcoholism Malabsorption	Tremor Ataxia Nystagmus Seizures Arrhythmias - torsade de pointes Cardiac arrest	Prolonged PR and QT Intervals ST-segment depression T-wave inversion Flattened P waves Increased QRS duration Torsade de pointes	Severe or symptomatic: 2 g 50% magnesium sulphate (4 ml; 8 mmol) IV over 15 min. Torsade de pointes: 2 g 50% magnesium sulphate (4 ml; 8 mmol) IV over 10 min. Seizure: 2 g 50% magnesium sulphate (4 ml; 8 mmol) IV over 10 min.

Table 12.1 Calcium and magnesium disorders

* A normal *total calcium* is about 2.2 to 2.6 mmol l^{-1}. A normal *ionized calcium* is about 1.1 to 1.3 mmol l^{-1}. Calcium values need to be interpreted with caution. Seek expert help if not sure. Total calcium depends on serum albumin values and will need to be corrected for low albumin values (corrected total calcium). Ionized calcium values are often measured by blood gas machines. It is important not to confuse ionized calcium, total calcium and corrected calcium values.

Poisoning

Poisoning is an infrequent cause of cardiac arrest, but remains a leading cause in victims younger than 40 years. It is also a common cause of non-traumatic coma in this age group.

Self-poisoning with therapeutic or recreational drugs is the main reason for hospital admission. Drug toxicity can also be caused by inappropriate dosing and drug interactions. Accidental poisoning is commonest in children. Homicidal poisoning is uncommon.

Industrial accidents, warfare or terrorism may cause chemical, biological, radiological or nuclear (CBRN) exposure. Decontamination and safe management for individual or mass casualty incidents is not part of this manual.

Initial treatment

Supportive care based on the ABCDE (Airway, Breathing, Circulation, Disability, Exposure) approach to prevent cardiorespiratory arrest whilst awaiting drug elimination is the mainstay of treatment. Airway obstruction and respiratory arrest secondary to a decreased conscious level is common. Alcohol excess is often present with self-poisoning.

- After opening and clearing the airway, check for breathing and a pulse (if trained to do so). Avoid mouth-to-mouth ventilation in the presence of toxins such as cyanide, hydrogen sulphide, corrosives and organophosphates. Ventilate the patient's lungs using a pocket mask or bag-mask and the highest possible concentration of oxygen. In paraquat poisoning, lung injury may be exacerbated by high concentrations of oxygen; adjust the inspired oxygen concentration according to pulse oximetry or arterial blood gases.

- There is a high incidence of pulmonary aspiration of gastric contents after poisoning. In unconscious patients who cannot protect their airway, use a rapid sequence induction with cricoid pressure to intubate the trachea and decrease the risk of aspiration. This must be undertaken by persons trained and competent in the technique.

- Provide standard basic and advanced life support if cardiac arrest occurs.

- Cardioversion is indicated for life-threatening tachyarrhythmia. Use the guidelines for peri-arrest arrhythmias (Chapter 11). Try to correct reversible causes.

- Drug-induced hypotension is common after self-poisoning. This usually responds to fluid therapy, but occasionally vasopressers (e.g. noradrenaline infusion) are required.

- Once resuscitation is under way, try to identify the poison(s). Relatives, friends and ambulance crews can usually provide useful information. Patient examination may give diagnostic clues such as odours, needle puncture marks, pinpoint pupils, tablet residues, signs of corrosion in the mouth, or blisters associated with prolonged coma.

- Measure the patient's temperature - hypo - or hyperthermia may occur after drug overdose.

- Patients with life-threatening features or at risk of further deterioration should be cared for in critical care settings.

- Consult a regional or national poisons centre for information on treatment of the poisoned patient. In the UK, specialist advice about specific poisons can be obtained by accessing TOXBASE® (www.toxbase.org). Similar centres exist in other countries. The World Health Organization lists poison centres at: www.who.int/ipcs/poisons/centre/directory/en/

Specific treatments

There are few specific therapies for poisons that are useful immediately. The emphasis is on intensive supportive therapy using the ABCDE approach, with correction of hypoxia, hypotension, acid/base, and electrolyte disorders.

Therapies include limiting absorption of ingested poisons, enhancing elimination, or the use of specific antidotes. Seek advice from a poisons centre for up-to-date guidance for severe or uncommon poisonings.

- Activated charcoal adsorbs certain drugs. Its value decreases over time after ingestion. There is little evidence that treatment with activated charcoal improves clinical outcome. Consider giving a single dose of activated charcoal to patients who have ingested a potentially toxic amount of a poison known to be adsorbed by activated charcoal up to one hour previously. Give only to patients with an intact or protected airway. Multiple doses may be beneficial in life-threatening poisoning with carbemazepine, dapsone, phenobarbital, quinine and theophylline.

- Gastric lavage followed by activated charcoal therapy is useful only within one hour of ingesting the poison. Generally, this should be carried out after tracheal intubation. Delayed gastric lavage has very little effect on drug absorption and may propel drugs further along the gastrointestinal tract.

- Whole-bowel irrigation can reduce drug absorption by cleansing the gastro-intestinal tract by enteral administration of a polyethylene glycol solution. Consider in potentially toxic ingestion of sustained release or enteric-coated drugs, oral iron poisoning, and the removal of ingested packets of illicit drugs.

- Laxatives (cathartics) or emetics (e.g. ipecacuanha) have no role in the management of the acutely poisoned patient and are not recommended.

- Urine alkalinisation (urine pH > 7.5) by giving IV sodium bicarbonate can be useful in moderate to severe salicylate poisoning in patients who do not need haemodialysis).

- Consider haemodialysis for poisoning with methanol, ethylene glycol, salicylates, and lithium. Charcoal haemoperfusion may be indicated for intoxication with carbamazepine, phenobarbital, phenytoin, or theophylline.

- Consider the use of lipid emulsion (Intralipid) for cardiac arrest caused by local anaesthetic toxicity (see below).

- Specific antidotes include: acetylcysteine for paracetamol; high-dose atropine for organophosphate insecticides; sodium nitrite, sodium thiosulfate, hydroxocobalamin, and amyl nitrite for cyanides; digoxin-specific Fab antibodies for digoxin; flumazenil for benzodiazepines; naloxone for opioids.

Specific antidotes

This section addresses only some causes of cardiac arrest from poisoning.

Opioid poisoning

Opioid poisoning causes respiratory depression, pinpoint pupils and coma followed by respiratory arrest. The opioid antagonist naloxone rapidly reverses these effects. There are fewer adverse events when the airway is opened and patients receive oxygen and ventilation (e.g. with pocket mask or bag-mask) before naloxone in opioid-induced respiratory depression; however, the use of naloxone may prevent the need for intubation.

The route for giving naloxone depends on the skills of the rescuer: intravenous (IV), intramuscular (IM), subcutaneous (SC), and intranasal (IN) routes can be used. The non-IV routes may be quicker because time is saved in not having to establish IV access, which can be extremely difficult in an IV drug abuser. The initial doses of naloxone are 400 mcg IV, 800 mcg IM, 800 mcg SC or

2 mg IN. Large opioid overdoses require titration to a total naloxone dose of 6 - 10 mg. The duration of action of naloxone is 45 - 70 min, but respiratory depression may persist for 4 - 5 h after opioid overdose. Thus, the clinical effects of naloxone may not last as long as those of a significant opioid overdose. Give increments of naloxone until the victim is breathing adequately and has protective airway reflexes.

Acute withdrawal from opioids produces a state of sympathetic excess and can cause complications such as pulmonary oedema, ventricular arrhythmia, and severe agitation. Use naloxone reversal of opioid intoxication with caution in patients suspected of opioid dependence.

Cardiac arrest is usually secondary to a respiratory arrest and associated with severe brain hypoxia. Prognosis is poor. Giving naloxone is unlikely to be harmful. Once cardiac arrest has occurred, follow standard resuscitation guidelines.

Benzodiazepines

Overdose of benzodiazepines can cause loss of consciousness, respiratory depression and hypotension. Flumazenil, a competitive antagonist of benzodiazepines, should be used only for reversal of sedation caused by a single ingestion of any of the benzodiazepines and when there is no history or risk of seizures. Reversal of benzodiazepine intoxication with flumazenil can cause significant toxicity (seizure, arrhythmia, hypotension, and withdrawal syndrome) in patients with benzodiazepine dependence or co-ingestion of proconvulsant medications such as tricyclic antidepressants. Do not use flumazenil routinely in the comatose overdose patient. There are no specific modifications required for cardiac arrest caused by benzodiazepines.

Tricyclic antidepressants

This includes tricyclic and related cyclic drugs (e.g. amitriptyline, desipramine, imipramine, nortriptyline, doxepin, and clomipramine). Self-poisoning with tricyclic antidepressants is common and can cause hypotension, seizures, coma and life-threatening arrhythmias. Cardiac toxicity mediated by anticholinergic and sodium channel-blocking effects can produce a broad-complex tachycardia (VT). Hypotension is exacerbated by alpha-1 receptor blockade. Anticholinergic effects include mydriasis, fever, dry skin, delirium, tachycardia, ileus, and urinary retention. Most life-threatening problems occur within the first 6 h after ingestion.

A widening QRS complex and right axis deviation indicates a greater risk of arrhythmias (Figure 12.2). Sodium bicarbonate should be considered for the treatment of tricyclic-induced ventricular conduction abnormalities. While no study has investigated the optimal target arterial pH with bicarbonate therapy, a pH of 7.45 - 7.55 has been commonly accepted.

Local anaesthetic toxicity

Local anaesthetic toxicity occurs typically in the setting of regional anaesthesia, when a bolus of local anaesthetic inadvertently enters an artery or vein. Systemic toxicity of local anaesthetics involves the central nervous system, and the cardiovascular system. Severe agitation, loss of consciousness, with or without tonic-clonic convulsions, sinus bradycardia, conduction blocks, asystole and ventricular tachyarrhythmia can all occur. Toxicity can be potentiated in pregnancy, extremes of age, or hypoxaemia.

Patients with both cardiovascular collapse and cardiac arrest attributable to local anaesthetic toxicity may benefit from treatment with intravenous 20% lipid emulsion in addition to standard advanced life support. Give an initial intravenous bolus of 1.5 ml kg⁻¹ 20% lipid emulsion followed by an infusion at 15 ml kg⁻¹ h⁻¹. Give up to three bolus doses of lipid at 5-minute intervals and continue the infusion until the patient is stable or has received up to a maximum of 12 ml kg⁻¹ of lipid emulsion (Figure 12.3).

Cocaine toxicity

Sympathetic overstimulation associated with cocaine toxicity may cause agitation, symptomatic tachycardia, hypertensive crisis, hyperthermia and myocardial ischaemia with angina. Small doses of intravenous benzodiazepines (midazolam, diazepam, lorazepam) are effective first-line drugs. Glyceryl trinitrate and phentolamine can reverse cocaine-induced coronary vasoconstriction. Use nitrates only as second-line therapy for myocardial ischaemia. Possible myocardial necrosis should be assessed using the ECG and cardiac markers (e.g. troponin) in patients with cocaine-related chest pain. If cardiac arrest occurs, follow standard resuscitation guidelines.

Drug-induced severe bradycardia

Severe bradycardia from poisoning or drug overdose may be refractory to standard ALS protocols because of prolonged receptor binding or direct cellular toxicity. Atropine can be life-saving in organophosphate, carbamate or nerve agent poisoning. Give atropine for bradycardia caused by acetylcholinesterase-inhibiting substances. Large (2 - 4 mg) and repeated doses may be required to achieve a clinical effect. Isoprenaline may be useful at high doses in refractory bradycardia induced by beta-receptor blockade. Heart block and ventricular arrhythmias associated with digoxin or digitalis glycoside poisoning may be treated effectively with digoxin-specific antibody fragments.

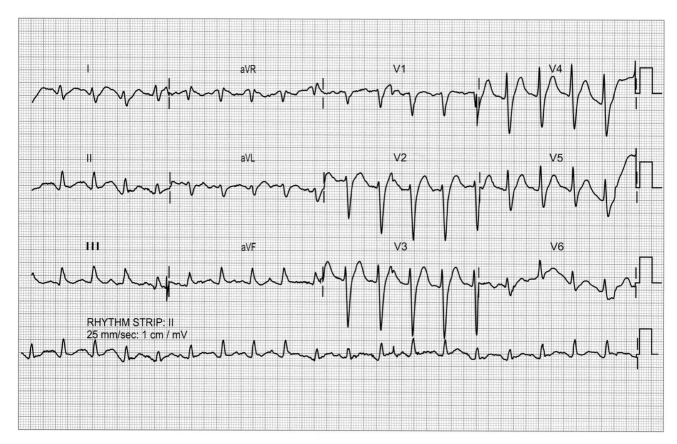

Figure 12.2 12-lead ECG showing features of severe tricyclic antidepressant toxicity

AAGBI Safety Guideline

Management of Severe Local Anaesthetic Toxicity

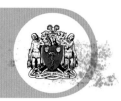

1 Recognition

Signs of severe toxicity:
- Sudden alteration in mental status, severe agitation or loss of consciousness, with or without tonic-clonic convulsions
- Cardiovascular collapse: sinus bradycardia, conduction blocks, asystole and ventricular tachyarrhythmias may all occur
- Local anaesthetic (LA) toxicity may occur some time after an initial injection

2 Immediate management

- Stop injecting the LA
- Call for help
- Maintain the airway and, if necessary, secure it with a tracheal tube
- Give 100% oxygen and ensure adequate lung ventilation (hyperventilation may help by increasing plasma pH in the presence of metabolic acidosis)
- Confirm or establish intravenous access
- Control seizures: give a benzodiazepine, thiopental or propofol in small incremental doses
- Assess cardiovascular status throughout
- Consider drawing blood for analysis, but do not delay definitive treatment to do this

3 Treatment

IN CIRCULATORY ARREST
- Start cardiopulmonary resuscitation (CPR) using standard protocols
- Manage arrhythmias using the same protocols, recognising that arrhythmias may be very refractory to treatment
- Consider the use of cardiopulmonary bypass if available

GIVE INTRAVENOUS LIPID EMULSION
(following the regimen overleaf)

- Continue CPR throughout treatment with lipid emulsion
- Recovery from LA-induced cardiac arrest may take >1 h
- Propofol is not a suitable substitute for lipid emulsion
- Lidocaine should not be used as an anti-arrhythmic therapy

WITHOUT CIRCULATORY ARREST
Use conventional therapies to treat:
- hypotension,
- bradycardia,
- tachyarrhythmia

CONSIDER INTRAVENOUS LIPID EMULSION
(following the regimen overleaf)

- Propofol is not a suitable substitute for lipid emulsion
- Lidocaine should not be used as an anti-arrhythmic therapy

4 Follow-up

- Arrange safe transfer to a clinical area with appropriate equipment and suitable staff until sustained recovery is achieved
- Exclude pancreatitis by regular clinical review, including daily amylase or lipase assays for two days
- Report cases as follows:
    in the United Kingdom to the National Patient Safety Agency (via **www.npsa.nhs.uk**)
    in the Republic of Ireland to the Irish Medicines Board (via **www.imb.ie**)
If Lipid has been given, please also report its use to the international registry at **www.lipidregistry.org**. Details may also be posted at **www.lipidrescue.org**

Your nearest bag of Lipid Emulsion is kept..

This guideline is not a standard of medical care. The ultimate judgement with regard to a particular clinical procedure or treatment plan must be made by the clinician in the light of the clinical data presented and the diagnostic and treatment options available.

© The Association of Anaesthetists of Great Britain & Ireland 2010

Figure 12.3 Management of severe local anaesthetic toxicity

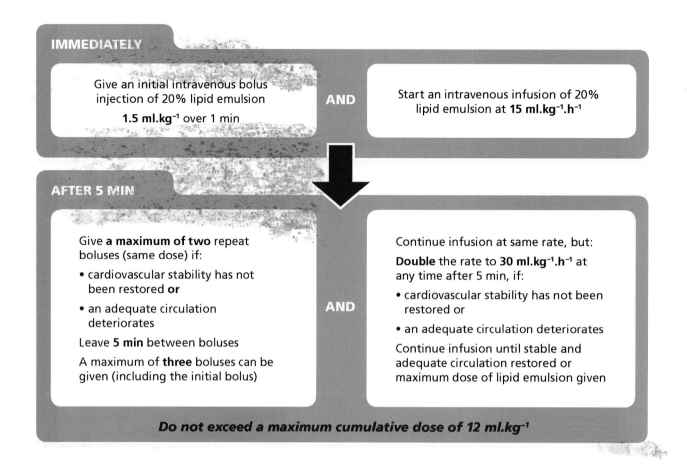

IMMEDIATELY

Give an initial intravenous bolus injection of 20% lipid emulsion **1.5 ml.kg⁻¹ over 1 min**

AND

Start an intravenous infusion of 20% lipid emulsion at **15 ml.kg⁻¹.h⁻¹**

AFTER 5 MIN

Give **a maximum of two** repeat boluses (same dose) if:

• cardiovascular stability has not been restored **or**

• an adequate circulation deteriorates

Leave **5 min** between boluses

A maximum of **three** boluses can be given (including the initial bolus)

AND

Continue infusion at same rate, but:

Double the rate to **30 ml.kg⁻¹.h⁻¹** at any time after 5 min, if:

• cardiovascular stability has not been restored or

• an adequate circulation deteriorates

Continue infusion until stable and adequate circulation restored or maximum dose of lipid emulsion given

Do not exceed a maximum cumulative dose of 12 ml.kg⁻¹

An approximate dose regimen for a 70-kg patient would be as follows:

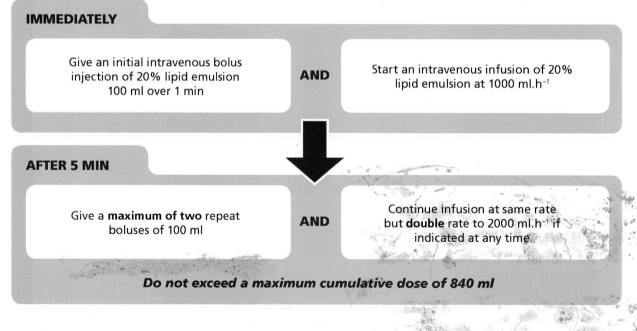

IMMEDIATELY

Give an initial intravenous bolus injection of 20% lipid emulsion 100 ml over 1 min

AND

Start an intravenous infusion of 20% lipid emulsion at 1000 ml.h⁻¹

AFTER 5 MIN

Give a **maximum of two** repeat boluses of 100 ml

AND

Continue infusion at same rate but **double** rate to 2000 ml.h⁻¹ if indicated at any time

Do not exceed a maximum cumulative dose of 840 ml

This AAGBI Safety Guideline was produced by a Working Party that comprised:
Grant Cave, Will Harrop-Griffiths (Chair), Martyn Harvey, Tim Meek, John Picard, Tim Short and Guy Weinberg.

This Safety Guideline is endorsed by the Australian and New Zealand College of Anaesthetists (ANZCA).

Figure 12.3 Management of severe local anaesthetic toxicity

Vasopressors, inotropes, calcium, glucagon, phosphodiesterase inhibitors and insulin-glucose may all be useful in beta-blocker and calcium channel blocker overdose. Transcutaneous pacing may be effective for severe bradycardia caused by poisoning and overdose (Chapters 10 and 11).

Further treatment and prognosis

A long period of coma in a single position can cause pressure sores and rhabdomyolysis. Measure electrolytes (particularly potassium), blood glucose and arterial blood gas values. Monitor temperature because thermoregulation is impaired. Both hypothermia and hyperthermia (hyperpyrexia) can occur after overdose of some drugs. Retain samples of blood and urine for analysis. Be prepared to continue resuscitation for a prolonged period, particularly in young patients, as the poison may be metabolised or excreted during extended life support measures.

Hypothermia

Definition

Hypothermia exists when the body core temperature is below 35°C and is classified arbitrarily as mild (32 - 35°C), moderate (28 - 32°C), or severe (< 28°C). The Swiss staging system based on clinical signs can be used by rescuers at the scene to describe victims: stage I - clearly conscious and shivering; stage II - impaired consciousness without shivering; stage III - unconscious; stage IV - no breathing and V - death due to irreversible hypothermia.

Diagnosis

Accidental hypothermia may be under-diagnosed in countries with a temperate climate. In people with normal thermoregulation, hypothermia can develop during exposure to cold environments, particularly wet or windy conditions, and in people who have been immobilised, or following immersion in cold water. When thermoregulation is impaired, for example, in the elderly and very young, hypothermia can follow a mild insult. The risk of hypothermia is also increased by drug or alcohol ingestion, exhaustion, illness, injury or neglect especially when there is a decrease in the level of consciousness. Hypothermia may be suspected from the clinical history or a brief external examination of a collapsed patient. A low-reading thermometer is needed to measure the core temperature and confirm the diagnosis. The core temperature measured in the lower third of the oesophagus correlates well with the temperature of the heart. 'Tympanic' measurement - using a thermistor technique - is a reliable alternative but may be lower than the oesophageal temperature if the environmental temperature is very cold, the probe is not well insulated, the external auditory canal is blocked or during cardiac arrest when there is no flow in the carotid artery. Widely available 'tympanic' thermometers based on infrared technique do not seal the ear canal and are often not suitable for low temperature readings.

Decision to resuscitate

Cooling of the human body decreases cellular oxygen consumption by about 6% per 1°C decrease in core temperature. In some cases, hypothermia can exert a protective effect on the brain and vital organs and intact neurological recovery is possible even after prolonged cardiac arrest if deep hypothermia develops before asphyxia.

Beware of diagnosing death in a hypothermic patient because cold alone may produce a very slow, small-volume, irregular pulse and unrecordable blood pressure. In a hypothermic patient, no signs of life (Swiss hypothermia stage IV) alone are unreliable for declaring death. At 18°C the brain can tolerate periods of circulatory arrest for ten times longer than at 37°C. Dilated pupils can be caused by a variety of insults and must not be regarded as a sign of death. Good quality survival has been reported after cardiac arrest and a core temperature of 13.7°C after immersion in cold water with prolonged CPR.

In the prehospital setting, resuscitation should be withheld only if the cause of a cardiac arrest is clearly attributable to a lethal injury, fatal illness, prolonged asphyxia, or if the chest is incompressible. In all other patients the traditional guiding principle that "no one is dead until warm and dead" should be considered. In remote wilderness areas, the impracticalities of achieving rewarming have to be considered. In the hospital setting involve senior doctors and use clinical judgment to determine when to stop resuscitating a hypothermic arrest victim.

Treatment of hypothermia

The standard principles of prevention and life support apply to the hypothermic patient. Do not delay urgent procedures, such as tracheal intubation and insertion of vascular catheters.

- Open the airway and, if there is no spontaneous respiratory effort, ventilate the patient's lungs with high concentrations of oxygen. If possible, use warmed (40 - 46°C) and humidified oxygen. Consider careful tracheal intubation when indicated according to the ALS algorithm. Procedures can precipitate VF. The advantages of adequate oxygenation and protection from aspiration outweigh the minimal risk of triggering VF by performing tracheal intubation.

- Palpate a major artery and, if available, look at the ECG for up to 1 min and look for signs of life before concluding that there is no cardiac output. Both the respiratory rate and pulse may be very slow in

ALS

severe hypothermia so more assessment time is necessary. Echocardiography or Doppler ultrasound can be used to establish if there is a cardiac output or peripheral blood flow.

- If the victim is pulseless, start chest compressions immediately. Use the same ventilation and chest compression rates as for a normothermic patient. Hypothermia can cause stiffness of the chest wall, making ventilation and chest compressions more difficult. If you are not experienced in patient assessment or if there is any doubt about whether a pulse is present, start chest compressions until more experienced help is available.

- Once resuscitation is under way, confirm hypothermia with a low reading thermometer. Use oesophageal, bladder, rectal, or tympanic temperature measurements. Try to use a consistent method to allow serial comparisons of temperature.

- The hypothermic heart may be unresponsive to cardio-active drugs, attempted electrical pacing, and attempted defibrillation. Drug metabolism is slowed, leading to potentially toxic plasma concentrations of any drugs given repeatedly. Withhold adrenaline and other drugs until the patient has been warmed to a temperature greater than about 30°C. Once 30°C has been reached, double the intervals between doses (twice as long as normal). As the patient's temperature returns towards normal (above 35°C), use the standard drug protocols.

- Give drugs via a central or large proximal vein if possible.

- Remember to rule out other primary causes of cardiorespiratory arrest (e.g. drug overdose, hypothyroidism or trauma) or reversible causes using the four Hs and four Ts approach.

- Monitor electrolytes, glucose and blood gases regularly during resuscitation and post-resuscitation care as rapid changes can occur.

- Blood gas analysers will give blood gas values for a temperature of 37°C unless the patient's temperature is entered in to the analyser. Oxygen and carbon dioxide partial pressures are lower in hypothermia because gases become more soluble as blood temperature decreases. In clinical practice it is much easier to make all the measurements at 37°C i.e. temperature uncorrected values. It is then only necessary to compare them with the well-known normal values for 37°C. This also enables comparison of serial results from blood gas samples taken during rewarming.

Arrhythmias

As the body core temperature decreases, sinus bradycardia tends to give way to atrial fibrillation (AF) followed by ventricular fibrillation (VF) and finally, asystole. Follow standard treatment protocols.

- Arrhythmias other than VF tend to revert spontaneously as the core temperature increases and usually do not require immediate treatment. Bradycardia can be physiological in severe hypothermia. Cardiac pacing is not indicated unless the bradycardia persists after rewarming.

- If VF/VT is detected, give a shock; if VF/VT persists after three shocks, delay further defibrillation attempts until the core temperature is above 30°C. If an AED is used, follow the AED prompts while rewarming the patient.

Rewarming

General measures for all victims include removal from the cold environment, prevention of further heat loss and rapid transfer to hospital. Rewarming may be passive, active external, or active internal.

- In the field, a patient with moderate or severe hypothermia should be immobilised and handled carefully, oxygenated adequately, monitored (including ECG and core temperature), and the whole body dried and insulated. Wet clothes should be cut off rather than stripped off; this will avoid excessive movement of the victim.

- Conscious victims can mobilise as exercise re-warms a person more rapidly than shivering. Exercise can increase any after-drop, i.e. further cooling after removal from a cold environment. Somnolent or comatose victims have a low threshold for developing VF or pulseless VT and should be immobilised and kept horizontal to avoid an after-drop or cardiovascular collapse.

- Passive rewarming is appropriate in conscious victims with mild hypothermia who are still able to shiver. This is best achieved by full body insulation with wool blankets, aluminium foil, a hat and warm environment. The application of chemical heat packs to the trunk is particularly helpful in moderate and severe hypothermia to prevent further heat loss in the prehospital setting.

- Rewarming in the field with heated intravenous fluids and warm humidified gases is not efficient. Intensive active rewarming must not delay transport to a hospital where advanced rewarming techniques, continuous monitoring and observation are available.

In general, alert hypothermic and shivering victims without an arrhythmia can be transported to the nearest hospital for passive rewarming and observation. Hypothermic victims with an altered consciousness should be taken to a hospital capable of active external and internal rewarming.

- Active external rewarming techniques include forced air rewarming and warmed (up to 42°C) intravenous fluids. These techniques are effective (rewarming rate 1 - 1.5°C h^{-1}) in patients with severe hypothermia and a perfusing rhythm.

- Active internal rewarming techniques include warm humidified gases; gastric, peritoneal, pleural or bladder lavage with warmed fluids (at 40°C), and extracorporeal rewarming.

- In a hypothermic patient with apnoea and cardiac arrest, extracorporeal rewarming is the preferred method of active internal rewarming because it provides sufficient circulation and oxygenation while the core body temperature is increased by 8 - 12°C h^{-1}. Survivors in one case series had an average of 65 min of conventional CPR before cardiopulmonary bypass. Unfortunately, facilities for extracorporeal rewarming are not always available and a combination of rewarming techniques may have to be used.

- During rewarming, patients will require large volumes of fluids as vasodilation causes expansion of the intravascular space. Continuous haemodynamic monitoring and warm IV fluids are essential.

Avalanche burial

In Europe and North America, there are about 150 snow avalanche deaths each year. Most are sports-related and involve skiers, snowboarders and snowmobilers. Death from avalanches is due to asphyxia, trauma and hypothermia. Avalanches occur in areas that are difficult to access by rescuers in a timely manner, and burials frequently involve multiple victims. Avalanche victims are not likely to survive when they are:

- buried > 35 min and in cardiac arrest with an obstructed airway on extrication;

- buried initially and in cardiac arrest with an obstructed airway on extrication, and an initial core temperature of < 32°C;

- buried initially and in cardiac arrest on extrication with an initial serum potassium of > 12 mmol l^{-1}.

Post-resuscitation care

Avoid hyperthermia during and after the warming period. Once ROSC has been achieved, use standard strategies for post-resuscitation care, including mild hypothermia if appropriate. There is no evidence for the routine use of steroids, barbiturates, or antibiotics.

Hyperthermia

Definition

Hyperthermia occurs when the body's ability to thermoregulate fails and core temperature exceeds that normally maintained by homeostatic mechanisms. Hyperthermia may be exogenous, caused by environmental conditions or secondary to endogenous heat production.

Environment-related hyperthermia occurs where heat, usually in the form of radiant energy, is absorbed by the body at a rate faster than can be lost by thermoregulatory mechanisms. Hyperthermia occurs along a continuum of heat-related conditions starting with heat stress, progressing to heat exhaustion, heat stroke and culminating in multi-organ dysfunction and cardiac arrest in some instances.

Malignant hyperthermia (MH) is a rare disorder of skeletal muscle calcium homeostasis characterised by muscle contracture and life-threatening hypermetabolic crisis following exposure of genetically predisposed individuals to halogenated anaesthetics and depolarising muscle relaxants.

Heat stroke

Heat stroke is a systemic inflammatory response with a core temperature > 40.6°C accompanied by mental state change and varying levels of organ dysfunction. There are two forms of heat stroke: classic non-exertional heat stroke occurs during high environmental temperatures and often affects the elderly during heat waves; exertional heat stroke occurs during strenuous physical exercise in high environmental temperatures and/or high humidity and usually effects healthy young adults. Mortality from heat stroke ranges between 10 - 50%.

Predisposing factors

The elderly are at increased risk for heat-related illness because of underlying illness, medication use, declining thermoregulatory mechanisms, and limited social support. There are several risk factors: lack of acclimatisation, dehydration, obesity, alcohol, cardiovascular disease, skin conditions (psoriasis, eczema, scleroderma, burn, cystic fibrosis) hyperthyroidism, phaeochromocytoma, and drugs (anticholinergics, diamorphine, cocaine, amphetamine, phenothiazines, sympathomimetics, calcium channel blockers, beta blockers).

Clinical Presentation

Heat stroke can resemble septic shock and may be caused by similar mechanisms. Features include:

- core temp 40.6°C or more;

- hot, dry skin (sweating is present in half cases of exertional heat stroke);

- early signs and symptoms include: extreme fatigue, headache, fainting, facial flushing, vomiting and diarrhoea;

- cardiovascular dysfunction including arrhythmias and hypotension;

- respiratory dysfunction including ARDS;

- central nervous system dysfunction including seizures and coma;

- liver and renal failure;

- coagulopathy;

- rhabdomyolysis.

Other clinical conditions need to be considered, including:

- drug toxicity;

- drug withdrawal syndrome;

- serotonin syndrome;

- neuroleptic malignant syndrome;

- sepsis;

- central nervous system infection;

- endocrine disorders e.g. thyroid storm, phaeochromocytoma.

Treatment

The mainstay of treatment is supportive therapy based on optimising the ABCDEs and rapidly cooling the patient.

- Start cooling before the patient reaches hospital. Aim to rapidly reduce the core temperature to approximately 39°C. Patients with severe heat stroke need to be managed in a critical care setting.

- Use haemodynamic monitoring to guide fluid therapy. Large volumes of fluid may be required. Correct electrolyte abnormalities.

- If cardiac arrest occurs, follow standard procedures for basic and advanced life support and cool the patient. Attempt defibrillation, if appropriate, according to current guidelines, while continuing to cool the patient. Animal studies suggest the prognosis is poor compared with normothermic cardiac arrest. The risk of unfavourable neurological outcome increases for each degree of body temperature > 37°C.

- Provide post-resuscitation care according to normal guidelines (Chapter 13).

Cooling techniques

Several cooling methods have been described but there are few formal trials on which method is best.

- Simple techniques include cool drinks, fanning the undressed patient and spraying tepid water on the patient. Ice packs over areas where there are large superficial blood vessels (axillae, groins, neck) are also useful. Surface cooling may cause shivering.

- In cooperative stable patients immersion in cold water is effective; however, this can cause peripheral vasoconstriction and reduce heat dissipation. Immersion is not practical in very sick patients.

- Use the same advanced cooling techniques as used for therapeutic hypothermia after cardiac arrest (Chapter 13). Consider the use of cold IV fluids, intravascular cooling catheters, surface cooling devices and extra corporeal circuits, e.g. continuous veno-veno haemofiltration or cardiopulmonary bypass.

- No specific drugs lower core temperature in heat stroke. There is no good evidence that antipyretics (e.g. non-steroidal anti-inflammatory drugs or paracetamol) are effective in heat stroke. Diazepam may be useful to treat seizures and facilitate cooling. Dantrolene (see below) has not been shown to be beneficial.

Malignant hyperthermia

Malignant hyperthermia is a life-threatening genetic sensitivity of skeletal muscles to volatile anaesthetics and depolarising neuromuscular blocking drugs occurring during or after anaesthesia. Stop triggering agents immediately; give oxygen, correct acidosis and electrolyte abnormalities. Start active cooling and give dantrolene. Other drugs such as 3,4-methylenedioxymethamphetamine (MDMA, 'ecstasy') and amphetamines also cause a condition similar to malignant hyperthermia and the use of dantrolene may be beneficial.

Drowning

Drowning is a common cause of accidental death. The most important detrimental consequence of drowning is hypoxia. Cardiac arrest is usually a secondary event. The duration of hypoxia is a critical factor in determining the victim's outcome; therefore, oxygenation, ventilation, and perfusion should be restored as rapidly as possible. Immediate resuscitation at the scene is essential for survival and neurological recovery after drowning. This will require bystander provision of CPR plus immediate activation of the EMS system. Patients who have spontaneous circulation and breathing when they reach hospital usually recover with good outcomes. Remember, some patients may have had a primary cardiac arrest (e.g. caused by myocardial infarction whilst swimming). Death from drowning is more common in young males, and is the leading cause of accidental death in Europe in this group.

Definition

Drowning is defined as a process resulting in primary respiratory impairment from submersion/immersion in a liquid medium. Implicit in this definition is that a liquid/air interface is present at the entrance of the victim's airway, preventing the victim from breathing air. The victim may live or die after this process, but whatever the outcome, he or she has been involved in a drowning incident. Immersion means to be covered in water. For drowning to occur, usually at least the face and airway must be immersed. Submersion implies that the entire body, including the airway, is under the water or other fluid.

Decision to resuscitate

Deciding whether to start or stop resuscitation of a drowning victim is notoriously difficult. No single factor predicts prognosis accurately.

- Start and continue resuscitation unless there is clear evidence that resuscitation attempts are futile (e.g. massive traumatic injuries, rigor mortis, putrefaction etc), or timely evacuation to a medical facility is not possible. Neurologically-intact survival has been reported in several victims submerged for > 60 min.

Treatment

Treatment of a drowning victim involves four phases. These comprise (i) aquatic rescue (ii) basic life support (iii) advanced life support (iv) post-resuscitation care.

Aquatic rescue and basic life support

- Ensure personal safety and minimise the danger to yourself at all times. If possible, attempt to save the drowning victim without entering the water. Talk to the victim, use a rescue aid (e.g. stick or clothing), or throw a rope or buoyant rescue aid if the victim is close to dry land. Alternatively, use a boat or other water vehicle to help with the rescue. Avoid entry into the water whenever possible. If entry into the water is essential, take a buoyant rescue aid or flotation device. It is safer to enter the water with two rescuers than alone.

- Remove the victim from the water and start resuscitation as quickly and safely as possible. Cervical spine injury is uncommon in drowning victims (approximately 0.5%). Spinal immobilisation is difficult in the water and delays removal from the water and adequate resuscitation of the victim. Consider cervical spine immobilisation if there is a history of diving, water slide use, signs of severe injury, or signs of alcohol intoxication. Despite potential spinal injury, if the victim is pulseless and apnoeic remove them from the water as quickly as possible (even if a back support device is not available) whilst attempting to limit neck flexion and extension.

- Try to remove the victim from the water in a horizontal position to minimise the risks of post-immersion hypotension and cardiovascular collapse.

Ventilation

- Prompt initiation of rescue breathing or positive pressure ventilation increases survival. If possible supplement ventilation with oxygen. Give five initial ventilations as soon as possible.

- Rescue breathing can be initiated whilst the victim is still in shallow water provided the safety of the rescuer is not compromised. It is likely to be difficult to pinch the victim's nose, so mouth-to-nose ventilation may be used as an alternative to mouth-to-mouth ventilation.

- If the victim is in deep water, open their airway and if there is no spontaneous breathing start in-water rescue breathing if trained to do so. In-water resuscitation is possible, but should ideally be performed with the support of a buoyant rescue aid. Give 10 - 15 rescue breaths over approximately 1 min. If normal breathing does not start spontaneously, and the victim is < 5 min from land, continue rescue breaths while towing. If more than an estimated 5 min from land, give rescue breaths over 1 min, then bring the victim to land as quickly as possible without further attempts at ventilation.

Chest compressions

As soon as the victim is removed from the water, check for breathing. If the victim is not breathing (or is making occasional gasps), start chest compressions immediately. Continue CPR in a ratio of 30 compressions to 2 ventilations. Most drowning victims will have sustained cardiac arrest secondary to hypoxia. In these patients, compression-only CPR is likely to be less effective and standard CPR should be used.

ALS

Defibrillation

Dry the victims chest before placing defibrillation electrodes. Standard procedures for defibrillation using an AED or manual defibrillator should be followed.

Regurgitation during resuscitation

- Regurgitation of stomach contents is common following resuscitation from drowning and makes airway management more difficult. If regurgitation occurs, turn the victim's mouth to the side and remove the regurgitated material using directed suction if possible. If spinal cord injury is suspected, log-roll the victim, keeping the head, neck, and torso aligned. Log rolling requires several rescuers. There is no need to clear the airway of aspirated water. Remove debris manually or when dry land has been reached with suction if available. Most drowning victims aspirate small amounts of water, and this is absorbed rapidly into the central circulation. Do not use abdominal thrusts or tip the victim head down to remove water from the lungs or stomach.

Advanced life support

Airway and breathing

- Give high-flow oxygen, ideally through an oxygen mask with reservoir bag, during the initial assessment of the spontaneously breathing drowning victim. Consider non-invasive ventilation or continuous positive airway pressure if the victim fails to respond to treatment with high-flow oxygen. Use pulse oximetry and arterial blood gas analysis to titrate the concentration of inspired oxygen.

- Consider early tracheal intubation and controlled ventilation for victims who fail to respond to these initial measures or who have a reduced level of consciousness. Take care to ensure optimal pre-oxygenation before intubation. Use a rapid-sequence induction with cricoid pressure to reduce the risk of aspiration. Pulmonary oedema fluid may pour from the airway and may need suctioning to enable a view of the larynx.

- After the tracheal tube is confirmed in position, titrate the inspired oxygen concentration to achieve a SaO_2 of 94 - 98%. High positive end-expiratory pressure (PEEP) levels may be required if the patients is severely hypoxaemic.

- In the event of cardiac arrest protect the airway of the victim early in the resuscitation attempt, ideally with a cuffed tracheal tube - reduced pulmonary compliance requiring high inflation pressures may limit the use of a supraglottic airway device.

Circulation and defibrillation

- Differentiating respiratory from cardiac arrest is

particularly important in the drowning victim. Delaying the initiation of chest compressions if the victim is in cardiac arrest will reduce survival.

- The typical post-arrest gasping is very difficult to distinguish from the initial respiratory efforts of a spontaneous recovering drowning victim. Palpation of the pulse as the sole indicator of the presence or absence of cardiac arrest is unreliable. When available additional diagnostic information should be obtained from other monitoring modalities such as ECG trace, $ETCO_2$, echocardiography to confirm the diagnosis of cardiac arrest.

- If the victim is in cardiac arrest, follow standard advanced life support protocols. If the victims core body temperature is less than 30°C, limit defibrillation attempts to three, and withhold IV drugs until the core body temperature increases above 30°C.

- During prolonged immersion, victims may become hypovolaemic from the hydrostatic pressure of the water on the body. Give IV fluid to correct hypovolaemia. After ROSC, use haemodynamic monitoring to guide fluid resuscitation.

Post-resuscitation care

- Victims of drowning are at risk of developing acute respiratory distress syndrome (ARDS) after submersion and standard ventilation strategies should be used.

- Pneumonia is common after drowning. Prophylactic antibiotics have not been shown to be of benefit, although they may be considered after submersion in grossly contaminated water such as sewage. Give broad-spectrum antibiotics if signs of infection develop subsequently.

- There are no differences in the treatment of victims of fresh or sea water drowning.

- If submersion occurs in icy water (< 5°C),hypothermia may develop rapidly and provide some protection against hypoxia. Once the victim is resuscitated it is unclear whether further therapeutic hypothermia is beneficial. A pragmatic approach might be to consider rewarming until a core temperature of 32 - 34°C is achieved, taking care to avoid hyperthermia (> 37°C) during the subsequent period of intensive care.

- Attempts have been made to improve neurological outcome following drowning with the use of barbiturates, intracranial pressure (ICP) monitoring, and steroids. None of these interventions has been shown to alter outcome.

- Cardiac arrhythmias may cause rapid loss of consciousness leading to drowning if the victim is in water at the time. Take a careful history in survivors of

ALS

a drowning incident to identify features suggestive of arrhythmic syncope. Symptoms may include syncope (whilst supine position, during exercise, with brief prodromal symptoms, repetitive episodes or associated with palpitations), seizures or a family history of sudden death. The absence of structural heart disease at post mortem does not rule the possibility of sudden cardiac death. Post mortem genetic analysis has proved helpful in these situations and should be considered if there is uncertainty over the cause of a drowning death.

Asthma

Worldwide, approximately 300 million people of all ages and ethnic backgrounds have asthma with a high prevalence in some European countries (United Kingdom, Ireland and Scandinavia). Annual worldwide deaths from asthma have been estimated at 250,000. Most deaths in the UK occur before hospital admission. Good asthma control and prevention of acute asthma is therefore important. The British Thoracic Society (BTS) and Scottish Intercollegiate Guidelines Network (SIGN) have published guidelines for the management of asthma available at www.brit-thoracic.org.uk

This guidance focuses on the treatment of patients with near-fatal asthma and cardiac arrest.

Patients at risk of asthma-related cardiac arrest

The risk of near-fatal asthma attacks is not necessarily related to asthma severity. Patients most at risk include those with:

- a history of near-fatal asthma requiring intubation and mechanical ventilation;

- a hospitalisation or emergency care for asthma in the past year;

- an increasing use and dependence of beta-2 agonists;

- anxiety, depressive disorders and/or poor compliance with therapy.

Causes of cardiac arrest

Cardiac arrest in the asthmatic is often a terminal event after a period of hypoxaemia; occasionally, it may be sudden. Cardiac arrest in asthmatics has been linked to:

- severe bronchospasm and mucous plugging leading to asphyxia;

- cardiac arrhythmias due to hypoxia, stimulant drugs (e.g. ß-adrenergic agonists, aminophylline) or electrolyte abnormalities;

- dynamic hyperinflation, i.e. auto-positive end-expiratory pressure (auto-PEEP), can occur in mechanically ventilated asthmatics. Auto-PEEP is caused by air trapping and 'breath stacking' (air entering the lungs and being unable to escape).

Gradual build-up of pressure occurs and reduces venous return and blood pressure;

- tension pneumothorax (often bilateral).

The 4 Hs and 4 Ts approach to reversible causes will help identify these causes in cardiac arrest.

Assessment and treatment

Use the ABCDE approach to assess severity and guide treatment. The severity of acute asthma is summarised in Table 12.2.

Asthma severity		
Near-fatal asthma	Raised PaCO$_2$ and/or mechanical ventilation with raised inflation pressures	
Life-threatening asthma	Any one of the following in a patient with severe asthma:	
	Clinical signs	**Measurements**
	Altered conscious level	PEF < 33% best or predicted
	Exhaustion	SpO$_2$ < 92%
	Arrhythmia	PaO$_2$ < 8 kPa
	Hypotension	'normal' PaCO$_2$ (4.6 - 6.0 kPa)
	Cyanosis	
	Silent chest	
	Poor expiratory effort	
Acute severe asthma	Any one of: - PEF 33 - 50% best or predicted - respiratory rate ≥ 25 min^{-1} - heart rate ≥ 110 min^{-1} - inability to complete sentences in one breath	
Moderate asthma exacerbation	- increasing symptoms - PEF > 50 - 75% best or predicted - no features of acute severe asthma	
Brittle asthma	- Type 1: wide PEF variability (> 40% diurnal variability for > 50% of time over a period of > 150 days) despite intensive therapy - Type 2: sudden severe attacks on a background of apparently well controlled asthma	

PEF = peak expiratory flow

Table 12.2 Severity of acute asthma exacerbations

(From British Thoracic Society/Scottish Intercollegiate Guidelines Network Guideline on the Management of Asthma - www.brit-thoracic.org.uk)

- Wheezing is a common physical finding, but severity does not correlate with the degree of airway obstruction. Other causes of wheezing include: pulmonary oedema, chronic obstructive pulmonary disease (COPD), pneumonia, anaphylaxis, foreign bodies, pulmonary embolism, bronchiectasis, subglottic mass.

- The patient with acute severe asthma requires aggressive medical management to prevent deterioration. Experienced clinicians should treat these patients in a critical care area.

- Use a concentration of inspired oxygen that will achieve an SpO_2 94 - 98%. High-flow oxygen by mask is sometimes necessary.

- Salbutamol (5 mg nebulised) is the main therapy for acute asthma. Repeated doses every 15 - 20 min, or continuous doses, may be needed. Nebuliser units that can be driven by high-flow oxygen should be used. Remember that nebulised drugs will not be delivered to the lungs effectively if the patient is tired and hypoventilating. If a nebuliser is not immediately available beta-2 agonists can be temporarily administered by repeating activations of a metered dose inhaler via a large volume spacer device.

- Give corticosteroids (prednisolone 30 - 40 mg orally or hydrocortisone 100 mg IV 6 -hourly) early. Oral formulations have a longer half-life but the IV route is easier to give in near fatal asthma.

- Nebulised anticholinergics (ipratropium 0.5 mg 4 - 6 hourly) produce additional bronchodilation in severe asthma and in those who do not respond to beta-agonists.

- Magnesium sulphate (2 g IV slowly = 8 mmol) is a bronchodilator and may be useful in severe or near-fatal asthma. Nebulised magnesium sulphate (250 mmol l^{-1}) in a volume of 2.5 - 5 ml is also safe and can be beneficial.

- Consider intravenous salbutamol (250 mcg IV slowly) in patients unresponsive to nebulised therapy or where nebulised / inhaled therapy is not possible (e.g. a patient receiving bag-mask ventilation). Use an infusion of 3 - 20 mcg min^{-1} if necessary.

- Aminophylline should be considered only in severe or near-fatal asthma. If after obtaining senior advice the decision is taken to administer IV aminophylline a loading dose of 5 mg kg^{-1} is given over 20 - 30 min (unless on maintenance therapy), followed by an infusion of 500 - 700 mcg kg^{-1} h^{-1}. Serum theophylline concentrations should be maintained below 20 mcg ml^{-1} to avoid toxicity.

- These patients are often dehydrated or hypovolaemic and will benefit from fluid replacement. Beta-2 agonists and steroids may induce hypokalaemia, which should be corrected with electrolyte supplements.

- Patients that fail to respond to initial treatment, or develop signs of life-threatening asthma, must be assessed by an intensive care specialist. These patients may benefit from tracheal intubation and ventilatory support.

Cardiac arrest

- Follow standard BLS and ALS protocols. Ventilation will be difficult because of increased airway resistance; try to avoid gastric inflation.

- Intubate the trachea early. There is a significant risk of gastric inflation and hypoventilation of the lungs when attempting to ventilate a severe asthmatic without a tracheal tube.

- The recommended respiratory rate (10 breaths min^{-1}) and tidal volume required for a normal chest rise during CPR should not cause dynamic hyperinflation of the lungs (gas trapping).

- If dynamic hyperinflation of the lungs is suspected during CPR, compression of the chest wall and/or a period of apnoea (disconnection of tracheal tube) may relieve gas-trapping. Although this procedure is supported by limited evidence, it is unlikely to be harmful in an otherwise desperate situation.

- Dynamic hyperinflation increases transthoracic impedance. In VF, consider higher shock energies for defibrillation if initial defibrillation attempts fail.

- Look for reversible causes using the 4 Hs and 4 Ts approach.

- Tension pneumothorax can be difficult to diagnose in cardiac arrest; it may be indicated by unilateral expansion of the chest wall, shifting of the trachea, and subcutaneous emphysema. Pleural ultrasound in skilled hands is faster and more sensitive than chest X-ray for the detection of pneumothorax. Early needle decompression (thoracocentesis) followed by chest drain insertion is needed. Needle decompression may fail due to inadequate needle length. In the ventilated patient, thoracostomy (a surgical hole in the chest wall and pleura) may be quicker to do and more effective for decompressing the chest (see trauma section).

- Always consider bilateral pneumothoraces in asthma-related cardiac arrest.

- Follow standard guidelines for post-resuscitation care.

Anaphylaxis

Definition

Anaphylaxis is a severe, life-threatening, generalised or systemic hypersensitivity reaction.

This is characterised by rapidly developing life-threatening airway and/or breathing and/or circulation problems usually associated with skin and mucosal changes.

This guidance is based on Emergency Treatment of Anaphylactic Reactions, Resuscitation Council UK, 2008 (For more details see www.resus.org.uk).

Aetiology

Anaphylaxis usually involves the release of inflammatory mediators from mast cells and, or basophils triggered by an allergen interacting with cell-bound immunoglobulin E (IgE). Non-IgE-mediated or non-immune release of mediators can also occur. Histamine and other inflammatory mediator release are responsible for the vasodilatation, oedema and increased capillary permeability.

Anaphylaxis is not always recognised, so studies may underestimate the incidence. Anaphylaxis is triggered by a broad range of triggers, with food, drugs and venom being the most common. Food triggers are commonest in children and drugs much more common in older people. Of foods, nuts are the most common cause; muscle relaxants, antibiotics, NSAIDs and aspirin are the most commonly implicated drugs. In many cases, no cause can be identified. A significant number of cases of anaphylaxis are idiopathic (non-IgE mediated).

The risk of death is increased in those with pre-existing asthma, particularly if the asthma is poorly controlled or in those asthmatics who fail to use, or delay treatment with, adrenaline. There are approximately 20 anaphylaxis deaths reported each year in the UK, although this may be a substantial under-estimate.

When anaphylaxis is fatal, death usually occurs very soon after contact with the trigger. Fatal food reactions cause respiratory arrest typically after 30 - 35 min; insect stings cause collapse from shock after 10 - 15 min; and deaths caused by intravenous medication occurred most commonly within 5 min. Death rarely occurs more than six hours after contact with the trigger.

Recognition

- Anaphylaxis is likely if a patient who is exposed to a trigger (allergen) develops a sudden illness (usually within minutes of exposure) with rapidly progressing skin changes and life-threatening airway and/or breathing and/or circulation problems. The reaction is usually unexpected.

- The lack of any consistent clinical manifestation and a range of possible presentations cause diagnostic difficulty. Patients have been given injections of adrenaline inappropriately for allergic reactions just involving the skin, or for vasovagal reactions or panic attacks. Guidelines for the treatment of an anaphylactic reaction must therefore take into account some inevitable diagnostic errors, with an emphasis on the need for safety.

Anaphylaxis is likely when all of the following three criteria are met:

- Sudden onset and rapid progression of symptoms

- Life-threatening Airway and/or Breathing and/or Circulation problems

- Skin and/or mucosal changes (flushing, urticaria, angioedema)

The following supports the diagnosis:

- Exposure to a known allergen for the patient

Remember:

- Skin or mucosal changes alone are not a sign of anaphylaxis

- Skin and mucosal changes can be subtle or absent in up to 20% of reactions (some patients can have only a decrease in blood pressure, i.e. a Circulation problem)

- There can also be gastrointestinal symptoms (e.g. vomiting, abdominal pain, incontinence)

Sudden onset and rapid progression of symptoms:

- The patient will feel and look unwell.

- Most reactions occur over several minutes. Rarely, reactions may be slower in onset.

- An intravenous trigger will cause a more rapid onset of reaction than stings which, in turn, tend to cause a more rapid onset than orally ingested triggers.

- The patient is usually anxious and can experience a "sense of impending doom".

ALS

Life-threatening Airway, Breathing and Circulation problems:

Use the ABCDE approach to recognise these.

Airway problems:

- Airway swelling, e.g. throat and tongue swelling (pharyngeal/laryngeal oedema). The patient has difficulty in breathing and swallowing and feels that the throat is closing up.

- Hoarse voice.

- Stridor - this is a high-pitched inspiratory noise caused by upper airway obstruction.

Breathing problems:

- Shortness of breath - increased respiratory rate.

- Wheeze.

- Patient becoming tired.

- Confusion caused by hypoxia.

- Cyanosis - this is usually a late sign.

- Respiratory arrest.

Circulation problems:

- Signs of shock - pale, clammy.

- Tachycardia.

- Hypotension - feeling faint, collapse.

- Decreased conscious level or loss of consciousness.

- Anaphylaxis can cause myocardial ischaemia and electrocardiograph (ECG) changes even in individuals with normal coronary arteries.

- Cardiac arrest.

Circulation problems (often referred to as anaphylactic shock) can be caused by direct myocardial depression, vasodilation and capillary leak, and loss of fluid from the circulation.

The above Airway, Breathing and Circulation problems can all alter the patient's neurological status (**Disability problems**) because of decreased brain perfusion. There may be confusion, agitation and loss of consciousness.

Skin and, or mucosal changes

These should be assessed as part of the **Exposure** when using the ABCDE approach.

- They are often the first feature and present in over 80% of anaphylactic reactions.

- They can be subtle or dramatic.

- There may be just skin, just mucosal, or both skin and mucosal changes.

- There may be erythema - a patchy, or generalised, red rash.

- There may be urticaria (also called hives, nettle rash, weals or welts), which can appear anywhere on the body. The weals may be pale, pink or red, and may look like nettle stings. They can be different shapes and sizes, and are often surrounded by a red flare. They are usually itchy.

- Angioedema is similar to urticaria but involves swelling of deeper tissues, most commonly in the eyelids and lips, and sometimes in the mouth and throat.

Although skin changes can be worrying or distressing for patients and those treating them, skin changes without life-threatening airway, breathing or circulation problems do not signify anaphylaxis.

Differential diagnosis

Life-threatening conditions:

- Sometimes an anaphylactic reaction can present with symptoms and signs that are very similar to life-threatening asthma.

- A low blood pressure (or normal in children) with a petechial or purpuric rash can be a sign of septic shock. Seek help early if there are any doubts about the diagnosis and treatment.

- Following the ABCDE approach will help with treating the differential diagnoses.

Non life-threatening conditions (these usually respond to simple measures):

- Faint (vasovagal episode).

- Panic attack.

- Breath-holding episode in child.

- Idiopathic (non-allergic) urticaria or angioedema.

There can be confusion between an anaphylactic reaction and a panic attack. Victims of previous anaphylaxis may be particularly prone to panic attacks if they think they have been re-exposed to the allergen that caused a previous problem. The sense of impending doom and breathlessness leading to hyperventilation are symptoms that resemble anaphylaxis in some ways. While there is no hypotension, pallor, wheeze, or urticarial rash or swelling, there may sometimes be flushing or blotchy skin associated with anxiety adding to the diagnostic difficulty. Diagnostic difficulty may also occur with vasovagal attacks after immunisation procedures, but the absence of rash, breathing difficulties, and swelling are useful distinguishing features, as is the slow pulse of a vasovagal attack compared with the rapid pulse of a severe anaphylactic episode. Fainting will usually respond to lying the patient down and raising the legs.

Treatment

As the diagnosis of anaphylaxis is not always obvious, all those who treat anaphylaxis must use the systematic ABCDE approach to the sick patient. Treat life-threatening problems as you find them. The key steps are described in the anaphylaxis algorithm (Figure 12.4).

- All patients should be placed in a comfortable position. Patients with airway and breathing problems may prefer to sit up as this will make breathing easier. Lying flat with or without leg elevation is helpful for patients with a low blood pressure (Circulation problem). If the patient feels faint, do not sit or stand them up - this can cause cardiac arrest. Patients who are breathing and unconscious should be placed on their side (recovery position).

- Removing the trigger for an anaphylactic reaction is not always possible. Stop any drug suspected of causing an anaphylactic reaction (e.g. stop intravenous infusion of a gelatin solution or antibiotic). Do not delay definitive treatment if removing the trigger is not feasible.

- Give the highest concentration of oxygen possible during resuscitation.

- Adrenaline is the most important drug for the treatment of an anaphylactic reaction. As an alpha-receptor agonist, it reverses peripheral vasodilation and reduces oedema. Its beta-receptor activity dilates the bronchial airways, increases the force of myocardial contraction, and suppresses histamine and leukotriene release. Adrenaline works best when given early after the onset of the reaction but it is not without risk, particularly when given intravenously. Adverse effects are extremely rare with correct doses injected intramuscularly (IM). Sometimes there has been uncertainty about whether complications (e.g. myocardial ischaemia) have been caused by the allergen itself or by the adrenaline given to treat it.

- The intramuscular (IM) route is the best for most individuals who have to give adrenaline to treat an anaphylactic reaction. Monitor the patient as soon as possible (pulse, blood pressure, ECG, pulse oximetry). This will help monitor the response to adrenaline.

- For adults give an initial IM adrenaline dose of 0.5 mg (0.5 ml of 1:1000 adrenaline = 0.5 mg = 500 mcg). Further doses can be given at about 5-min intervals according to the patient's response.

- The best site for IM injection is the anterolateral aspect of the middle third of the thigh. The needle used for injection needs to be sufficiently long to ensure that the adrenaline is injected into muscle.

- The use of IV adrenaline applies only to those experienced in the use and titration of vasopressors in their normal clinical practice (e.g. anaesthetists, emergency physicians, intensive care doctors). In patients with a spontaneous circulation, intravenous adrenaline can cause life-threatening hypertension, tachycardia, arrhythmias, and myocardial ischaemia. Patients who are given IV adrenaline must be monitored - continuous ECG and pulse oximetry and frequent non-invasive blood pressure measurements as a minimum.

- Titrate IV adrenaline using 50 mcg boluses according to response. If repeated adrenaline doses are needed, start an IV adrenaline infusion. The pre-filled 10 ml syringe of 1:10,000 adrenaline contains 100 mcg ml^{-1}. A dose of 50 mcg is 0.5 ml, which is the smallest dose that can be given accurately. Do not give the undiluted 1:1000 adrenaline concentration IV.

- Auto-injectors are often given to patients at risk of anaphylaxis for their own use. Healthcare professionals should be familiar with the use of the most commonly available auto-injector devices. If an adrenaline auto-injector is the only available adrenaline preparation when treating anaphylaxis, healthcare providers should use it.

- Give a rapid IV fluid challenge (500 - 1000 ml in an adult) and monitor the response; give further doses as necessary. There is no evidence to support the use of colloids over crystalloids in this setting. Consider colloid infusion as a cause in a patient receiving a colloid at the time of onset of an anaphylactic reaction and stop the infusion. Hartmann's solution or 0.9% saline are suitable fluids for initial resuscitation. A large volume of fluid may be needed.

- Antihistamines are a second line treatment for an anaphylactic reaction. Antihistamines (H1-antihistamine) may help counter histamine-mediated vasodilation and bronchoconstriction. They may not help in reactions depending in part on other mediators but they have the virtue of safety. Used alone, they are unlikely to be life-saving in a true anaphylactic reaction. Give chlorphenamine 10 mg IM or IV slowly.

- Corticosteroids may help prevent or shorten protracted reactions. Inject hydrocortisone 200 mg IM or IV slowly.

ALS

Anaphylaxis algorithm

Anaphylactic reaction?

↓

Airway, Breathing, Circulation, Disability, Exposure

↓

Diagnosis - look for:
- Acute onset of illness
- Life-threatening Airway and/or Breathing and/or Circulation problems [1]
- And usually skin changes

↓

- **Call for help**
- Lie patient flat
- Raise patient's legs

↓

Adrenaline [2]

↓

When skills and equipment available:

- Establish airway
- High flow oxygen
- IV fluid challenge [3]
- Chlorphenamine [4]
- Hydrocortisone [5]

Monitor:
- Pulse oximetry
- ECG
- Blood pressure

---

[1] Life-threatening problems:

Airway:	swelling, hoarseness, stridor
Breathing:	rapid breathing, wheeze, fatigue, cyanosis, $SpO_2 < 92\%$, confusion
Circulation:	pale, clammy, low blood pressure, faintness, drowsy/coma

[2] Adrenaline (give IM unless experienced with IV adrenaline)
IM doses of 1:1000 adrenaline (repeat after 5 min if no better)
- Adult   500 micrograms IM (0.5 mL)
- Child more than 12 years: 500 micrograms IM (0.5 mL)
- Child 6 -12 years: 300 micrograms IM (0.3 mL)
- Child less than 6 years: 150 micrograms IM (0.15 mL)

Adrenaline IV to be given **only by experienced specialists**
Titrate: Adults 50 micrograms; Children 1 microgram/kg

[3] IV fluid challenge:

Adult - 500 – 1000 mL
Child - crystalloid 20 mL/kg

Stop IV colloid
if this might be the cause
of anaphylaxis

	[4] Chlorphenamine (IM or slow IV)	[5] Hydrocortisone (IM or slow IV)
Adult or child more than 12 years	10 mg	200 mg
Child 6 - 12 years	5 mg	100 mg
Child 6 months to 6 years	2.5 mg	50 mg
Child less than 6 months	250 micrograms/kg	25 mg

March 2008

Figure 12.4 Anaphylaxis algorithm

- If the patient has asthma-like features alone, treat as for asthma. As well as the drugs listed above, consider further bronchodilator therapy with salbutamol (inhaled or IV), ipratropium (inhaled), aminophylline (IV) or magnesium (IV). Remember that intravenous magnesium is a vasodilator and can cause hot flushes and make hypotension worse.

- Adrenaline remains the first line vasopressor for the treatment of anaphylactic reactions. Consider other vasopressors and inotropes (noradrenaline, vasopressin, metaraminol and glucagon) when initial resuscitation with adrenaline and fluids has not been successful. Only use these drugs in specialist settings (e.g. intensive care units) where there is experience in their use. Glucagon can be useful to treat an anaphylactic reaction in a patient taking a beta-blocker.

- If cardiorespiratory arrest occurs, as well as standard ALS, consider the use of steroids, antihistamines (if not given already) and large volumes of intravenous fluids. Prolonged resuscitation may be necessary.

- Airway obstruction may occur rapidly in severe anaphylaxis, particularly in patients with angioedema. Warning signs are swelling of the tongue and lips, hoarseness and oropharyngeal swelling.

- Consider early tracheal intubation; delay may make intubation extremely difficult. As airway obstruction progresses, supraglottic airway devices (e.g. LMA) are likely to be difficult to insert. Attempts at tracheal intubation may exacerbate laryngeal oedema. Early involvement of a senior anaesthetist is mandatory when managing these patients. A surgical airway may be required if tracheal intubation is not possible.

Investigations

The specific test to help confirm a diagnosis of an anaphylactic reaction is measurement of mast cell tryptase. In anaphylaxis, mast cell degranulation leads to markedly increased blood tryptase concentrations.

Mast cell tryptase sample timing

The time of onset of the anaphylactic reaction is the time when symptoms were first noticed.

a) Minimum: one sample at 1 - 2 h after the start of symptoms.

b) Ideally: Three **timed** samples:

  1) Initial sample as soon as feasible after resuscitation has started - do not delay resuscitation to take sample.

  2) Second sample at 1 - 2 h after the start of symptoms

  3) Third sample either at 24 h or in convalescence. This provides baseline tryptase levels - some individuals have an elevated baseline level.

c) Use a serum or clotted blood ('liver function test' bottle) sample.

d) *Record the timing of each sample accurately* on the sample bottle and request form.

e) Consult your local laboratory if you have any queries.

Discharge and follow-up

Patients who have had a suspected anaphylactic reaction should be treated and then observed for at least 6 h in a clinical area with facilities for treating life-threatening ABC problems. Patients with a good response to initial treatment should be warned of the possibility of an early recurrence of symptoms and in some circumstances should be kept under observation for up to 24 h. This caution is particularly applicable to:

- Severe reactions with slow onset caused by idiopathic anaphylaxis.

- Reactions in individuals with severe asthma or with a severe asthmatic component.

- Reactions with the possibility of continuing absorption of allergen.

- Patients with a previous history of biphasic reactions.

- Patients presenting in the evening or at night, or those who may not be able to respond to any deterioration.

- Patients in areas where access to emergency care is difficult.

The exact incidence of biphasic reactions is unknown. There is no reliable way of predicting who will have a biphasic reaction. It is therefore important that decisions about discharge are made for each patient by an experienced clinician.

Before discharge from hospital all patients must be:

- Given clear instructions to return to hospital if symptoms return.

- Considered for anti-histamines and oral steroid therapy for up to 3 days. This is helpful for treatment of urticaria and may decrease the chance of further reaction.

- Have a plan for follow-up, including contact with the patient's general practitioner.

- *All patients* presenting with anaphylaxis should be referred to an allergy clinic to identify the cause, and thereby reduce the risk of future reactions and prepare the patient to manage future episodes themselves.

Cardiac arrest following cardiac surgery

After major cardiac surgery, cardiac arrest is relatively common in the immediate post-operative phase, with a reported incidence of 0.7% - 2.9%. Cardiac arrest is usually preceded by physiological deterioration, although it may occur suddenly in stable patients. Continuous monitoring on the intensive care unit (ICU) enables immediate intervention at the time of arrest. Survival to hospital discharge of patients having a cardiac arrest during the first 24 h after cardiac surgery is reported as 54 - 79% in adults and 41% in children.

Aetiology

There are usually specific causes of cardiac arrest that are all potentially reversible. The main causes of cardiac arrest in the initial post-operative period include:

- cardiac tamponade;

- myocardial ischaemia;

- haemorrhage causing hypovolaemic shock;

- disconnection of the pacing system in a pacing-dependent patient;

- tension pneumothorax;

- electrolyte disturbances (particularly hypo/hyperkalaemia).

Diagnosis

An immediate decision on the likely cause of cardiac arrest must be made to enable rapid intervention and successful resuscitation. Patients in the ICU are highly monitored and an arrest is most likely to be signalled by monitoring alarms where absence of pulsation or perfusing pressure on the arterial line, loss of pulse oximeter trace, pulmonary artery (PA) trace, or end-tidal CO_2 trace and rapid assessment of the patient can be sufficient to indicate cardiac arrest without the need to palpate a central pulse. Call for senior help early including a cardiothoracic surgeon and cardiac anaesthetist.

Treatment

- Start external chest compressions immediately in all patients who collapse without an output. Consider reversible causes using the 4 Hs and 4 Ts approach: hypoxia - check tube position, ventilate with 100% oxygen; tension pneumothorax - clinical examination, thoracic ultrasound; hypovolaemia, pacing failure.

- In asystole, secondary to a loss of cardiac pacing, chest compression can be delayed momentarily as long as the surgically inserted temporary pacing wires can be connected rapidly and pacing re-established (DDD [Dual chamber pacing, Dual chamber sensing and Dual chamber response] at 100 min^{-1} at maximum amplitude).

- The effectiveness of compressions may be verified by looking at the arterial trace. Inability to attain a perfusing blood pressure during compressions (e.g. systolic pressure of 80 mmHg) may indicate tamponade, tension pneumothorax, or severe haemorrhage and should precipitate emergency resternotomy.

- Intra-aortic balloon pumps should be changed to pressure triggering during CPR.

- In PEA, switch off the pacemaker as it may potentially hide underlying VF.

- External chest compressions can cause sternal disruption or cardiac damage. In the post cardiac surgery ICU, a witnessed and monitored VF/VT cardiac arrest should be treated immediately with up to three quick successive (stacked) defibrillation attempts.

- Three failed shocks in the post cardiac surgery setting should trigger the need for emergency resternotomy. Further defibrillation is attempted as indicated in the ALS algorithm and should be performed with internal paddles at 20 J if resternotomy has been performed.

- Use adrenaline very cautiously and titrate to effect (intravenous doses of 100 mcg or less in adults).

- Emergency resternotomy is an integral part of resuscitation after cardiac surgery, once all other reversible causes have been excluded. Once an adequate airway and ventilation has been established, and if three attempts at defibrillation have failed in VF/VT, undertake resternotomy without delay. Emergency resternotomy is also indicated in asystole or PEA, when other treatments have failed. Resuscitation teams should be well rehearsed in this technique so that it can be performed safely within 5 min of the onset of cardiac arrest. Resternotomy equipment should be prepared as soon as an arrest is identified.

- Consider re-instituting cardiopulmonary bypass if necessary.

Traumatic cardiorespiratory arrest

Cardiac arrest secondary to traumatic injury has a very high mortality, with an overall survival of 5.6% (range 0 - 17%). In survivors, neurological disability is common.

Cardiac arrest from a primary medical problem (e.g. cardiac arrhythmia, hypoglycaemia, seizure) can cause a secondary traumatic event (e.g. fall, road traffic accident). Despite the initial reported mechanism, traumatic injuries may not be the primary cause of a cardiorespiratory arrest and standard advanced life support, including chest compressions, are appropriate. Survival usually depends on early resuscitation by experienced rescuers.

Causes of cardiac arrest in trauma patients include: severe traumatic brain injury, hypovolaemia from massive blood loss, hypoxia from respiratory arrest, direct injury to vital organs and major vessels, tension pneumothorax, and cardiac tamponade.

Commotio cordis is actual or near cardiac arrest caused by a blunt impact to the chest wall over the heart. A blow to the chest can cause VF. Commotio cordis occurs mostly during sports (most commonly baseball) and recreational activities and victims are usually teenage males. Follow standard CPR guidelines. Early defibrillation is important for survival.

Treatment

- Survival from traumatic cardiac arrests is correlated with duration of CPR and pre-hospital time. Prolonged CPR is associated with a poor outcome. Treatment on scene should focus on high-quality CPR, advanced life support and exclusion of reversible causes using the 4 Hs and 4 Ts.

- Undertake only essential life-saving interventions on scene and, if the patient has signs of life, transfer rapidly to the nearest appropriate hospital. Do not delay for spinal immobilisation.

- Effective airway management is essential to maintain oxygenation of the severely compromised trauma patient. Early tracheal intubation by experienced rescuers can be beneficial. Use basic airway management manoeuvres and alternative airways to maintain oxygenation if tracheal intubation cannot be accomplished immediately. If these measures fail, a surgical airway is indicated.

- In low cardiac output conditions, positive pressure ventilation causes further circulatory depression, or even cardiac arrest, by impeding venous return to the heart. Monitor ventilation with continuous waveform capnography and adjust to achieve normocapnia. This may enable slow respiratory rates and low tidal volumes and the corresponding decrease in transpulmonary pressure may increase venous return and cardiac output.

- Treatment of reversible causes:

  - Hypoxaemia - (oxygenation, ventilation).

  - Hypovolaemia - compressible haemorrhage (pressure, pressure dressings, tourniquets, novel haemostatic agents) or non-compressible haemorrhage (splints, intravenous fluid).

  - Tension pneumothorax - decompress quickly by lateral or anterior thoracostomy (incision in chest wall through to the pleural cavity). This is likely to be more effective than needle thoracostomy and quicker than inserting a chest tube.

  - Cardiac tamponade - immediate thoracotomy.

- Chest compressions may not be effective in hypovolaemic cardiac arrest but most survivors of traumatic cardiac arrest do not have hypovolaemia and standard advanced life support may be lifesaving.

- If available, ultrasound will help diagnose rapidly haemoperitoneum, haemopneumothorax, tension pneumothorax and cardiac tamponade. This requires a trained operator and should not delay treatment.

- Give intravenous fluids conservatively until bleeding is controlled. In the presence of uncontrolled bleeding, excessive fluid will increase the bleeding. The choice of fluid and blood products will depend on local practice. In the UK, the National Institute for Health and Clinical Excellence (NICE) has published guidelines on pre-hospital fluid replacement in trauma. The recommendations include giving 250 ml boluses of crystalloid solution until a radial pulse is achieved and not delaying rapid transport of trauma victims for fluid infusion in the field.

Emergency thoracotomy

- Consider on-scene resuscitative thoracotomy in cardiac arrest caused by penetrating chest trauma if it can be accomplished within 10 min after the loss of the pulse. This requires a trained rescuer.

- Consider emergency department thoracotomy (EDT) in the following circumstances:

  - After blunt trauma EDT should be limited to those with vital signs on arrival and a witnessed cardiac arrest (estimated survival rate 1.6%).

  - Penetrating cardiac injuries who arrive at hospital after a short on scene and transport time with witnessed signs of life or ECG activity are candidates for EDT (estimated survival rate 31%).

  - Penetrating non-cardiac thoracic injuries even though survival rates are low.

○ EDT should be undertaken in patients with exsanguinating abdominal vascular injury even though survival rates are low. This procedure should be used as an adjunct to definitive repair of abdominal vascular injury.

Pregnancy

Mortality related to pregnancy in developed countries is rare, occurring in an estimated 1:30,000 deliveries. The mother and fetus must be considered in emergencies during pregnancy. Effective resuscitation of the mother is often the best way to optimise fetal outcome. Significant physiological changes occur during pregnancy; for example, cardiac output, circulatory volume, minute ventilation, and oxygen consumption all increase. The gravid uterus can cause compression of iliac and abdominal vessels when the mother is in the supine position, resulting in reduced cardiac output and hypotension. Resuscitation guidelines for pregnancy are based largely on case series, extrapolation from non-pregnant arrests, manikin studies and expert opinion based on the physiology of pregnancy and changes that occur in normal labour.

Causes of cardiac arrest in pregnancy

Cardiac arrest in pregnancy is most commonly caused by:

- Cardiac disease
- Pulmonary embolism
- Psychiatric disorders
- Hypertensive disorders of pregnancy
- Sepsis
- Haemorrhage
- Amniotic fluid embolism
- Ectopic pregnancy.

Pregnant women can also have the same causes of cardiac arrest as females of the same age group (e.g. anaphylaxis, drug overdose, trauma).

Treatment

Key interventions to prevent cardiac arrest

In an emergency, use the ABCDE approach. Many cardiovascular problems associated with pregnancy are caused by compression of the inferior vena cava. Treat a distressed or compromised pregnant patient as follows.

- Place the patient in the left lateral position or manually and gently displace the uterus to the left.

- Give high-flow oxygen guided by pulse oximetry.

- Give a fluid bolus if there is hypotension or evidence of hypovolaemia.

- Immediately re-evaluate the need for any drugs being given.

- Seek expert help early. Obstetric and neonatal specialists should be involved early in the resuscitation.

- Identify and treat the underlying cause.

Modifications for cardiac arrest

- In cardiac arrest, all the principles of basic and advanced life support apply.

- Summon help immediately. For effective resuscitation of mother and fetus, expert help must be obtained; this should include an obstetrician and neonatologist.

- Start CPR according to standard guidelines. Ensure good quality chest compressions with minimal interruptions.

- After 20 weeks gestation the pregnant woman's uterus can press down against the inferior vena cava and the aorta, impeding venous return, cardiac output and uterine perfusion. Caval compression limits the effectiveness of chest compressions.

- The potential for caval compression suggests that intravenous access should ideally be established above the diaphragm.

- Manually displace the uterus to the left to remove caval compression. Add left lateral tilt only if this is feasible i.e. tilting table - the optimal angle of tilt is unknown. Aim for between 15 and 30 degrees. Even a small amount of tilt may be better than no tilt. The angle of tilt used needs to allow high quality chest compressions and if needed permit Caesarean delivery of the fetus (see below). If tilting on a firm surface is not possible then maintain left uterine displacement and continue effective chest compressions with patient supine.

- The method used for tilting will depend on where the patient is and what is available. The patient's body will need to be supported on a firm surface to allow effective chest compressions. Methods for tilting include:

  ○ if the patient is already on a spinal board, the board can be tilted to provide a left lateral tilt

  ○ operating table which can be manually or electronically tilted.

- Start preparing for emergency Caesarean section (see below) - the fetus will need to be delivered if initial resuscitation efforts fail.

- There is an increased risk of pulmonary aspiration of gastric contents in pregnancy. Early tracheal intubation decreases this risk. Tracheal intubation can be more difficult in the pregnant patient. Expert help, a failed intubation drill, and the use of alternative airway devices may be needed.

- Attempt defibrillation using standard energy doses. Left lateral tilt and large breasts can make it difficult to place an apical defibrillator pad.

Reversible causes

Look for reversible causes using the 4 Hs and 4 Ts approach. Abdominal ultrasound by a skilled operator to detect possible causes during cardiac arrest can be useful. It can also permit an evaluation of fetal viability, multiple pregnancy and placental localisation. It should not however delay treatments. Specific reversible causes of cardiac arrest in pregnancy are:

- **Haemorrhage:** This can occur both antenatally and postnatally. Causes include ectopic pregnancy, placental abruption, placenta praevia and uterine rupture. Maternity units should have a massive haemorrhage protocol. Treatment is based on the ABCDE approach. The key step is to stop the bleeding. Consider the following: fluid resuscitation including use of a rapid transfusion system and cell salvage, correction of coagulopathy, oxytocin, ergometrine and prostaglandins to correct uterine atony, uterine compression sutures, intrauterine balloon devices, radiological embolisation of a bleeding vessel, and surgical control including aortic cross clamping/compression and hysterectomy. Placenta percreta may require extensive intra-pelvic surgery.

- **Drugs:** Overdose can occur in women with eclampsia receiving magnesium sulphate, particularly if the patient becomes oliguric. Give calcium to treat magnesium toxicity (see life-threatening electrolyte abnormalities). Central neural blockade for analgesia or anaesthesia can cause problems due to sympathetic blockade (hypotension, bradycardia) or local anaesthetic toxicity (see poisoning section).

- **Cardiovascular disease:** Myocardial infarction and aneurysm or dissection of the aorta or its branches, and peripartum cardiomyopathy cause most deaths from acquired cardiac disease. Patients with known cardiac disease need to be managed in a specialist unit. Pregnant women may develop an acute coronary syndrome, typically in association with risk factors such as obesity, older age, higher parity, smoking, diabetes, pre-existing hypertension and a family history of ischaemic heart disease. Pregnant patients can have atypical features such as epigastric pain and vomiting. Percutaneous coronary intervention (PCI) is the reperfusion strategy of choice for ST-elevation myocardial infarction in pregnancy. Thrombolysis should be considered if urgent PCI is unavailable. Increasing numbers of women with congenital heart disease are becoming pregnant. Pregnant women with known congenital heart disease should be managed in specialist centres.

- **Pre-eclampsia and eclampsia:** Eclampsia is defined as the development of convulsions and/or

unexplained coma during pregnancy or postpartum in patients with signs and symptoms of pre-eclampsia. Magnesium sulphate treatment may prevent eclampsia developing in labour or immediately postpartum in women with pre-eclampsia.

- **Amniotic fluid embolism** usually presents around the time of delivery often in the labouring mother with sudden cardiovascular collapse, breathlessness, cyanosis, arrhythmias, hypotension and haemorrhage associated with disseminated intravascular coagulopathy. Treatment is supportive based on the ABCDE approach and correction of coagulopathy. There is no specific therapy.

- **Pulmonary embolus** causing cardiopulmonary collapse can present throughout pregnancy. CPR should be started with modifications as necessary. The use of fibrinolysis (thrombolysis) needs considerable thought, particularly if a peri-mortem Caesarean section is being considered. If the diagnosis is suspected and maternal cardiac output has not returned it should be given.

Peri-mortem Caesarean section

When initial resuscitation attempts fail, delivery of the fetus may improve the chances of successful resuscitation of both the mother and fetus. The best survival rate for infants over 24 - 25 weeks gestation occurs when delivery of the infant is achieved within 5 min after the mother's cardiac arrest. This requires that Caesarean section starts at about 4 min after cardiac arrest. Delivery relieves caval compression and may improve the likelihood of resuscitating the mother by permitting an increase in venous return during the CPR attempt. Delivery also enables access to the abdominal cavity so that aortic clamping or compression is possible. Internal cardiac massage is also possible. Once the fetus has been delivered resuscitation of the newborn child can also begin.

In the supine position, the gravid uterus begins to compromise blood flow in the inferior vena cava and abdominal aorta at approximately 20 weeks' gestation; however, fetal viability currently begins at approximately 24 weeks.

- **Gestational age < 20 weeks.** Urgent Caesarean delivery need not be considered, because a gravid uterus of this size is unlikely to compromise maternal cardiac output and fetal viability is not an issue.

- **Gestational age approximately 20 - 23 weeks.** Initiate emergency delivery of the fetus to permit successful resuscitation of the mother, not survival of the delivered infant, which is unlikely at this gestational age.

- **Gestational age approximately > 24 weeks.** Initiate emergency delivery to help save the life of both the mother and the infant.

Planning for resuscitation in pregnancy

Advanced life support in pregnancy requires co-ordination of maternal resuscitation, Caesarean delivery of the fetus, and newborn resuscitation within 5 min. To achieve this, units likely to deal with cardiac arrest in pregnancy should:

- have in place plans and equipment for resuscitation of both the pregnant patient and the newborn child;

- ensure early involvement of obstetric and neonatal teams;

- ensure regular training of staff in obstetric emergencies.

Electrocution

Electrical injury is a relatively infrequent but potentially devastating multi-system injury with high morbidity and mortality. Most electrical injuries in adults occur in the workplace and are associated generally with high voltage, whereas children are at risk primarily at home, where the voltage is lower (220 V in Europe, Australia, Asia; 110 V in the USA and Canada). Electrocution from lightning strikes is rare, but causes about 1000 deaths worldwide each year.

Factors influencing the severity of electrical injury include whether the current is alternating (AC) or direct (DC), voltage, magnitude of energy delivered, resistance to current flow, pathway of current through the patient, and the area and duration of contact. Skin resistance is decreased by moisture, which increases the likelihood of injury. Electric current follows the path of least resistance; conductive neurovascular bundles within limbs are particularly prone to damage.

Contact with AC may cause tetanic contraction of skeletal muscle, which may prevent release from the source of electricity. Myocardial or respiratory failure may cause immediate death:

- **Respiratory arrest** may be caused by central respiratory depression or paralysis of the respiratory muscles.

- Current may precipitate **VF** if it traverses the myocardium during the vulnerable period (analogous to an R-on-T phenomenon). Electrical current may also cause myocardial ischaemia because of coronary artery spasm.

- **Asystole** may be primary, or secondary to asphyxia following respiratory arrest.

Current that traverses the myocardium is more likely to be fatal. A transthoracic (hand to hand) pathway is more likely to be fatal than a vertical (hand to foot) or straddle (foot to foot) pathway. There may be extensive tissue destruction along the current pathway.

Lightning strikes deliver as much as 300 kV over a few milliseconds. Most of the current from a lightning strike passes over the surface of the body in a process called external flashover. Both industrial shocks and lightning strikes cause deep burns at the point of contact - in industry the points of contact are usually on the upper limbs, hands and wrists, whilst with lightning they are mostly on the head, neck and shoulders. Injury may also occur indirectly through ground current or current 'splashing' from a tree or other object that is hit by lightning. Explosive force generated by a lightning strike may cause blunt trauma.

The pattern and severity of injury from a lightning strike varies considerably. As with industrial and domestic electric shock, death is caused by cardiac or respiratory arrest. In those who survive the initial shock, extensive catecholamine release or autonomic stimulation may occur, causing hypertension, tachycardia, nonspecific ECG changes (including prolongation of the QT interval and transient T wave inversion), and myocardial necrosis. Creatine kinase may be released from myocardial and skeletal muscle. Lightning also causes various central and peripheral neurological problems.

Treatment

Ensure that any power source is switched off and do not approach the victim until it is safe. High voltage (above domestic mains) electricity can arc and conduct through the ground for up to a few metres around the victim. It is safe to approach and handle casualties after lightning strike, although it would be wise to move to a safer environment. Follow standard resuscitation guidelines.

- Airway management can be difficult if there are electrical burns around the face and neck. Intubate the trachea early in these cases as soft tissue oedema can cause subsequent airway obstruction. Consider cervical spine immobilisation. This should not delay airway management.

- Muscular paralysis, especially after high voltage, may persist for several hours; ventilatory support is required during this period.

- Ventricular fibrillation is the commonest initial arrhythmia after high voltage AC shock; treat with prompt attempted defibrillation. Asystole is more common after DC shock; use standard guidelines for treatment of this and of other arrhythmias.

- Remove smouldering clothing and shoes to prevent further thermal injury.

- Give fluids if there is significant tissue destruction. Maintain a good urine output to increase excretion of myoglobin, potassium and other products of tissue damage.

- Consider early surgical intervention in patients with severe thermal injuries.

- Conduct a thorough secondary survey to exclude injuries caused by tetanic muscular contraction or from the person being thrown by the force of the shock.

- Electrocution can cause severe, deep soft tissue injury with relatively minor skin wounds because current tends to follow neurovascular bundles; look carefully for features of compartment syndrome, which will necessitate fasciotomy.

Further treatment and prognosis

Immediate resuscitation in young victims of cardiac arrest due to electrocution can result in survival. Successful resuscitation has been reported after prolonged life support. All those who survive electrical injury should be monitored in hospital if they have a history of cardiorespiratory problems or have suffered:

- loss of consciousness;

- cardiac arrest;

- electrocardiographic abnormalities;

- soft tissue damage and burns.

Severe burns (thermal or electrical), myocardial necrosis, the extent of central nervous system injury, and secondary multiple system organ failure, determine the morbidity and long-term prognosis. There is no specific therapy for electrical injury, and the management is symptomatic. Prevention remains the best way to minimise the prevalence and severity of electrical injury.

Key learning points

- The conditions described in this chapter account for a large proportion of cardiac arrests in younger patients.

- Use the ABCDE approach for early recognition and treatment to prevent cardiac arrest

- High quality CPR and treatment of reversible causes is the mainstay of treatment of cardiac arrest from any cause.

- Call for expert help early when specialist procedures are needed - e.g. delivery of fetus for cardiac arrest in pregnancy.

Further reading

Alfonzo AV, Isles C, Geddes C, Deighan C. Potassium disorders—clinical spectrum and emergency management. Resuscitation 2006;70:10-25.

Alfonzo AV, Simpson K, Deighan C, Campbell S, Fox J. Modifications to advanced life support in renal failure. Resuscitation 2007;73:12-28.

Bouchama A, Knochel JP. Heat stroke. N Engl J Med 2002;346:1978-88.

Deakin CD, Morrison LJ, Morley PT, et al. 2010 International Consensus on Cardiopulmonary Resuscitation and Emergency Cardiovascular Care Science with Treatment Recommendations. Part 8: Advanced Life Support. Resuscitation 2010;81:e93-e169.

Deakin CD, Nolan JP, Soar J, et al. European Resuscitation Council Guidelines for Resuscitation 2010. Section 4. Adult Advanced Life Support. Resuscitation 2010;81:1305-52.

Dijkman A, Huisman CM, Smit M, et al. Cardiac arrest in pregnancy: increasing use of perimortem caesarean section due to emergency skills training? BJOG 2010;117:282-7.

Dunning J, Fabbri A, Kolh PH, et al. Guideline for resuscitation in cardiac arrest after cardiac surgery. Eur J Cardiothorac Surg 2009;36:3-28.

Idris AH, Berg RA, Bierens J, et al. Recommended guidelines for uniform reporting of data from drowning: The "Utstein style". Resuscitation 2003;59:45-57.

Katz V, Balderston K, DeFreest M. Perimortem cesarean delivery: were our assumptions correct? Am J Obstet Gynecol 2005;192:1916-20; discussion 20-1.

Levy ML, Thomas M, Small I, Pearce L, Pinnock H, Stephenson P. Summary of the 2008 BTS/SIGN British Guideline on the management of asthma. Prim Care Respir J 2009;18 Suppl 1:S1-16.

Lewis G. The Confidential Enquiry into Maternal and Child Health (CEMACH). Saving Mothers' Lives: Reviewing maternal deaths to make motherhood safer – 2003-2005. The Seventh Report of the Confidential Enquiries into Maternal Deaths in the United Kingdom. London: CEMACH; 2007.

Management of Severe Local Anaesthetic Toxicity. Association of Anaesthetists of Great Britain and Ireland, 2010. (Accessed 28 June 2010, www.aagbi.org)

National Institute for Clinical Excellence. Pre-hospital initiation of fluid replacement therapy for trauma. London: National Institute for Clinical Excellence; 2004.

Soar J, Perkins GD, Abbas G, et al. European Resuscitation Council Guidelines for Resuscitation 2010. Section 8. Cardiac arrest in special circumstances: electrolyte abnormalities, poisoning, drowning, accidental hypothermia, hyperthermia, asthma, anaphylaxis, cardiac surgery, trauma, pregnancy, electrocution. Resuscitation 2010;81:1400-33.

Soar J, Pumphrey R, Cant A, et al. Emergency treatment of anaphylactic reactions—guidelines for healthcare providers. Resuscitation 2008;77:157-69.

Zafren K, Durrer B, Herry JP, Brugger H. Lightning injuries: prevention and on-site treatment in mountains and remote areas. Official guidelines of the International Commission for Mountain Emergency Medicine and the Medical Commission of the International Mountaineering and Climbing Federation (ICAR and UIAA MEDCOM). Resuscitation 2005;65:369-72.

Zimmerman JL. Poisonings and overdoses in the intensive care unit: General and specific management issues. Crit Care Med 2003;31:2794-801.

Post-resuscitation Care

Introduction

Return of a spontaneous circulation (ROSC) is an important step in the continuum of resuscitation. However, the next goal is to return the patient to a state of normal cerebral function, and to establish and maintain a stable cardiac rhythm and normal haemodynamic function. This requires further treatment, tailored to each patient's individual needs. The quality of treatment provided in this post-resuscitation phase - the final ring in the Chain of Survival - significantly influences the patient's ultimate outcome. The post-resuscitation phase starts at the location where ROSC is achieved but, once stabilised, the patient needs transfer to the most appropriate high-care area (e.g. intensive care unit (ICU), coronary care unit (CCU)) for continued monitoring and treatment.

The post-cardiac arrest syndrome

The post-cardiac arrest syndrome, which comprises post-cardiac arrest brain injury, post-cardiac arrest myocardial dysfunction, the systemic ischaemia/reperfusion response, and persistence of the precipitating pathology, often complicates the post-resuscitation phase. The severity of this syndrome will vary with the duration and cause of cardiac arrest. It may not occur at all if the cardiac arrest is brief. Post-cardiac arrest brain injury manifests as coma, seizures, myoclonus, varying degrees of neurological dysfunction and brain death. Post-cardiac arrest brain injury may be exacerbated by microcirculatory failure, impaired autoregulation, hypercarbia, hypoxaemia and hyperoxaemia, pyrexia, hyperglycaemia and seizures. Significant myocardial dysfunction is common after cardiac arrest but typically recovers by 2 - 3 days. The whole body ischaemia/reperfusion that occurs with resuscitation from cardiac arrest activates immunological and coagulation pathways contributing to multiple organ failure and increasing the risk of infection. Thus, the post-cardiac arrest syndrome has many features in common with sepsis, including intravascular volume depletion and vasodilation.

Continued resuscitation

In the immediate post-resuscitation phase, pending transfer to an appropriate high-care area, treat the patient by following the ABCDE approach (Figure 13.1).

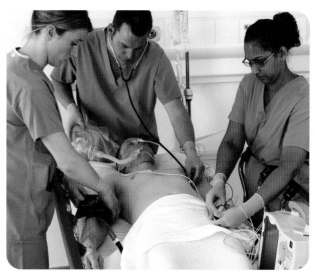

Figure 13.1 Immediate post-resuscitation care using the ABCDE approach

Airway and breathing

Patients who have had a brief period of cardiac arrest and have responded immediately to appropriate treatment (e.g. witnessed ventricular fibrillation (VF) reverting to sinus rhythm after early defibrillation) may achieve a rapid return of normal cerebral function. These patients do not require tracheal intubation and ventilation, but should be given oxygen by face mask to maintain a normal arterial oxygen saturation.

Hypoxaemia and hypercarbia both increase the likelihood of a further cardiac arrest and may contribute to secondary brain injury. Several animal studies indicate that hyperoxaemia causes oxidative stress and harms post-ischaemic neurones. One clinical study has shown that post-resuscitation hyperoxaemia is associated with worse outcome, compared with both normoxaemia and hypoxaemia. As soon as arterial blood oxygen saturation can be monitored reliably (by blood gas analysis and/or pulse oximetry [SpO_2]), titrate the inspired oxygen concentration to maintain the arterial blood oxygen saturation in the range of 94 - 98%. Consider tracheal intubation, sedation and controlled ventilation in any patient with obtunded cerebral function. Adjust ventilation to achieve normocarbia and monitor this using the end-tidal carbon dioxide ($ETCO_2$) with waveform capnography and arterial blood gas values.

Examine the patient's chest and look for symmetrical chest movement. Listen to ensure that the breath sounds are equal on both sides. A tracheal tube that has been inserted too far will tend to go down the right main bronchus and fail to ventilate the left lung. If ribs have been fractured during chest compression there may be a pneumothorax (reduced or absent breath sounds) or a flail segment. Listen for evidence of pulmonary oedema or pulmonary aspiration of gastric contents. Insert a gastric tube - this will decompress the stomach following mouth-to-mouth or bag-mask ventilation, prevent splinting of the diaphragm, and enable drainage of gastric contents.

If the intubated patient regains consciousness soon after ROSC, and is cooperative and breathing normally, consider immediate extubation: coughing on the tracheal tube will increase the patient's plasma catecholamine concentrations significantly, which may provoke arrhythmias and/or hypertension. Ensure that rigid suction is available. If immediate or early extubation is not possible sedate the patient to ensure the tracheal tube is tolerated, and provide ventilatory support.

Circulation

Cardiac rhythm and haemodynamic function are likely to be unstable following a cardiac arrest. Continuous monitoring of the ECG is essential. Seek evidence of poor cardiac function. Record the pulse and blood pressure and assess peripheral perfusion: warm, pink digits with a rapid capillary refill usually imply adequate perfusion. Grossly distended neck veins when the patient is semi-upright may indicate right ventricular failure, but in rare cases could indicate pericardial tamponade. Left ventricular failure may be indicated by fine inspiratory crackles heard on auscultation of the lung fields, and the production of pink frothy sputum. Try to optimise right and left heart filling pressures: measurement of central venous pressure will guide this. If the facility for direct continuous arterial blood pressure monitoring is available (e.g. in the emergency department) insert an arterial cannula to enable reliable monitoring during transfer. Once in a high-care area, the use of non-invasive cardiac output monitoring devices may be valuable. Infusion of fluids may be required to increase right heart filling pressures or conversely, diuretics and vasodilators may be needed to treat left ventricular failure.

Record a 12-lead ECG as soon as possible. Acute ST-segment elevation or new left bundle branch block in a patient with a typical history of acute myocardial infarction (AMI) is an indication for treatment to try to re-open an occluded coronary artery (reperfusion therapy), either with fibrinolytic therapy or by emergency percutaneous coronary intervention (PCI) (Chapter 4). Primary PCI is the preferred treatment for STEMI if it can be performed by an experienced team in a timely manner. If primary PCI is not feasible in an appropriate time frame (within 90 min of first medical contact), give fibrinolytic therapy (Chapter 4). Cardiopulmonary resuscitation, even if prolonged, is not a contraindication to fibrinolytic therapy.

In post-cardiac arrest patients, chest pain and/or ST elevation are relatively poor predictors of acute coronary occlusion; for this reason primary PCI should be considered in all post-cardiac arrest patients who are suspected of having coronary artery disease as the cause of their arrest, even if they are sedated and mechanically ventilated. Several studies indicate that the combination of therapeutic hypothermia (see below) and PCI is feasible and safe after cardiac arrest caused by AMI.

Disability and exposure

Although cardiac arrest is frequently caused by primary cardiac disease, other precipitating conditions must be excluded, particularly in hospital patients (e.g. massive blood loss, respiratory failure, pulmonary embolism). Assess the other body systems rapidly so that further resuscitation can be targeted at the patient's needs. To examine the patient properly full exposure of the body may be necessary.

Although it may not be of immediate significance to the patient's management, assess neurological function rapidly and record the Glasgow Coma Scale score (Table 13.1). The maximum score possible is 15; the minimum score possible is 3.

Glasgow Coma Scale score		
Eye Opening	Spontaneously	4
	To speech	3
	To pain	2
	Nil	1
Verbal	Orientated	5
	Confused	4
	Inappropriate words	3
	Incomprehensible sounds	2
	Nil	1
Best Motor Response	Obeys commands	6
	Localises	5
	Normal flexion	4
	Abnormal flexion	3
	Extension	2
	Nil	1

Table 13.1 The Glasgow Coma Scale score

Consider the need for inducing mild hypothermia in any patient that remains comatose after initial resuscitation from cardiac arrest (see below). When therapeutic hypothermia is considered an appropriate treatment, it should be started as soon as possible - do not wait until the patient is in the ICU before starting to cool.

Further Assessment

History

Obtain a comprehensive history as quickly as possible. Those involved in caring for the patient immediately before the cardiac arrest may be able to help (e.g. emergency medical personnel, general practitioner, and relatives). Specifically, symptoms of cardiac disease should be sought. Consider other causes of cardiac arrest if there is little to suggest primary cardiac disease (e.g. drug overdose, subarachnoid haemorrhage). Make a note of any delay before the start of resuscitation, and the duration of the resuscitation; this may have prognostic significance, although is generally unreliable and certainly should not be used alone to predict outcome. The patient's baseline physiological reserve (before the cardiac arrest) is one of the most important factors taken into consideration by the ICU team when determining whether prolonged multiple organ support is appropriate.

Monitoring

Continuous monitoring of ECG, arterial and possibly central venous blood pressures, respiratory rate, pulse oximetry, capnography, core temperature and urinary output is essential to detect changes during the period of instability that follows resuscitation from cardiac arrest. Monitor continuously the effects of medical interventions (e.g. assisted ventilation, diuretic therapy).

Investigations

Several physiological variables may be abnormal immediately after a cardiac arrest and urgent biochemical and cardiological investigations should be undertaken (Table 13.2).

Arterial blood gases

Guidance on the interpretation of arterial blood gas values is given in Chapter 15.

Hypoperfusion during the period of cardiac arrest will usually cause a metabolic acidosis. This will cause a low pH (acidaemia), low standard bicarbonate and a base deficit. The rate at which the acidaemia resolves in the post-resuscitation period is an important guide to the adequacy of tissue perfusion. The most effective way of correcting any acidaemia is by addressing the underlying cause. For example, poor peripheral perfusion is treated best by giving fluid and inotropic drugs and not by giving sodium bicarbonate.

The normal physiological response to a metabolic acidosis is to reduce the $PaCO_2$ by an increase in ventilation (respiratory compensation). The patient who is breathing spontaneously may fail to achieve this if ventilation is depressed by sedatives, a reduced conscious level, or significant pulmonary disease. In these cases, the $PaCO_2$ may increase, causing a combined respiratory and metabolic acidosis and profound acidaemia.

Giving bicarbonate may, paradoxically, increase intracellular acidosis, as it is converted to CO_2 with the release of hydrogen ions within the cell. Indications for bicarbonate include cardiac arrest associated with hyperkalaemia or tricyclic overdose. Do not give bicarbonate routinely to correct acidaemia after cardiac arrest.

Full blood count

- To exclude anaemia as contributor to myocardial ischaemia and provide baseline values.

Biochemistry

- To assess renal function.
- To assess electrolyte concentrations (K^+, Mg^{2+}, and Ca^{2+}).*
- To ensure normoglycaemia.
- To commence serial cardiac troponin measurements.
- To provide baseline values.

12-lead ECG

- To record cardiac rhythm.**
- To look for evidence of acute coronary syndrome.
- To look for evidence of old myocardial infarction.
- To provide a baseline record.

Chest radiograph

- To establish the position of a tracheal tube, a gastric tube, and/or a central venous catheter.
- To check for evidence of pulmonary oedema.
- To check for evidence of pulmonary aspiration.
- To exclude pneumothorax.
- To assess cardiac contour (accurate assessment of heart size requires standard PA erect radiograph - not always practicable in the post-resuscitation situation).

Arterial blood gases

- To ensure adequacy of ventilation and oxygenation.
- To ensure correction of acid/base imbalance.

Echocardiography

- To identify contributing causes to cardiac arrest.
- To assess LV and RV structure and function.

*Immediately after a cardiac arrest there is typically a period of hyperkalaemia. However endogenous catecholamine release promotes influx of potassium into cells and may cause hypokalaemia. Hypokalaemia may cause ventricular arrhythmias. Give potassium to maintain the serum potassium between 4.0 - 4.5 mmol l^{-1}.

**Normal sinus rhythm is required for optimal cardiac function. Atrial contraction contributes significantly to ventricular filling, especially in the presence of myocardial disease and valve disease. Loss of the sequential atrial and ventricular contraction of sinus rhythm may reduce cardiac output substantially in some patients.

Table 13.2 Investigations after restoration of circulation

ALS

Patient transfer

Following the period of initial post-resuscitation care and stabilisation, the patient will need to be transferred to an appropriate critical care environment (e.g. ICU or CCU). The decision to transfer a patient from the place where stabilisation has been achieved should be made only after discussion with senior members of the admitting team. Continue all established monitoring during the transfer and secure all cannulae, catheters, tubes and drains. Make a full re-assessment immediately before the patient is transferred. Ensure that portable suction apparatus, an oxygen supply and a defibrillator/monitor accompany the patient and transfer team.

The transfer team should comprise individuals capable of monitoring the patient and responding appropriately to any change in patient condition, including a further cardiac arrest. The Intensive Care Society (UK) has published guidelines for the transport of the critically ill adult (www.ics.ac.uk). These outline the requirements for equipment and personnel when transferring critically ill patients.

Optimising organ function

The extent of secondary organ injury after ROSC depends on the ability to minimise the harmful consequences of post-cardiac arrest syndrome (Figure 13.2). There are opportunities to limit the insult to organs following cardiac arrest.

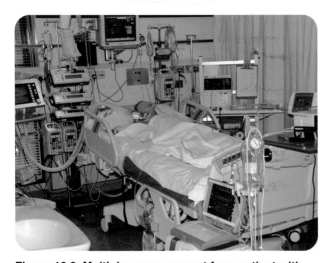

Figure 13.2 Multiple organ support for a patient with the post-cardiac arrest syndrome

Heart and cardiovascular system

Post-cardiac arrest myocardial dysfunction causes haemodynamic instability, which manifests as hypotension, a low cardiac output and arrhythmias. Early echocardiography will enable the degree of myocardial dysfunction to be quantified. In the ICU an arterial line for continuous blood pressure monitoring is essential. Treatment with fluid, inotropes and vasopressors may be guided by blood pressure, heart rate, urine output, and rate

of plasma lactate clearance and central venous oxygen saturations. Non-invasive cardiac output monitors may help to guide treatment but there is no evidence that their use affects outcome. If treatment with fluid resuscitation and vasoactive drugs is insufficient to support the circulation, consider insertion of an intra-aortic balloon pump. Infusion of relatively large volumes of fluids is tolerated remarkably well by patients with post-cardiac arrest syndrome.

In the absence of definitive data supporting a specific goal for blood pressure, target the mean arterial blood pressure to achieve an adequate urine output (1 ml kg^{-1} h^{-1}) and normal or decreasing plasma lactate values, taking into consideration the patient's normal blood pressure, the cause of the arrest and the severity of any myocardial dysfunction. Importantly, hypothermia (see below) may increase urine output and impair lactate clearance.

Referral for implantable cardioverter defibrillator

Consider the possible requirement for an implantable cardioverter defibrillator (ICD) in any patient who has been resuscitated from cardiac arrest in a shockable rhythm outside the context of proven acute ST segment elevation myocardial infarction. All such patients should be referred before discharge from hospital for assessment by a cardiologist with expertise in heart rhythm disorders (Chapter 10).

Brain: optimising neurological recovery

Cerebral perfusion

Immediately after ROSC there is a period (about 15 min) of cerebral hyperaemia. After asphyxial cardiac arrest, brain oedema may occur transiently after ROSC but it is associated only rarely with clinically relevant increases in intracranial pressure. Autoregulation of cerebral blood flow is impaired for some time after cardiac arrest, which means that cerebral perfusion varies with cerebral perfusion pressure instead of being linked to neuronal activity. Following ROSC, maintain mean arterial pressure near the patient's normal level.

Sedation

Although it has been common practice to sedate and ventilate patients for at least 24 h after ROSC, there are no data to support a defined period of ventilation, sedation and neuromuscular blockade after cardiac arrest. Patients need to be well-sedated during treatment with therapeutic hypothermia, and the duration of sedation and ventilation is therefore influenced by this treatment. There are no data to indicate whether or not the choice of sedation influences outcome, but a combination of opioids and hypnotics is usually used. Short-acting drugs (e.g. propofol, alfentanil, remifentanil) will enable earlier neurological assessment. Adequate sedation will reduce oxygen consumption. During hypothermia, optimal sedation can reduce or prevent shivering, which enables the target temperature to be achieved more rapidly.

Control of seizures

Seizures or myoclonus or both occur in 5% - 15% of adult patients who achieve ROSC and 10% - 40% of those who remain comatose. Seizures increase cerebral metabolism by up to three-fold and may cause cerebral injury: treat promptly and effectively with benzodiazepines, phenytoin, sodium valproate, propofol, or a barbiturate. Myoclonus can be particularly difficult to treat; phenytoin is often ineffective. Clonazepam is the most effective antimyoclonic drug, but sodium valproate, levetiracetam and propofol may also be effective. Start maintenance therapy after the first event once potential precipitating causes (e.g. intracranial haemorrhage, electrolyte imbalance) are excluded. No studies directly address the use of prophylactic anticonvulsant drugs after cardiac arrest in adults.

Glucose control

There is a strong association between high blood glucose after resuscitation from cardiac arrest and poor neurological outcome. However, severe hypoglycaemia is associated with increased mortality in critically ill patients, and comatose patients are at particular risk from unrecognised hypoglycaemia. Based on the available data and expert consensus, following ROSC, blood glucose should be maintained at ≤10 mmol l⁻¹. Hypoglycaemia (< 4.0 mmol l⁻¹) must be avoided. Strict glucose control (4.5 - 6.0 mmol l⁻¹) should not be implemented in adult patients with ROSC after cardiac arrest because of the increased risk of hypoglycaemia.

Temperature control

Treatment of hyperpyrexia

A period of hyperthermia (hyperpyrexia) is common in the first 48 h after cardiac arrest. Several studies document an association between post-cardiac arrest pyrexia and poor outcome. Although the effect of elevated temperature on outcome is not proved, treat any hyperthermia occurring after cardiac arrest with antipyretics or active cooling.

Therapeutic hypothermia

Mild hypothermia is neuroprotective and improves outcome after a period of global cerebral hypoxia-ischaemia. Cooling suppresses many of the pathways leading to delayed cell death, including apoptosis (programmed cell death). Hypothermia decreases the cerebral metabolic rate for oxygen by about 6% for each 1°C reduction in temperature and this may reduce the release of excitatory amino acids and free radicals.

Which post-cardiac arrest patients should be cooled?

All studies of post-cardiac arrest therapeutic hypothermia have included only patients in coma. There is good evidence supporting the use of induced hypothermia in comatose survivors of out-of-hospital cardiac arrest caused by VF. Two randomised trials demonstrated improved neurological outcome at hospital discharge or at 6 months in comatose patients after out-of-hospital VF cardiac arrest. Cooling was initiated within minutes to hours after ROSC and a temperature range of 32 - 34°C was maintained for 12 - 24 h. Extrapolation of these data to other cardiac arrests (e.g. other initial rhythms, in-hospital arrests, children) seems reasonable but is supported only by data derived from non-randomised trials.

Based on the evidence available and expert consensus, consider therapeutic hypothermia for any mechanically ventilated patient admitted to the ICU for post resuscitation organ support.

How to cool

The practical application of therapeutic hypothermia is divided into three phases: induction, maintenance, and rewarming. Animal data indicate that earlier cooling after ROSC produces better outcome. External and/or internal cooling techniques can be used to initiate cooling. An infusion of 30 ml kg⁻¹ of 4°C 0.9% sodium chloride or Hartmann's solution decreases core temperature by approximately 1.5°C and this technique can be used to initiate cooling prehospital. Other methods of inducing and/or maintaining hypothermia include:

- Simple ice packs and/or wet towels are inexpensive; however, these methods may be more time consuming for nursing staff, may result in greater temperature fluctuations, and do not enable controlled rewarming.

- Ice-cold fluids alone cannot be used to maintain hypothermia, but even the addition of simple ice packs may control the temperature adequately.

- Cooling blankets or pads.

- Water or air circulating blankets.

- Transnasal evaporative cooling.

- Water circulating gel-coated pads.

- Intravascular heat exchanger, placed usually in the femoral or subclavian veins.

- Cardiopulmonary bypass.

In most cases, it is easy to cool patients initially after ROSC because the temperature usually decreases spontaneously within this first hour. Initial cooling is facilitated by neuromuscular blockade and sedation, which will prevent shivering. Magnesium sulphate (e.g. 5 g infused over 5 h), can also be given to reduce the shivering threshold.

In the maintenance phase, a cooling method with effective temperature monitoring that avoids temperature fluctuations is preferred. This is achieved best with external or internal cooling devices that include continuous temperature feedback to achieve a set target temperature. The temperature is typically monitored from a thermistor placed in the bladder and/or oesophagus. There are no data indicating that any specific cooling technique increases survival when compared with any other cooling technique; however, internal devices enable more precise temperature control compared with external techniques. Once the temperature is in the target range (32 - 34°C), maintain this temperature for 24 h. Rewarming must be achieved slowly: the optimal rate is not known, but expert consensus supports about 0.25 - 0.5 °C of warming per hour and strict avoidance of hyperthermia. Plasma electrolyte concentrations, effective intravascular volume and metabolic rate can change rapidly during rewarming, as they do during cooling.

Physiological effects and complications of hypothermia

The well-recognised physiological effects of hypothermia need to be managed carefully.

- Shivering will increase metabolic and heat production, thus reducing cooling rates - strategies to reduce shivering are discussed above.

- Mild hypothermia increases systemic vascular resistance, causes arrhythmias (usually bradycardia).

- Hypothermia causes a diuresis and electrolyte abnormalities such as hypophosphataemia, hypokalaemia, hypomagnesaemia and hypocalcaemia.

- Hypothermia decreases insulin sensitivity and insulin secretion, hyperglycaemia, which will need treatment with insulin (see glucose control).

- Mild hypothermia impairs coagulation and increases bleeding although this has not been confirmed in many clinical studies.

- Hypothermia can impair the immune system and increase infection rates.

- The serum amylase concentration is commonly increased during hypothermia but the significance of this unclear.

- The clearance of sedative drugs and neuromuscular blockers is reduced by up to 30% at a core temperature of 34°C.

Contraindications to hypothermia

Generally recognised contraindications to therapeutic hypothermia, but which are not applied universally,

include: severe systemic infection, established multiple organ failure, and pre-existing medical coagulopathy (fibrinolytic therapy is not a contraindication to therapeutic hypothermia).

Prognostication

Two thirds of those dying after admission to ICU following out-of-hospital cardiac arrest die from neurological injury. A quarter of those dying after admission to ICU following in-hospital cardiac arrest die from neurological injury. A means of predicting neurological outcome that can be applied to individual patients immediately after ROSC is required. Many studies have focused on prediction of poor long term outcome (severe cerebral disability or death), based on clinical or test findings that indicate irreversible brain injury, to enable clinicians to limit care or withdraw organ support. The implications of these prognostic tests are such that they should have 100% specificity or zero false positive rate, i.e. no individuals should have a 'good' long-term outcome if predicted to have a poor outcome.

Clinical examination

There are no clinical neurological signs that predict reliably poor outcome (severe cerebral disability or death) less than 24 h after cardiac arrest. In adult patients who are comatose after cardiac arrest, and who have not been treated with hypothermia and who do not have confounding factors (such as hypotension, sedatives or muscle relaxants) the absence of both pupillary light and corneal reflex at ≥ 72 h predicts poor outcome reliably. Absence of vestibulo-ocular reflexes at ≥ 24 h and a GCS motor score of 2 or less (extension or no response to pain) at ≥ 72 h are less reliable. Other clinical signs, including myoclonus, are not recommended for predicting poor outcome. The presence of myoclonic status in adults is strongly associated with poor outcome but rare cases of good neurological recovery from this situation have been described and accurate diagnosis of myoclonic status is problematic.

Biochemical markers

Serum (e.g. neuronal specific enolase, S100 protein) or cerebrospinal fluid (CSF) biomarkers alone are insufficient as predictors of poor outcomes in comatose patients after cardiac arrest with or without treatment with therapeutic hypothermia.

Neurophysiological studies

No neurophysiological study predicts outcome for a comatose patient reliably within the first 24 h after cardiac arrest. If somatosensory evoked potentials (SSEPs) are measured after 24 h in comatose cardiac arrest survivors not treated with therapeutic hypothermia, bilateral absence of the N20 cortical response to median nerve stimulation predicts poor outcome. Very few hospitals in the UK have the resources to enable SSEPs to be measured.

Imaging studies

Many imaging modalities (magnetic resonance imaging [MRI], computed tomography [CT], single photon emission computed tomography [SPECT], cerebral angiography, transcranial Doppler, nuclear medicine, near infra-red spectroscopy [NIRS]) have been studied to determine their utility for prediction of outcome in adult survivors of cardiac arrest. Based on the available evidence, none of these imaging modalities will predict reliably outcome of comatose cardiac arrest survivors.

Impact of therapeutic hypothermia on prognostication

Most prognostication studies have been undertaken before implementation of therapeutic hypothermia and there is evidence that this therapy makes these tests less reliable even when undertaken after normothermia has been restored. Potentially reliable predictors of poor outcome in patients treated with therapeutic hypothermia after cardiac arrest include bilateral absence of N20 peak on SSEP ≥ 24 h after cardiac arrest and the absence of both corneal and pupillary reflexes 3 or more days after cardiac arrest. Given the limited available evidence, decisions to limit care should not be made based on the results of a single prognostication tool.

Organ donation

Post-cardiac arrest patients who do not survive should be considered as potential organ donors, either after brain death or as non-heart-beating donors.

Care of the resuscitation team

Audit all resuscitation attempts and, ideally, send these data to the National Cardiac Arrest Audit (Chapter 2). Feedback for the resuscitation team should be constructive and not based on a fault/blame culture. Whether the resuscitation attempt was successful or not, the patient's relatives will require considerable support. Consider the pastoral needs of all those associated with the arrest.

Key learning points

- After cardiac arrest, return of spontaneous circulation is just the first stage in a continuum of resuscitation.

- The quality of post-resuscitation care will influence significantly the patient's final outcome.

- These patients require appropriate monitoring, safe transfer to a critical care environment, and continued organ support.

- The post-cardiac arrest syndrome comprises post-cardiac arrest brain injury, post-cardiac arrest myocardial dysfunction, the systemic ischaemia/reperfusion response, and persistence of precipitating pathology.

- Our ability to predict the final neurological outcome for those patients remaining comatose after cardiopulmonary resuscitation remains very poor.

Further reading

Deakin CD, Nolan JP, Soar J, et al. European Resuscitation Council Guidelines for Resuscitation 2010. Section 4. Adult Advanced Life Support. Resuscitation 2010;81: 1305-52.

Deakin CD, Morrison LJ, Morley PT, et al. 2010 International Consensus on Cardiopulmonary Resuscitation and Emergency Cardiovascular Care Science with Treatment Recommendations. Part 8: Advanced Life Support. Resuscitation 2010;81: e93-e169.

Laver S, Farrow C, Turner D, Nolan J. Mode of death after admission to an intensive care unit following cardiac arrest. Intensive Care Med 2004;30: 2126-8.

Nolan JP, Laver SR, Welch CA, Harrison DA, Gupta V, Rowan K. Outcome following admission to UK intensive care units after cardiac arrest: a secondary analysis of the ICNARC Case Mix Programme Database. Anaesthesia 2007;62:1207-16.

Nolan JP, Morley PT, Vanden Hoek TL, Hickey RW. Therapeutic hypothermia after cardiac arrest. An advisory statement by the Advanced Life Support Task Force of the International Liaison Committee on Resuscitation. Resuscitation 2003;57:231-5.

Nolan JP, Neumar RW, Adrie C, et al. Post-cardiac arrest syndrome: epidemiology, pathophysiology, treatment, and prognostication. A Scientific Statement from the International Liaison Committee on Resuscitation; the American Heart Association Emergency Cardiovascular Care Committee; the Council on Cardiovascular Surgery and Anesthesia; the Council on Cardiopulmonary, Perioperative, and Critical Care; the Council on Clinical Cardiology; the Council on Stroke. Resuscitation 2008;79:350-79.

Polderman KH, Herold I. Therapeutic hypothermia and controlled normothermia in the intensive care unit: practical considerations, side effects, and cooling methods. Crit Care Med 2009;37:1101-20.

Learning outcomes

To understand:

▶ **The role of telephone-advised cardiopulmonary resuscitation (CPR)**

▶ **The current position on CPR versus defibrillation first**

▶ **How to change over efficiently from an AED to a manual defibrillator**

▶ **Principles of prehospital airway management**

▶ **The importance of effective handover to hospital staff**

▶ **Rules for stopping resuscitation**

▶ **The potential role of cardiac arrest centres**

Introduction

A prehospital section has been included for the first time in the Resuscitation Council (UK) Advanced Life Support (ALS) course manual. The aim is to bring together resuscitation topics of specific relevance to the pre-hospital emergency medical services (EMS). The increased emphasis on the importance of minimally interrupted high-quality chest compressions and reducing the pre-shock pause by continuing chest compressions while the defibrillator is charged demands a well structured, monitored training programme for prehospital EMS practitioners. This should include comprehensive competency-based training and regular opportunities to refresh skills. It is recognised that in most cases prehospital resuscitation has to be managed by fewer practitioners than would normally be present at an in-hospital arrest; also transportation to a receiving centre adds an extra dimension. This emphasises the need for a structured and disciplined approach. The Resuscitation Council (UK) ALS course provides the ideal platform to develop and practise resuscitation skills and strengthen the multidisciplinary team approach.

Telephone-advised CPR

Telephone-advised CPR has been included in the 2010 Resuscitation Council (UK) Guidelines because:

- there is widespread use of telephone triage systems that include advice for a rescuer attending a cardiac arrest victim before professional help arrives;

- the wide availability of mobile phones makes it likely that there will be a phone available at the site where the victim has collapsed;

- there is robust research examining best practice of both the diagnosis of cardiac arrest by telephone and also the content and delivery of subsequent instructions provided to rescuers;

- in adults, telephone-advised compression-only CPR produces better survival rates than telephone-advised conventional CPR (chest compressions and mouth-to-mouth ventilation);

- it has been acknowledged that the time to first compression can be reduced significantly if a lay bystander can deliver chest compressions while waiting for professionals to arrive.

The aims of providing guidance on telephone advice are:

- to enable an early correct diagnosis of cardiac arrest to be made;

- to enable the lay rescuer to start early, effective CPR, minimising the time from collapse to the first effective chest compression, and to continue correctly performed CPR until help arrives.

Telephone triage guidelines

The use of telephone triage to grade the urgency of emergency calls to the EMS is used throughout the UK and is becoming an integral part of the Chain of Survival for victims of cardiac arrest. As part of the call, if appropriate, call handlers will offer CPR instructions to the caller. After out-of-hospital cardiac arrest, help from the EMS will be accessed by telephone and because of the widespread use of mobile phones it is common for a phone to be available at the point where resuscitation is taking place. The opportunity to provide instructions by phone on how to give CPR enables the time to the first chest compression to be reduced dramatically, compared with waiting for the arrival of the EMS. The shorter the time until chest compressions are commenced, the higher the survival rate. However, significant delays in giving advice over the phone and/or poor quality CPR will limit the benefits.

Standardised advice to bystanders should increase the chance that the cardiac arrest will be diagnosed and treated correctly. Further research on this topic will help to improve outcome.

Telephone triage systems

In the UK, call handlers who answer 999 calls may have no background medical training apart from that provided when they were trained to use the system. They read the triage questions from a screen and the deviation allowed from the precise wording in either the question or the advice supplied, varies from supplier to supplier according to licence.

Diagnosis

The diagnosis of cardiac arrest may be difficult over the telephone. Palpation of the carotid pulse by laypeople is unreliable for the diagnosis of cardiac arrest. Absence of breathing can be a better indicator of cardiac arrest, but many cardiac arrest victims gasp initially (agonal breathing) and this is often misinterpreted by the lay rescuer as breathing. Consequently, the call handler should ask if the victim is "breathing normally" instead of simply "breathing". A few cardiac arrest victims will have seizures. Seizure activity as a feature of cardiac arrest can cause confusion and delay the correct diagnosis. Asking whether the patient is a known epileptic may help to reduce the risk of patients with epilepsy receiving bystander CPR inappropriately.

Telephone-advised compression-only CPR

When EMS response times are short (< 5 min), there is some evidence that compression-only CPR produces at least equivalent outcomes to conventional CPR (chest compressions and mouth-to-mouth ventilation). In adults, telephone-advised compression-only CPR produces better survival rates than telephone-advised conventional CPR. Rescuers may be more willing to give resuscitation if they do not have to provide ventilation. In children, 70% of out-of-hospital cardiac arrests are asphyxial in origin and survival rates are better if they are provided with both chest compressions and ventilations. However, even in children, after cardiac arrest from a primary cardiac cause, there is no difference in survival after compression-only or conventional CPR - either technique produces better survival rates than no CPR. Telephone-advised CPR guidelines provide instruction in compression-only CPR for both adults and children because it is quicker and easier to describe.

Defibrillation

CPR versus defibrillation first

Defibrillation is a key link in the Chain of Survival and is one of the few interventions that has been shown to improve outcome from ventricular fibrillation/pulseless ventricular tachycardia (VF/VT) cardiac arrest. The probability of successful defibrillation and subsequent survival to hospital discharge declines rapidly with time and the ability to deliver early defibrillation is one of the most important factors in determining survival from cardiac arrest.

Several studies have examined whether a period of CPR before defibrillation is beneficial, particularly in patients with an unwitnessed arrest or prolonged collapse without resuscitation. A review of evidence for the 2005 guidelines resulted in the recommendation that it was reasonable for EMS personnel to give a period of about 2 min of CPR (i.e. about five cycles at 30:2) before defibrillation in patients with prolonged collapse (> 5 min). This recommendation was based on clinical studies in which response times exceeded 4 - 5 min and in which a period of 1.5 - 3 min of CPR by paramedics or EMS physicians before shock delivery, compared with immediate defibrillation, improved return of spontaneous circulation (ROSC), survival to hospital discharge and one-year survival for adults with out-of-hospital VF/VT. *not recommended see 2nd paragraph below*

In contrast, in two randomised controlled trials, a period of 1.5 - 3 min of CPR by EMS personnel before defibrillation did not improve ROSC or survival to hospital discharge in patients with out-of-hospital VF/VT, regardless of EMS response interval. Four other studies have also failed to demonstrate significant improvements in overall ROSC or survival to hospital discharge with an initial period of CPR.

The duration of collapse is frequently difficult to estimate accurately and there is evidence that performing chest compressions while preparing and charging a defibrillator improves the probability of survival. For these reasons, in any cardiac arrest that they have not witnessed, EMS personnel should provide high-quality CPR while a defibrillator is prepared, applied and charged, but routine delivery of a specified period of CPR (e.g. 2 - 3 min) before rhythm analysis and shock delivery is no longer recommended.

Transition from AED to manual defibrillator

In many situations, an automated external defibrillator (AED) is used to provide initial defibrillation but is subsequently swapped for a manual defibrillator on arrival of EMS personnel. If such a swap is done without considering the phase of the AED cycle, the next shock may be delayed, which may compromise outcome. For this reason, EMS personnel should leave the AED connected while securing the airway and IV access. The AED can be left attached for the next rhythm analysis and, if indicated, shock delivery, before being swapped for the manual defibrillator.

One shock versus three-shock sequence

A three-stacked shock strategy (as opposed to a single shock) may be considered when a conscious patient has a witnessed arrest when already connected to a manual defibrillator with self-adhesive defibrillation pads.

Although there are no data supporting a three-shock strategy in any circumstances, it is unlikely that chest compressions will improve the already very high chance of ROSC when defibrillation occurs early in the electrical phase, immediately after onset of VF.

Prehospital airway management

There is insufficient evidence to support or refute the use of any specific technique to maintain an airway and provide ventilation in adults with prehospital or in-hospital cardiac arrest. Tracheal intubation has been perceived as the optimal method of providing and maintaining a clear and secure airway during cardiac arrest but data are accumulating on the challenges associated with prehospital intubation. It is now strongly recommended that tracheal intubation should be used only when trained personnel are available to carry out the procedure with a high level of skill and confidence. In the absence of experienced personnel the use of supraglottic airway devices (SADs) during CPR is probably more rational. However, there are only poor-quality data on the pre-hospital use of these devices during cardiac arrest. The use of SADs is discussed in more detail in Chapter 7.

Tracheal intubation

The perceived advantages of tracheal intubation over bag-mask ventilation include: enabling ventilation without interrupting chest compressions, enabling effective ventilation (particularly when lung and/or chest compliance is poor), minimising gastric inflation and therefore the risk of regurgitation, protection against pulmonary aspiration of gastric contents, and the potential to free a rescuer's hands for other tasks.

Use of the bag-mask is more likely to cause gastric distension, which, theoretically, is more likely to cause regurgitation and aspiration. However, there are no reliable data to indicate that the incidence of aspiration is any higher in cardiac arrest patients ventilated using a bag-mask compared with those ventilated via a tracheal tube.

The disadvantages of tracheal intubation over bag-valve-mask ventilation include:

- The risk of an unrecognised misplaced tracheal tube in patients with out-of-hospital cardiac arrest, the documented incidence ranges from 0.5 - 17%.

- A prolonged period without chest compressions while intubation is attempted: in a study of prehospital intubation by paramedics during 100 cardiac arrests, the total duration of the interruptions in CPR associated with tracheal intubation attempts was 110 s and in 25% the interruptions were for > 3 min.

- A comparatively high failure rate: intubation success rates correlate with the experience of the intubator.

Healthcare personnel who undertake prehospital intubation should do so only within a structured, monitored programme, which should include comprehensive competency-based training and regular opportunities to refresh skills. Rescuers must weigh the risks and benefits of intubation against the need to provide effective chest compressions. The intubation attempt may require some interruption of chest compressions but, once an advanced airway is in place, ventilation will not require interruption of chest compressions and the patient may be attached to a mechanical ventilator device initially set to deliver a tidal volume of 6 - 7 ml kg^{-1} at 10 breaths min^{-1}. Personnel skilled in advanced airway management should be able to undertake laryngoscopy without stopping chest compressions; a brief pause in chest compressions will be required only as the tube is passed between the vocal cords. Alternatively, to avoid any interruptions in chest compressions, the intubation attempt may be deferred until ROSC. No intubation attempt should interrupt chest compressions for > 10 s. After intubation, confirm correct tube placement and secure the tube adequately.

With the increasing availability of efficient intraosseous (IO) devices, and the lack of efficacy of tracheal drug administration, tracheal administration of drugs is no longer recommended.

Confirmation of the correct placement of the tracheal tube

Unrecognised oesophageal intubation is the most serious complication of attempted tracheal intubation. Routine use of primary and secondary techniques to confirm correct placement of the tracheal tube should reduce this risk. Primary assessment should include observation of bilateral chest expansion, bilateral auscultation in the axillae (breath sounds should be equal and adequate), and auscultation over the epigastrium (breath sounds should not be heard). Clinical signs of correct tube placement (condensation in the tube, chest rise, breath sounds on auscultation of lungs, and inability to hear gas entering the stomach) are not completely reliable. Secondary confirmation of tracheal tube placement by an ETCO$_2$ or oesophageal detector device should reduce the risk of unrecognised oesophageal intubation. If there is doubt about correct tube placement, use the laryngoscope and look directly to see if the tube passes through the vocal cords. None of the secondary confirmation techniques will differentiate between a tube placed in a main bronchus and one placed correctly in the trachea.

Waveform capnography is the most sensitive and specific way to confirm and monitor continuously the position of a tracheal tube in victims of cardiac arrest. Existing portable monitors may make capnographic initial confirmation and continuous monitoring of tracheal tube position feasible in almost all settings where intubation is performed, including out of hospital. In the absence of a waveform capnograph it may be preferable to use a supraglottic airway device when advanced airway management is indicated.

CPR during transportation to hospital

During transportation to hospital, manual CPR is often performed poorly; mechanical CPR can maintain high quality CPR during transfer by land ambulance or helicopter. Mechanical devices also have the advantage of allowing defibrillation without interrupting chest compressions. However, these devices have to be applied efficiently if prolonged interruption to chest compressions is to be avoided. Ongoing multicentre prospective trials should eventually provide the data to determine the precise role of mechanical devices in prehospital resuscitation.

Hospital handover

If a cardiac arrest victim is transported to hospital, clear and accurate communication and documentation are essential elements of the handover to hospital staff. Vital information may be lost or misinterpreted if communication between EMS practitioners and hospital staff is not effective.

If resuscitation is continuing en route to hospital, a pre-alert message is essential to ensure that emergency department staff and/or the hospital resuscitation team are ready to receive the patient. This gives time for the hospital resuscitation team to elect a team leader and assign roles to team members. Specific interventions to treat potentially reversible causes or specialist intervention can be arranged.

Emergency medical services personnel need to be completely focused on communicating vital information about the patient, the circumstances surrounding the resuscitation and actions taken. This has to be done against a background of considerable activity and with the added pressure of time. Hospital staff will be focused on beginning their own assessment and treatment of the patient, but this must not prevent them from listening to the vital information provided by the EMS personnel. A structured approach will enhance the handover and make the transition as rapid and effective as possible. Communication failure has been cited as a contributory factor in cases of error and harm to patients. A British Medical Association document *Safe Handover; Safe Patients* gives guidance to ensure that the risks involved in the process of transferring clinical responsibility are minimised (http://www.bma.org.uk/employmentandcontracts/working_arrangements/Handover.jsp).

The ALS course enables prehospital and hospital staff to understand each other's role and develops the multidisciplinary team approach.

Rules for stopping resuscitation

Following out-of-hospital cardiac arrest, failure of ALS-trained EMS personnel to achieve ROSC at the scene is associated with an extremely low probability of survival. The rare exception, where the transfer to hospital of a patient with ongoing CPR results in long-term good quality survival, is usually associated with special circumstances, such as pre-existing hypothermia or drug overdose. For this reason, attempts have been made to formulate and validate rules for stopping resuscitation that allow EMS personnel to stop the resuscitation attempt and pronounce life extinct without transporting the victim to hospital. One such rule recommends stopping CPR when there is no ROSC, no shocks are administered, and the arrest is not witnessed by EMS personnel. However, this rule was validated with defibrillation-only emergency medical technicians in Canada and may not apply to an EMS system staffed by paramedics. In the UK, guidelines from the Joint Royal Colleges Ambulance Service Liaison Committee (2006), advise that ambulance clinicians may stop resuscitation if all of the following criteria are met:

- 15 min or more has passed since the onset of collapse;

- no bystander CPR was given before arrival of the ambulance;

- there is no suspicion of drowning, hypothermia, poisoning/overdose, or pregnancy;

- asystole is present for > 30 s on the ECG monitor screen;

Pre-hospital resuscitation attempts are generally discontinued also if the rhythm remains asystole despite 20 min ALS except in cases of drowning and hypothermia.

Regionalisation of post-resuscitation care

Several studies with historical control groups have shown improved survival after implementation of a comprehensive package of post-resuscitation care that includes therapeutic hypothermia and percutaneous coronary intervention. There is also evidence of improved survival after out-of-hospital cardiac arrest in large hospitals with cardiac catheter facilities compared with smaller hospitals with no cardiac catheter facilities. Several studies of out-of-hospital adult cardiac arrest failed to demonstrate any effect of transport interval from the scene to the receiving hospital on survival to hospital discharge if ROSC was achieved at the scene and transport intervals were short (3 - 11 min). This implies that it may be safe to bypass local hospitals and transport the post-cardiac arrest patient to a regional cardiac arrest centre. There is indirect evidence that regional cardiac resuscitation systems of care improve outcome after ST elevation myocardial infarction (STEMI).

The implication from all these data is that specialist cardiac arrest centres and systems of care may be effective but, as yet, there is no direct evidence to support this hypothesis.

Key learning points

- In adults, telephone-advised compression-only CPR produces better survival rates than telephone-advised conventional CPR.

- EMS personnel should provide high-quality CPR while preparing, applying and charging a defibrillator, but a routine, specified period of CPR before shock delivery is not recommended.

- Tracheal intubation should be attempted only by those with a high level of skill and experience with the technique.

- Waveform capnography is the most sensitive and specific method for confirming the position of a tracheal tube in victims of cardiac arrest.

Further reading

Deakin CD, Nolan JP, Soar J, et al. European Resuscitation Council Guidelines for Resuscitation 2010. Section 4. Adult Advanced Life Support. Resuscitation 2010;81:1305-52.

Deakin CD, Nolan JP, Sunde K, Koster RW. European Resuscitation Council Guidelines for Resuscitation 2010. Section 3. Electrical Therapies: Automated External Defibrillators, Defibrillation, Cardioversion and Pacing. Resuscitation 2010;81:1293-1304.

Hupfl M, Selig HF, Nagele P. Chest-compression-only versus standard cardiopulmonary resuscitation: a meta-analysis. Lancet 2010;376:1552-57.

Nichol G, Aufderheide TP, Eigel B, et al. Regional systems of care for out-of-hospital cardiac arrest: A policy statement from the American Heart Association. Circulation 2010;121:709-29.

Rea TD, Fahrenbruch C, Culley L, et al. CPR with chest compresssions alone or with rescue breathing. New England Journal of Medicine 2010;363:423-33.

Svensson L, Bohm K, Castren M, et al. Compression-only CPR or standard CPR in out-of-hospital cardiac arrest. New England Journal of Medicine 2010;363:434-42.

ALS

Blood Gas Analysis and Pulse Oximetry

Introduction

Interpreting the analysis of an arterial blood sample to determine a patient's acid-base status and respiratory gas exchange is a key component in the management of any ill patient and, in particular, in the peri-arrest situation. Although there is often a great temptation to try and analyse the numerical data in isolation, it is essential to have a system to ensure that nothing is overlooked or misinterpreted; as when reading an ECG, this starts with asking "how is the patient?" This should include any known history along with details of current oxygen therapy and medications.

There are usually four key pieces of information contained in the results of analysis of an arterial blood sample:

- pH
- $PaCO_2$ (partial pressure of carbon dioxide in arterial blood)
- Bicarbonate and base excess
- PaO_2 (partial pressure of oxygen in arterial blood)

In order to interpret these results, we first need to understand what each means. Normal ranges are given in the text; however, these will vary slightly between institutions.

pH

The acidity or alkalinity of the blood (or any solution) is determined by the concentration of hydrogen ions [H^+]; the greater the concentration, the more acid the solution. In the body, the concentration of hydrogen ions is extremely low, normally around 40 nanomoles per litre (nmol l^{-1}), where a nanomole is 1 billionth of a mole (a mole is the molecular weight of a substance in grams, i.e. for hydrogen it would be 2 g). To put this into perspective,

sodium ions (Na^+) are present in a concentration of 135 millimoles per litre (mmol l^{-1}), i.e. 3 million times greater. In order to make dealing with such small numbers easier, we use the pH scale; this is a logarithmic scale expressing the hydrogen ion concentration between 1 and 14. The pH of a normal arterial blood sample lies between 7.35 and 7.45, or [H^+] 44 - 36 nmol l^{-1}. There are two key points to remember about the pH scale:

1. The numerical value of pH changes inversely with hydrogen ion concentration. Consequently a **decrease in blood pH below 7.35** indicates an increase in [H^+] above normal, a condition referred to as an **acidaemia**. Conversely, an **increase in blood pH above 7.45** indicates a reduction in [H^+] below normal, a condition referred to as an **alkalaemia**. Clinicians often use the terms acidosis and alkalosis respectively to describe these situations. Strictly speaking, these terms refer to the processes that lead to the changes in pH, and it is in this context that they will be used in this manual.

2. Small changes in pH represent big changes in hydrogen ion [H^+] concentration. For example, a pH change from 7.4 to 7.1 means that the hydrogen ion concentration has increased from 40 nmol l^{-1} to 80 nmol l^{-1}, i.e. it has doubled for a pH change of 0.3.

Many of the complex reactions within cells are controlled by enzymes that function only within a very narrow pH range; hence, normal pH is controlled tightly between 7.35 and 7.45. However, each day during normal activity we produce massive amounts of hydrogen ions (approximately 14 500 000 000 nmol), which if unchecked would cause a substantial decrease in pH (acidaemia) before they could be excreted. To prevent this happening the body has a series of substances known as buffers that take up hydrogen ions and thereby prevent the development of an acidaemia. The major intracellular buffers are proteins, phosphate and haemoglobin (within red blood cells) and the extracellular buffers are plasma proteins and bicarbonate (see below).

Clearly the buffering system is only a temporary solution to the production of acids; ultimately they will all be consumed and acids will start to accumulate. A system is therefore required to eliminate the acids and thereby regenerate the buffers. This is achieved by the lungs and kidneys.

Partial pressure

We normally use percentages to describe the composition of a mixture of gases, a good example being air: 21% oxygen, 78% nitrogen, 0.04% carbon dioxide. However, a better indication of the number of molecules of a gas in a mixture is better described by referring to its partial pressure. The partial pressure is the contribution each gas in a mixture makes to the total pressure. The importance of using this measure is best demonstrated by the fact that if we double the total pressure of a mixture, the partial pressures of the constituents are doubled, but the percentages remain the same. We breathe gases at atmospheric pressure or 1 atmosphere, very close to a pressure of 100 kiloPascals (kPa) or 750 mmHg (1 kPa = 7.5 mmHg). As a result, when breathing air, the contribution (partial pressure) of nitrogen is 78% of 100 kPa or 78 kPa and oxygen 21% of 100 kPa or 21 kPa. When breathing 40% oxygen, the partial pressure of the oxygen in the inspired gas is 40 kPa.

At atmospheric pressure, the partial pressure of a gas in a mixture (in kPa) is numerically the same as the percentage (%) of the gas by volume.

When a gas is dissolved in a liquid (e.g. blood) the partial pressure within the liquid is the same as in the gas in contact with the liquid. This enables us to measure the partial pressure of oxygen and carbon dioxide in blood.

In summary, the partial pressure of a gas is a measure of the concentration of the gas in the medium it is in and is expressed as $P_{medium}Gas$, e.g. $PaCO_2$ is the partial pressure (P) of carbon dioxide (CO_2) in arterial blood (a).

$PaCO_2$

Carbon dioxide (CO_2) is an important waste product of metabolism. Under normal circumstances, it is transported in the blood to the lungs where it is excreted during expiration. For transport to the lungs, it is either combined with protein or haemoglobin, or is dissolved in plasma where it reacts with water to form hydrogen ions and bicarbonate (HCO_3^-):

$$CO_2 + H_2O \rightleftharpoons H^+ + HCO_3^-$$

The normal $PaCO_2$ is 5.3 kPa with a range of 4.7 - 6.0 kPa.

In the lungs, the reaction proceeds in reverse: CO_2 is generated and expired. From this reaction, we can see that CO_2 behaves as an acid: any increase in $PaCO_2$ will cause the reaction to move to the right and increase the hydrogen ion concentration with the subsequent development of an acidaemia. There will, of course, be the same increase in bicarbonate concentration but, as this is only nanomoles, it has little effect on the overall total concentration of 22 - 26 mmol l^{-1}. If the metabolic production of CO_2 is constant, the only factor that affects the amount in the blood is the rate at which it is removed

by alveolar ventilation. A **decrease in alveolar ventilation** will reduce excretion of CO_2 causing an increase in $PaCO_2$ and the production of more hydrogen ions. If the pH decreases below 7.35 an acidaemia has been produced. As the primary cause of the acidaemia is a problem with the respiratory system, we call this process a **respiratory acidosis**.

Conversely, an **increase in alveolar ventilation** that removes CO_2 faster than it is generated reduces $PaCO_2$ and moves the reaction to the left, reducing the concentration of hydrogen ions. As a result the pH will increase and if it exceeds 7.45 an alkalaemia has been produced. Again, the primary cause is the respiratory system and we call this process a **respiratory alkalosis**.

It is easy to understand therefore how even brief periods of apnoea, as occurs during cardiac arrest, result in a respiratory acidosis. However, under normal circumstances, the respiratory centre in the brain stem is very sensitive to blood $[H^+]$ and within a few minutes rapidly increases alveolar ventilation. This increases CO_2 excretion, reduces $PaCO_2$, decreases $[H^+]$ and returns pH to normal.

The lungs are the primary mechanism by which $[H^+]$ is adjusted by regulating $PaCO_2$.

Bicarbonate and base excess

Bicarbonate

Bicarbonate (HCO_3^-) is the most important buffer. It is generated by the kidneys and is measured easily in an arterial blood sample. It can be thought of as the opposite of an acid and as such is also called a base. When bicarbonate buffers hydrogen ions, carbon dioxide and water are produced, and it is via this route that the vast majority of acids (90%) are excreted each day. However, the acids not eliminated by the respiratory system can also be buffered as shown below. The reaction below moves to the right and bicarbonate neutralises the effect of the H^+ and prevents a decrease in plasma pH. In the kidneys, the reaction proceeds to the left, the H^+ is excreted in the urine and bicarbonate filtered and returned to the plasma. Depending on the acid load, the kidneys will excrete either acid or alkaline urine.

$$H^+ + HCO_3^- \rightleftharpoons H_2CO_3$$

Under normal circumstances, the concentration of bicarbonate is 22 - 26 mmol l^{-1}.

If there is an acute increase in the acid load, although the respiratory system will try and increase excretion of carbon dioxide, bicarbonate will decrease as it buffers the extra H^+. Once the reserves of bicarbonate are used, H^+ will accumulate decreasing the pH. Unlike the respiratory system, the kidneys respond slowly and it takes several days for additional bicarbonate to be produced to meet the demand to buffer the extra acid. If the kidneys fail to produce sufficient bicarbonate the resultant **metabolic acidosis** will lead to a decrease in pH below 7.35 (acidaemia).

Occasionally, there is an excess of bicarbonate. This will have the effect of excessive buffering of hydrogen ions and will produce a **metabolic alkalosis** and increase the pH above 7.45 (alkalaemia).

Base excess

This is a measure of the amount of excess acid or base is in the blood as a result of a metabolic derangement. It is calculated as the amount of strong acid or base that would have to be added to a blood sample with an abnormal pH to restore it to normal (pH 7.4). Consequently, a patient with a **base excess** of 8 mmol l^{-1} would require 8 mmol l^{-1} of **strong acid** to return their pH to normal; that is they have a metabolic alkalosis (compare with bicarbonate which would be raised, so both move in the same direction). Conversely, a patient with a **base deficit** of 8 mmol l^{-1} will require the addition of 8 mmol l^{-1} of **strong base** to normalise their pH (again, compare with bicarbonate which would be reduced). Unfortunately, the term "negative base excess" is used instead of base deficit and in the example above, the patient would have a negative base excess of -8 mmol l^{-1}.

As a result, the normal values of base excess are +2 to -2 mmol l^{-1}.

A base excess more negative than -2 mmol l^{-1} indicates a metabolic acidosis.

A base excess greater than +2 mmol l^{-1} indicates a metabolic alkalosis.

The respiratory - metabolic link

From the above we can see that the body has two systems for ensuring a stable internal environment and preventing the development of an acidosis. Additional protection is provided by the fact that the two systems are linked and can compensate for derangements in each other. This link is provided by the presence of carbonic acid (H_2CO_3), which is dependent on the presence of an enzyme called carbonic anhydrase, present in both red blood cells and the kidneys, and ideally situated to facilitate the link between the two systems.

$$CO_2 + H_2O \rightleftharpoons H_2CO_3 \rightleftharpoons H^+ + HCO_3^-$$

Although this link exists, the ability of each system to compensate for the other is not instantaneous, but becomes more marked when the initial disturbance in one system is prolonged. A typical example demonstrating the link between the two systems is a patient with chronic obstructive pulmonary disease (COPD). This condition results in diminished capacity to excrete carbon dioxide and a respiratory acidosis. If left uncompensated, this would result in a persistent acidaemia, but the increase in carbon dioxide drives the reaction above to the right, with the production of carbonic acid (H_2CO_3). In the kidneys this has the effect of increasing H^+ ions which are excreted in the urine while at the same time increasing bicarbonate production to buffer the H^+ ions in the plasma. As a result the patient has a respiratory acidosis (increased $PaCO_2$) with a compensatory metabolic alkalosis (increased bicarbonate) and the pH will return close to normal.

A different example is a diabetic in ketoacidosis (strictly speaking ketoacidaemia). When the excess ketoacids exceed the kidney's ability for excretion, they are buffered, which consumes plasma bicarbonate. Increasing bicarbonate production takes several days. However, the reaction above can also move to the left by increasing ventilation and reducing $PaCO_2$; in effect, converting the H^+ to CO_2. Consequently, the patient has a metabolic acidosis (reduced bicarbonate) with a compensatory respiratory alkalosis (reduced $PaCO_2$).

PaO_2

The concentration of oxygen in inspired air is 21% - representing a partial pressure of 21 kPa. This is gradually reduced as the air passes down the respiratory tract, firstly because of the addition of water vapour and, in the alveoli, by the addition of carbon dioxide so that here it is normally around 13 kPa. However, the partial pressure of oxygen in arterial blood (PaO_2) is always lower than alveolar; the extent of this gradient is determined largely by the presence of any lung disease. In a healthy individual breathing air, the PaO_2 is normally higher than 11 kPa i.e. about 10 kPa lower than the inspired partial pressure. This can be used as a rule of thumb to estimate the PaO_2 for any given inspired concentration, in that it should be numerically about 10 less than the inspired concentration (%). For example, 40% inspired oxygen should result in a PaO_2 of approximately 30 kPa. With increasing lung injury, the gap between inspired concentration and PaO_2 increases. This is important to recognise because for someone breathing 50% oxygen a PaO_2 of 13 kPa is not 'normal'.

Interestingly, PaO_2 also decreases slightly with age, reaching 10 kPa at around 75 years, but then climbs again and plateaus at around 11 kPa at 85 years.

Interpreting the results

Interpretation of the result of blood gas analysis is achieved best by following strictly five steps. For clarity, only changes in base excess are discussed; however, bicarbonate will also change numerically in the same direction.

ALS

Step 1

How is the patient? This will often provide useful clues to help with interpretation of the results. For example, one might reasonably predict that analysis of arterial blood shortly after successful resuscitation would show signs of a respiratory acidosis caused by a period of inadequate ventilation and a metabolic acidosis due to the period of anaerobic respiration during the arrest producing lactic acid. Consequently, we would expect the patient to have a very low pH with changes in both $PaCO_2$ and base excess. A patient with a well-compensated, chronic condition will usually display clues about the primary cause and secondary compensation. Without the clinical history, the results of a blood gas analysis from a patient with COPD could be misinterpreted as a primary metabolic alkalosis with a compensatory respiratory acidosis.

Step 2

Is the patient hypoxaemic?
The PaO_2 while breathing room air should be 10.0 - 13.0 kPa. However, if the patient is receiving supplemental oxygen, the PaO_2 must be interpreted in light of the inspired oxygen concentration. As discussed above, the inspired partial pressure of oxygen can be regarded as the numerical equivalent of the inspired concentration (%). If there is a difference of greater than 10 between the two values, there is a defect in oxygenation, proportional to the magnitude of the difference.

Step 3

Is the patient acidaemic (pH < 7.35) or alkalaemic (pH> 7.45)? If the pH is within or very close to the normal range then this suggests normality or a chronic condition with full compensation. In principle, the body never overcompensates and this should enable the primary problem to be determined. If necessary, seek more clinical information about the patient.

Step 4

What has happened to the PaCO₂? In other words, is the abnormality wholly or partially due to a defect in the respiratory system?

If the pH is <7.35 (acidaemia):
4a. Is the $PaCO_2$ increased (>6.0 kPa)?
If so, there is a **respiratory acidosis** that may be accounting for all or part of the derangement. There could also be a metabolic component, see Step 5a.

If the pH is > 7.45 (alkalaemia):
4b. Is the $PaCO_2$ reduced (<4.7 kPa)?
If so, there is a **respiratory alkalosis**, but this is an unusual isolated finding in a patient breathing spontaneously, with a normal respiratory rate. It is seen more often in patients who are being mechanically

ventilated with excessively high rates and/or tidal volumes. As a result, $PaCO_2$ decreases, there is a reduction in H^+ and an alkalosis develops.

Step 5

What has happened to the base excess or bicarbonate? In other words, is the abnormality wholly or partially due to a defect in the metabolic system?

If the pH is <7.35 (acidaemia):
5a. Is the base excess reduced (more negative than minus 2 mmol l⁻¹), and /or the bicarbonate reduced (<22 mmol l⁻¹)? If so, there is **a metabolic acidosis** accounting for all or part of the derangement. There could be a respiratory component if the $PaCO_2$ is also increased - see Step 4a, a situation commonly seen after a cardiac arrest.

If the pH is > 7.45 (alkalaemia):
5b. Is the base excess increased (> +2 mmol l⁻¹) and/or the bicarbonate increased (>26 mmol l⁻¹)?
If so, there is a **metabolic alkalosis** accounting for all or part of the derangement. There could be a respiratory component if the $PaCO_2$ is also decreased - see Step 4b, but this would be very unusual.

Example cases

Using the above, work through cases 1 - 3 at the end of this chapter. These are based on clinical cases to highlight key points.

Derangements of both PaCO₂ and base excess or bicarbonate - compensation

In addition to the combined changes seen in case 3, the results may show changes in both the respiratory and metabolic components, but with minimal disturbance of the pH. This is the result of compensation; both the respiratory and metabolic systems are capable of reacting to changes in the other, the aim being to minimise long term changes in pH. Four examples follow:

Example 1
pH <7.40, with a increased $PaCO_2$ (> 6.0 kPa) and increased base excess (>+2 mmol l⁻¹) or bicarbonate (>26 mmol l⁻¹).

The tendency towards an acidaemia indicates that this is the primary problem and the increased $PaCO_2$ indicates that it is a **respiratory acidosis**. The increased base excess/bicarbonate represents a **compensatory metabolic alkalosis,** bringing the pH back towards normality.

Example 2
pH <7.40, with a decreased base excess (<-2 mmol l⁻¹) or bicarbonate (<22 mmol l⁻¹) and decreased $PaCO_2$ (<4.7 kPa).

The tendency towards an acidaemia indicates that this is the primary problem and the decreased base excess/bicarbonate suggests that it is a **metabolic acidosis**. The decrease in $PaCO_2$ represents a **compensatory respiratory alkalosis,** bringing the pH back towards normality.

Example 3
pH > 7.40, with increased base excess (>+2 mmol l^{-1}) or bicarbonate (>26 mmol l^{-1}) and increased $PaCO_2$ (>6.0 kPa).

The tendency towards an alkalaemia indicates that this is the primary problem and the increase in base excess/bicarbonate suggests that it is primarily a **metabolic alkalosis**. The increased $PaCO_2$ is **respiratory compensation** bringing the pH back towards normality. This picture may be seen where there is loss of acid from the body e.g. prolonged vomiting of gastric contents (hydrochloric acid) and also occurs in chronic hypokalaemia. In this case, the body compensates by moving potassium from intracellular to extracellular in exchange for hydrogen ions. The pH increases and CO_2 is retained to try and compensate.

Example 4
pH > 7.40, with a decreased $PaCO_2$ (<4.7 kPa) and decreased base excess (<-2 mmol l^{-1}) or bicarbonate (<22 mmol l^{-1}).

The tendency towards an alkalaemia indicates that this is the primary problem and the decrease in $PaCO_2$ suggests that this is primarily a **respiratory alkalosis**. The decrease in base excess/bicarbonate is the **metabolic compensation** bringing the pH back towards normality. This is not a common finding, but may be seen after a few days when hyperventilation is used to help control intracranial pressure in patients with brain injury.

Using the above, work through cases 4 and 5 at the end of this chapter.

There is one final situation that deserves mention and is important to identify: an ill patient with a pH <7.4, a normal $PaCO_2$ (4 - 6.0 kPa) and a decreased base excess (<-2 mmol l^{-1}) or bicarbonate (< 22 mmol l^{-1}).

This is most likely to represent the situation of a metabolic acidosis in a patient with chronic carbon dioxide retention. The patient is trying to compensate by lowering their carbon dioxide (to cause a compensatory respiratory alkalosis), but they are starting from a higher $PaCO_2$. Their lung disease will limit the amount of CO_2 they can excrete, thereby preventing it decreasing any further. Once again it illustrates the importance of having information about the patient as identified at the beginning.

Practical aspects of blood gas analysis during resuscitation

During cardiac arrest, arterial blood gas values are of limited use because they correlate poorly with the severity of hypoxaemia, hypercarbia and acidosis in the tissues. Indeed, during cardiac arrest, venous blood gases may reflect more accurately the acid-base state of the tissues. These are interpreted using the same 5-step approach, however, the normal range of values will be different to arterial blood and they should be interpreted cautiously.

Once return of spontaneous circulation (ROSC) is achieved, arterial blood gas analysis will provide a useful guide to post cardiac arrest treatment, such as the optimal fractional inspired oxygen (FiO_2) and minute ventilation. Arterial lactate concentration can also be used to indicate adequacy of tissue oxygenation, normal arterial blood lactate concentration being 0.7 - 1.8 mmol l^{-1}. Immediately after cardiac arrest, concentrations are high, reflecting the lactic acidosis that has been caused by inadequate oxygenation of the tissues during the period of cardiac arrest. After ROSC a progressively decreasing lactate value is another indicator of adequate tissue oxygenation.

In the peri-arrest setting, it may be easiest to obtain a sample of arterial blood (into a heparinised syringe) from the femoral artery. The radial artery may be preferable once the patient has an adequate cardiac output and blood pressure. The radial artery is also the best site for insertion of an arterial cannula; this enables continuous monitoring of blood pressure and frequent blood sampling in the post cardiac arrest period.

Pulse oximetry

Role

Pulse oximetry is a vital adjunct to the assessment of hypoxaemia. Clinical recognition of decreased arterial oxygen saturation of haemoglobin (SaO_2) is subjective and unreliable, with the classic sign of cyanosis appearing late when arterial oxygen saturation is between 80 - 85%. Pulse oximetry is simple to use, relatively cheap, non-invasive and provides an immediate, objective measure of arterial blood oxygen saturation. It is now used widely in all in-hospital settings and increasingly in both primary care and the prehospital environment. Oxygen saturation, 'the fifth vital sign', now also forms a component of many early warning systems to identify the deteriorating patient.

Principles

The pulse oximeter probe containing light-emitting diodes (LEDs) and a photoreceptor situated opposite, is placed across tissue, usually a finger or earlobe. Some of the light is transmitted through the tissues while some is absorbed. The ratio of transmitted to absorbed light is used to generate the peripheral arterial oxygen saturation (SpO_2) displayed as a digital reading, waveform, or both. As a result of rapid sampling of the light signal, the displayed reading will alter every 0.5 - 1 s, displaying the average SpO_2 over the preceding 5 - 10 s. Most pulse oximeters are accurate to within +/- 2% above an SaO_2 of 90%.

ALS

Tissue thickness should be optimally between 5 - 10 mm. Poor readings may be improved by trying different sites, warming sites or applying local vasodilators.

Pulse oximeters often provide an audible tone related to the SpO$_2$, with a decreasing tone reflecting increasing degrees of hypoxaemia. Information about pulse rate and waveform (plethysmographic waveform) may also be provided. A poor signal may indicate a low blood pressure or poor tissue perfusion - reassess the patient.

Pulse oximetry provides only a measure of oxygen saturation, not content, and thus gives no indication of actual tissue oxygenation. Furthermore, it provides no information on the partial pressure of carbon dioxide in the body (PaCO$_2$) and is not a measure of adequacy of ventilation. In cases of critical illness, or when type II respiratory failure (see below) is suspected (e.g. known COPD, congenital heart disease) arterial blood gas sampling must be performed. Readings from a pulse oximeter must not be used in isolation: it is vital to interpret them in light of the clinical picture and alongside other investigations, and potential sources of error.

Limitations

The relationship between oxygen saturation and arterial oxygen partial pressure (PaO$_2$) is demonstrated by the oxyhaemoglobin dissociation curve (Figure 15.1). The sinusoid shape of the curve means that an initial decrease from a normal PaO$_2$ is not accompanied by a drop of similar magnitude in the oxygen saturation of the blood, and early hypoxaemia may be masked. At the point where the SpO$_2$ reaches 90-92%, the PaO$_2$ will have decreased to around 8 kPa. In other words, the partial pressure of oxygen in the arterial blood will have decreased by almost 50% despite a reduction in oxygen saturation of only 6-8%.

The output from a pulse oximeter relies on a comparison between current signal output and standardised reference data derived from healthy volunteers. Readings provided are thus limited by the scope of the population included in these studies, and become increasingly unreliable with increasing hypoxaemia. Below 70% the displayed values are highly unreliable.

There are several acknowledged sources of error with pulse oximetry:

- Presence of other haemoglobins: carboxyhaemoglobin (carbon monoxide poisoning), methaemoglobin (congenital or acquired), fetal haemoglobins and sickling red cells (sickle cell disease)

- Surgical and imaging dyes: methylene blue, indocyanine green and indigo carmine cause falsely low saturation readings

Oxygen dissociation curve

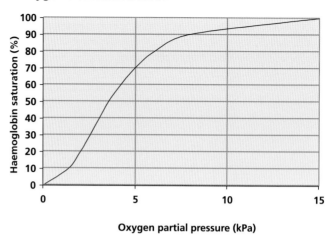

Figure 15.1 Oxyhaemoglobin dissociation curve

- Nail varnish (especially blue, black and green)

- High-ambient light levels (fluorescent and xenon lamps)

- Motion artefact

- Reduced pulse volume:

  - Hypotension

  - Low cardiac output

  - Vasoconstriction

  - Hypothermia

Pulse oximeters are not affected by:

- Anaemia (reduced haemoglobin)

- Jaundice (hyperbilirubinaemia)

- Skin pigmentation

Pulse oximetry does not provide a reliable signal during CPR.

Uses

Pulse oximetry has four main uses:

1. detection of/screening for hypoxaemia;

2. targeting oxygen therapy;

3. routine monitoring during anaesthesia;

4. diagnostic (e.g. sleep apnoea).

Targeted oxygen therapy

In critically ill patients, those presenting with acute hypoxaemia (initial SpO_2 < 85%), or in the peri-arrest situation, give high-concentration oxygen immediately. Give this initially with an oxygen mask and reservoir ('non-rebreathing' mask) and an oxygen flow of 15 l min^{-1}. During cardiac arrest use 100% inspired oxygen concentration to maximise arterial oxygen content and delivery to the tissues.

Once ROSC has been achieved and the oxygen saturation of arterial blood can be monitored reliably, adjust the inspired oxygen concentration to maintain a SpO_2 of 94 - 98%. If pulse oximetry (with a reliable reading) is unavailable, continue oxygen via a reservoir mask until definitive monitoring or assessment of oxygenation is available. All critically ill patients will need arterial blood gas sampling and analysis as soon as possible. Evidence suggests both hypoxaemia and hyperoxaemia (PaO_2 > 20 kPa) in the post-resuscitation phase may lead to worse outcomes than those in whom normoxaemia is maintained.

Special clinical situations

Patients with respiratory failure can be divided into two groups:

- Type I: low PaO_2 (< 8 kPa), normal $PaCO_2$ (< 6 - 7 kPa). In these patients it is safe to give a high concentration of oxygen initially with the aim of returning their PaO_2 to normal and then once clinically stable, adjusting the inspired oxygen concentration to maintain an SpO_2 of 94 - 98%.

- Type II: low PaO_2 (< 8 kPa), increased $PaCO_2$ (> 6 - 7 kPa). This is often described as hypercapnic respiratory failure and is usually caused by COPD. If given excessive oxygen, these patients may develop worsening respiratory failure with further increases in $PaCO_2$ and the development of a respiratory acidosis. If unchecked, this will eventually lead to unconsciousness, and respiratory and cardiac arrest. **The target oxygen saturation in this at risk population should be 88 - 92%.** However, when critically ill, give these patients high-flow oxygen initially; then analyse the arterial blood gases and use the results to adjust the inspired oxygen concentration. When clinically stable and a reliable pulse oximetry reading is obtained, adjust the inspired oxygen concentration to maintain an SpO_2 of 88 - 92%.

In patients with a myocardial infarction or an acute coronary syndrome, and who are not critically or seriously ill, aim to maintain an SpO_2 of 94 - 98% (or 88 - 92% if the patient is at risk of hypercapnic respiratory failure). This may be achievable without supplementary oxygen, and represents a change from previously accepted practice.

Key learning points

- The results of arterial blood gas analysis should be interpreted systematically using the 5-step approach.

- Pulse oximetry enables arterial blood oxygen saturation to be monitored continuously.

- During CPR use an inspired oxygen concentration of 100% until return of spontaneous circulation (ROSC) is achieved.

- After ROSC is achieved, and once the SpO_2 can be monitored reliably, titrate the inspired oxygen concentration to keep the SpO_2 in the range 94 - 98% (or 88 - 92% in patients at risk of hypercapnic respiratory failure).

Further reading

A Simple Guide to Blood Gas Analysis. Eds. Driscoll P, Brown T, Gwinnutt C, Wardle T. BMJ Publishing Group. London 1997.

O'Driscoll BR, Howard LS, Davison AG. BTS guideline for emergency oxygen use in adult patients. Thorax 2008;63 Suppl 6:vi1-68.

Example cases

Case 1:

21 year old woman, thrown from her horse at a local event. On the way to hospital, she has become increasingly drowsy and the paramedics have inserted an oropharyngeal airway and given high-flow oxygen via a face mask with a reservoir. On arrival at hospital, an arterial blood sample shows:

PaO_2	18.8 kPa (FiO_2 85%)
pH	7.19
$PaCO_2$	10.2 kPa
Bicarbonate	23.6 mmol l^{-1}
Base excess	-2.4 mmol l^{-1}

Step 1: From the history we would predict the reduction in level of consciousness to impair ventilation, decreasing oxygenation and increasing $PaCO_2$, causing a respiratory acidosis. There is unlikely to be much compensation because the situation is acute.

Step 2: Although the PaO_2 is just above the normal range, breathing 85% oxygen we would expect a PaO_2 around 75 kPa. Therefore there is a significant impairment in oxygenation.

Step 3: The patient clearly has an acidaemia with a pH well below normal.

Step 4: The $PaCO_2$ is increased, consistent with the low pH and the patient has a respiratory acidosis.

Step 5: The base excess is just below the normal limit and the bicarbonate is within normal limits. This confirms that there is no significant metabolic contribution or compensation.

In summary, the patient has an acute respiratory acidosis with impaired oxygenation.

Case 2:

A 19 year old man with asthma is bought to the emergency department (ED) by his parents. Over the past 4 h he has become increasingly wheezy with no response to his inhalers. He is now very distressed, tachypnoeic and has audible wheeze. He is receiving oxygen at 15 l min^{-1} via a face mask with reservoir and analysis of an arterial blood sample shows:

PaO_2	23.6 kPa (FiO_2 85%)
pH	7.57
$PaCO_2$	3.4 kPa
Bicarbonate	23.1 mmol l^{-1}
Base excess	+1.8 mmol l^{-1}

Step 1: From the history we would predict the bronchospasm to impair oxygenation and the hyperventilation to reduce his $PaCO_2$ causing a respiratory alkalosis. There is unlikely to be much compensation because the situation is acute.

Step 2: Although the PaO_2 is above the normal range, breathing 85% oxygen we would expect a PaO_2 around 75 kPa. Therefore there is a significant impairment in oxygenation.

Step 3: The patient clearly has an alkalaemia with a pH above the normal range.

Step 4: The $PaCO_2$ is decreased, consistent with the raised pH and the patient has a respiratory alkalosis.

Step 5: The base excess and bicarbonate are within normal limits. This confirms that there is no significant metabolic contribution or compensation.

In summary, the patient has an acute respiratory alkalosis with impaired oxygenation.

Case 3:

A 52 year old man, complaining of crushing central chest pain is bought to the ED by his wife. He is attached to an ECG monitor, given oxygen 40% by face mask, and sublingual GTN; an intravenous cannua is inserted and he is given aspirin and morphine. After about 5 minutes he suddenly has a cardiac arrest. After 4 minutes of resuscitation he has a palpable pulse and starts to breathe spontaneously. Analysis of an arterial blood sample shows:

PaO_2	8.9 kPa (FiO_2 40%)
pH	7.11
$PaCO_2$	7.2 kPa
Bicarbonate	14 mmol l^{-1}
Base excess	-10.6 mmol l^{-1}

Step 1: From the history we would predict the impaired ventilation to result in hypoxaemia, an increased $PaCO_2$ and respiratory acidosis. The impaired circulation will cause an increase in anaerobic respiration, production of lactate and a metabolic acidosis that will consume bicarbonate. The failure of circulation is likely to prevent any degree of compensation.

Step 2: The patient is hypoxaemic and breathing 40% oxygen. We would expect a PaO_2 around 30 kPa. Therefore there is a significant impairment in oxygenation.

Step 3: The patient clearly has a severe acidaemia, with a very low pH.

Step 4: The $PaCO_2$ is increased, consistent with the low pH and the patient has a respiratory acidosis.

Step 5: The base excess and bicarbonate are both reduced. This is consistent with a metabolic acidosis.

In summary, the patient has a mixed respiratory and metabolic acidosis with impaired oxygenation.

Case 4:

A 68 year old man with a long history of COPD is reviewed on the medical ward before discharge. Analysis of an arterial blood sample shows:

PaO_2	8.9 kPa (FiO_2 40%)
pH	7.34
$PaCO_2$	7.3 kPa
Bicarbonate	30.2 mmol l^{-1}
Base excess	5.3 mmol l^{-1}

Step 1: From the history we would predict the patient to have a chronically raised $PaCO_2$ causing a respiratory acidosis. However, there is likely to be significant compensation in the form of a metabolic alkalosis. Oxygenation is likely to be impaired.

Step 2: The PaO_2 is significantly reduced. Breathing 40% oxygen we would expect a PaO_2 around 30 kPa. Therefore there is a significant impairment in oxygenation.

Step 3: The patient has a borderline acidaemia with a pH just below the normal range.

Step 4: The $PaCO_2$ is increased, causing a respiratory acidosis. However, the increase is probably greater than we would expect from the minimal reduction in pH.

Step 5: The base excess and bicarbonate are both increased confirming that there is a metabolic alkalosis. This compensation has helped minimise or compensate for the pH disturbance caused by the respiratory acidosis.

In summary, the patient has a chronic respiratory acidosis with a compensatory metabolic alkalosis, with significantly impaired oxygenation.

Case 5:

A 22 year old male, recently diagnosed with insulin dependent diabetes mellitus presents to the ED having been unwell for 48 h and with a gradually increasing blood sugar concentration, despite taking his insulin. He is notably tachypnoeic and tachycardic and a point-of-care measurement of his blood glucose is 23 mmol l^{-1}. Analysis of an arterial blood sample while breathing oxygen, 6 l min^{-1} via a facemask shows:

PaO_2	22.2 kPa (FiO_2 40%)
pH	7.34
$PaCO_2$	3.8 kPa
Bicarbonate	19.1 mmol l^{-1}
Base excess	-7.9 mmol l^{-1}

Step 1: From the history the most likely problem is that the patient is developing a diabetic ketoacidosis i.e. a metabolic acidosis. However, the fact that he is tachypnoeic suggests that he is trying to compensate by reducing his $PaCO_2$. This will cause a respiratory alkalosis. If there are no abnormal signs in his chest, oxygenation should be relatively normal.

Step 2: Breathing 40% oxygen we would expect a PaO_2 around 30 kPa. However, with a tachypnoea, the facemask is probably delivering less than 40% oxygen and so his oxygenation is unimpaired.

Step 3: The patient has a borderline acidaemia with a pH just below the normal range.

Step 4: The $PaCO_2$ is decreased, causing a respiratory alkalosis and therefore not the cause of the primary disturbance.

Step 5: The base excess and bicarbonate are both decreased confirming that there is a metabolic acidosis. However, the pH is not as low as would be expected for this degree of change.

In summary, the patient has a metabolic acidosis (as a result of impaired glucose metabolism and the production of ketoacids) with a compensatory respiratory alkalosis.

ALS

Decisions Relating to Resuscitation

CHAPTER 16

Learning outcomes

To understand:

▶ **Ethical principles**

▶ **Advance decisions to refuse treatment**

▶ **When not to start cardiopulmonary resuscitation (CPR)**

▶ **Discussing CPR decisions with patients and those close to them**

▶ **Who should make decisions about CPR**

▶ **When to stop resuscitation attempts**

Introduction

Successful resuscitation attempts have brought extended, useful and precious life to many individuals. However, only a minority of people survive and make a complete recovery after attempted resuscitation from cardiac arrest. Attempted resuscitation carries a risk of causing suffering and prolonging the process of dying. It is not an appropriate goal of medicine to prolong life at all costs. Ideally, decisions about whether or not it is appropriate to start cardiopulmonary resuscitation (CPR) should be made in advance, as part of the overall concept of advance care planning. Detailed guidance has been published by the British Medical Association (BMA), Resuscitation Council (UK) {RC(UK)} and Royal College of Nursing (RCN) and also by the General Medical Council (GMC). As an ALS provider, you should read and be familiar with that guidance and follow the principles that it contains.

It is incumbent on all healthcare practitioners to practice within the law. The law as it relates to CPR varies from country to country. Even within the UK there are some differences between countries. This is addressed within the joint statement by the BMA, RC(UK) and RCN. As an ALS provider you should be familiar with the relevant aspects of law in the country where you live and work. Guidance on the legal status of those who attempt resuscitation has been published by the RC(UK).

Discussing decisions about CPR can be difficult and distressing for patients and relatives, and for healthcare providers. These decisions may be influenced by various factors including personal beliefs and opinions, cultural or religious influences, ethical and legal considerations, and by social or economic circumstances. Some patients with capacity decide that they do not want treatment and record their wishes in an advance decision to refuse treatment (formerly known as 'living wills'). As an ALS provider you should understand the ethical and legal principles as well as the clinical aspects involved before undertaking discussions or making a decision about CPR.

Principles

The four key principles of medical ethics are summarised in the box:

> **Beneficence** requires provision of benefit while balancing benefit and risks. Commonly this will involve attempting CPR but if risks clearly outweigh any likely benefit it will mean withholding CPR. Beneficence includes also responding to the overall needs of the community, such as establishing a programme of public access defibrillation.
>
> **Non-maleficence** means doing no harm. CPR should not be attempted in people in whom it will not succeed, where no benefit is likely but there is a clear risk of harm.
>
> **Justice** implies a duty to spread benefits and risks equally within a society. If CPR is provided, it should be available to all who may benefit from it; there should be no discrimination purely on the grounds of factors such as age or disability.
>
> **Autonomy** relates to people making their own informed decisions rather than healthcare professionals making decisions for them. Autonomy requires that a person with capacity is adequately informed, is free from undue pressure, and that there is consistency in their preferences.

Advance decisions to refuse CPR

Advance decisions to refuse treatment have been introduced in many countries and emphasise the importance of patient autonomy. Resuscitation must not be attempted if CPR is contrary to the recorded, sustained wishes of an adult who had capacity and was aware of the implications at the time of making that advance decision. However, it is important to ensure that an advance decision is valid and that the circumstances in which the decision is applied are those that were envisaged or defined at the time that it was made.

The term 'advance decision' may apply to any expression of patient preferences. Refusal does not have to be in writing in order to be valid. If patients have expressed clear and consistent refusal verbally, this is likely to have the same status as a written advance decision. People should ensure that their healthcare team and those close to them are aware of their wishes.

In sudden out-of-hospital cardiac arrest, those attending usually do not know the patient's situation and wishes and, even if an advance decision has been recorded, it may not be available. In these circumstances CPR can be started immediately and any further information obtained when possible. There is no ethical difficulty in stopping a resuscitation attempt that has started if the healthcare professionals are presented later with a valid advance decision refusing the treatment that has been started.

There is still considerable international variation in the medical attitude to written advance decisions. In some countries, such as the UK, a written advance decision is legally binding. Where no explicit advance decision has been made and the express wishes of the patient are unknown there is a presumption that healthcare professionals will, if appropriate, make all reasonable efforts to resuscitate the patient.

When to withhold CPR

While patients have a right to refuse treatment, they do not have an automatic right to demand treatment; they cannot insist that resuscitation must be attempted in any circumstance. Doctors cannot be required to give treatment that is contrary to their clinical judgement. This type of decision is often complex and should be undertaken by senior, experienced members of the medical team.

The decision to make no resuscitation attempt raises several ethical and moral questions. What constitutes futility? What exactly should be withheld? Who should decide and who should be consulted? Who should be informed?

What constitutes futility?

Futility may be considered to exist if resuscitation will not prolong life of a quality that would be acceptable to the patient. Although predictors of non-survival after attempted resuscitation have been published, none has sufficient predictive value when applied to an independent validation group. Furthermore, the outcome for a cohort undergoing attempted resuscitation is dependent on system factors such as time to CPR and time to defibrillation. It is difficult to predict how these factors will impact on the outcome of individuals.

Inevitably, judgements will have to be made, and there will be grey areas where subjective opinions are required in patients with comorbidity such as heart failure, chronic respiratory disease, asphyxia, major trauma, head injury and neurological disease. The age of the patient may feature in the decision but is only a relatively weak independent predictor of outcome; however, the elderly commonly have significant comorbidity, which influences outcome.

What exactly should be withheld?

Do not attempt resuscitation (DNAR) means that in the event of cardiac or respiratory arrest, CPR should not be started - nothing more than that. Other treatment should be continued, including pain relief and sedation, as required. Treatment such as ventilation and oxygen therapy, nutrition, antibiotics, fluid and vasopressors, is also continued as indicated. If not, orders not to continue or initiate any such treatments should be made independently of DNAR orders.

In the past, in many countries, doctors would make a DNAR decision without consulting with the patient, the relatives, or other members of the health care team. Many countries have now published clear guidelines on how these decisions should be taken. In most cases, this guidance emphasises involvement by the patient and/or relatives.

Who should decide not to attempt resuscitation and who should be consulted?

The overall responsibility for this decision rests with the senior healthcare professional in charge of the patient after appropriate consultation with other healthcare professionals involved in the patient's care.

People have ethical and legal rights to be involved in decisions that relate to them and if the patient has capacity their views should be sought unless there is a clearly justifiable reason to indicate otherwise. It is not necessary to initiate discussion about CPR with every patient, for example if there is no reason to expect cardiac arrest to occur, or if the patient is in the final stage of an irreversible illness in which CPR would be inappropriate as it would offer no benefit.

It is good practice to involve relatives in decisions although they have no legal status in terms of actual decision-making. A patient with capacity should give their consent before involving the family in a DNAR discussion. Refusal from a patient with capacity to allow information to be disclosed to relatives must be respected.

If patients who lack capacity have previously appointed a welfare attorney with power to make such decisions on their behalf, that person must be consulted when a decision has to be made balancing the risks and burdens of CPR. There are slight differences in the law relating to patients who lack capacity in England & Wales, in Scotland and in Northern Ireland, so it is essential to be familiar with the law that applies in your locality.

In some circumstances there are legal requirements to involve others in the decision-making process when a patient lacks capacity. For example the Mental Capacity Act 2005, which applies in England and Wales requires appointment of an Independent Mental Capacity Advocate (IMCA) to act on behalf of the patient who lacks capacity. However, when decisions have to be made in an emergency, there may not be time to appoint and contact an IMCA and decisions must be made in the patient's best interests, and the basis for such decisions documented clearly and fully.

When differences of opinion occur between the healthcare team and the patient or their representatives these can usually be resolved with careful discussion and explanation, or if necessary by obtaining a second clinical opinion. In general, decisions by legal authorities are often fraught with delays and uncertainties, especially if there is an adversarial legal system, and formal legal judgement should be sought only if there are irreconcilable differences between the parties involved. In particularly difficult cases, the senior doctor may wish to consult his/her own medical defence society for a legal opinion.

Who should be informed?

Once the decision has been made it must be communicated clearly to all who may be involved, including the patient. Unless the patient refuses, the decision should also be communicated to the patient's relatives. The decision, the reasons for it, and a record of who has been involved in the discussions should be recorded in the medical notes - ideally on a special DNAR form - and should clearly document the date the decision was made. The decision should be recorded in the nursing records, if these are separate. The decision must be communicated to all those involved in the patient's care.

Communicating decisions about CPR to patients and those close to them

Whilst it is generally advisable to explain to patients and those close to them any decisions that have been taken about their treatment, and the reasons for those decisions, it is important that this is not done without careful consideration. This topic is also covered in the BMA, RC(UK) and RCN joint statement, which emphasises that it is not necessary to inform every patient about a decision not to attempt CPR because it would not be successful, where discussing that decision would be unnecessarily distressing and of little or no value to the patient. Any discussion with those close to patients must respect the patient's wishes in relation to confidentiality.

Communicating decisions about CPR to the healthcare team

Good communication within the team is an essential component of high quality, safe healthcare. When a decision is made not to attempt CPR, the basis for that decision, details of those involved in making it, and details of discussions with patients and those close to them should

be recorded. The decision itself should be recorded in a way that is immediately available and recognisable to those present, should the patient suffer sudden cardiac arrest. The RC(UK) has defined standards for the recording of decisions relating to CPR and has developed a model form for recording decisions not to attempt CPR in any individual. Such decisions were referred to at one time as 'Do Not Resuscitate' (DNR) decisions. DNR was replaced by DNAR ('Do Not Attempt Resuscitation') to emphasise the reality that many resuscitation attempts will not be successful. Unfortunately some healthcare providers have mistakenly and inappropriately interpreted the recording of these decisions as indicating that other treatment can or should be withheld. To discourage this it has been suggested that the term DNACPR should be used, to try to emphasise that the recorded decision refers only to the use of CPR and not to any other aspect of treatment that the patient may need. As an ALS provider you should ensure that you record decisions about CPR fully, clearly and accurately, and that these decisions do not (through your actions or those of others) lead to withholding from patients other treatment that they may need. Whilst the term 'DNAR' is used throughout RC(UK) material, it is interchangeable and identical in definition with the term 'DNACPR' which is also in common use.

When to stop CPR

Most of resuscitation attempts do not succeed and in those that are unsuccessful a decision has to be made to stop CPR. This decision can be made when it is clear that continuing CPR will not be successful. Factors influencing the decision will include the patient's medical history and prognosis, the cardiac arrest rhythm that is present, the response or lack of response to initial resuscitation measures, and the duration of the resuscitation attempt (particularly if the rhythm is asystole - see below). Sometimes, during a resuscitation attempt, further information becomes available that was not known at the time CPR was started, and that indicates that further CPR will not succeed. It is appropriate to stop CPR in those circumstances.

In general, CPR should be continued as long as a shockable rhythm or other reversible cause for cardiac arrest persists. It is generally accepted that asystole for more than 20 min in the absence of a reversible cause (see below), and with all advanced life support measures in place, is unlikely to respond to further CPR and is a reasonable basis for stopping CPR.

A decision to abandon CPR is made by the team leader, but this should be after consultation with the other team members. Ultimately, the decision is based on a clinical judgement that further advanced life support will not re-start the heart and breathing.

Decision making by non-doctors

Many cases of out-of-hospital cardiac arrest are attended by emergency medical technicians or paramedics, who face similar dilemmas about when CPR will not succeed and when it should be stopped. In general CPR will be started in out-of-hospital cardiac arrest unless there is a valid advance decision refusing it or a valid DNAR order or it is clear that CPR would be futile, for example, in cases of mortal injuries such as decapitation or hemicorporectomy, known prolonged submersion, incineration, rigor mortis, and dependent lividity. In such cases, the non-doctor can identify that death has occurred but does not certify the cause of death (which in most countries can be done only by a physician or coroner).

But when should a decision be made to abandon a resuscitation attempt? For example, should ALS trained paramedics be able to declare death when the patient remains in asystole after 20 min despite ALS interventions? In some countries, including the UK, paramedics may cease a resuscitation attempt in this situation. Their strict protocol requires that certain conditions that might indicate a remote chance of survival (e.g. hypothermia) are absent. The presence of asystole must also be established beyond reasonable doubt and documented on ECG recordings (see Chapter 14).

Similar decisions about initiating resuscitation or recognising that death has occurred and is irreversible may be made by experienced nurses, working in the community or in establishments that provide care for people who are terminally or chronically ill. Whenever possible in such settings, decisions about CPR should be considered before they are needed, as part of advance care planning. In some situations it will be appropriate for experienced nurses to undertake any necessary discussions and to make and record a DNAR order on behalf of the patient and their healthcare team.

Special circumstances

Certain circumstances, e.g. hypothermia at the time of cardiac arrest, will enhance the chances of recovery without neurological damage. In such situations do not use the usual prognostic criteria (such as asystole persisting for more than 20 min) and continue CPR until the reversible problem has been corrected (e.g. re warming has been achieved).

Withdrawal of other treatment after a resuscitation attempt

Prediction of the likely clinical and neurological outcome in people who remain unconscious after regaining a spontaneous circulation is difficult during the first 3 days. In general, other supportive treatment should be continued during this period, after which the prognosis can be assessed with greater confidence. This topic is covered in more detail in Chapter 13.

Key learning points

- In the event of cardiac arrest, CPR should be started promptly and effectively.

- If a valid advance decision refusing CPR has been made, do not attempt CPR.

- When CPR will not re-start the heart and breathing, CPR is not appropriate.

- If continuing CPR will not be successful, make the decision to stop.

- Decisions relating to CPR should be made carefully, recorded fully, and communicated effectively.

- Decisions relating to CPR should not prevent patients from receiving any other treatment needed.

Further reading

Baskett PJ, Lim A. The varying ethical attitudes towards resuscitation in Europe. Resuscitation 2004;62:267-73.

British Medical Association, Resuscitation Council (UK) and Royal College of Nursing. Decisions relating to cardiopulmonary resuscitation. 2007. www.resus.org.uk

General Medical Council. Treatment and care towards the end of life. 2010. www.gmc-uk.org

Lippert FK, Raffay V, Georgiou M, Steen PA, Bossaert L. European Resuscitation Council Guidelines for Resuscitation 2010. Section 10. The ethics of resuscitation and end-of-life decisions. Resuscitation 2010;81: 1445-51.

Resuscitation Council (UK). The legal status of those who attempt resuscitation. 2010. www.resus.org.uk

Supporting the Relative in Resuscitation Practice

Throughout this chapter, the term 'relatives' includes close friends/significant others.

Introduction

In many cases of out-of-hospital cardiac arrest, the person who performs CPR will be a close friend or relative and they may wish to remain with the patient.

Many relatives find it more distressing to be separated from their family member during these critical moments than to witness attempts at resuscitation. In keeping with the move to more open clinical practice, healthcare professionals should take the preferences of patients and relatives into account.

If the resuscitation attempt fails, relatives perceive a number of advantages of being present during resuscitation:

- It helps them come to terms with the reality of death, avoiding prolonged denial and contributing to a healthier bereavement.

- The relative can speak while there is still a chance that the dying person can hear.

- They are not distressed by being separated from a loved one at a time when they feel the need to be present.

- They can see that everything possible was done for the dying person, which assists with their understanding of the reality of the situation.

- They can touch and speak with the deceased whilst the body is warm.

There are potential disadvantages of relatives being present:

- The resuscitation attempt may prove distressing, particularly if the relatives are not kept informed.

- Relatives can physically, or emotionally, hinder the staff involved in the resuscitation attempt. Observed actions or remarks by medical or nursing staff may offend grieving family members.

- Relatives may be disturbed by the memory of events, although evidence indicates that fantasy is worse than fact. The staff should take into account the expectations of the bereaved and their cultural background during and following death.

- Relatives may demonstrate their emotions vocally or physically whilst others may wish to sit quietly or read religious text. The staff must have sufficient insight, knowledge and skills to anticipate these needs and identify potential problems.

The involvement of relatives and friends

Care and consideration of the relative during resuscitation becomes increasingly important as procedures become more invasive. Support should be provided by an appropriately qualified healthcare professional whose responsibility is to care for family members witnessing cardiopulmonary resuscitation. The following safeguards should be used:

- Acknowledge the difficulty of the situation. Ensure that they understand that they have a choice of whether or not to be present during resuscitation. Avoid provoking feelings of guilt whatever their decision.

- Explain that they will be looked after whether or not they decide to witness the resuscitation attempt. Ensure that introductions are made and names are known.

- Give a clear explanation of what has happened in terms of the illness or injury and what they can expect to see when they enter the resuscitation area.

- Ensure that the relatives understand that they will be able to leave and return at any time, and will always be accompanied.

- Ask the relative not to interfere with the resuscitation process but offer them the opportunity to touch the patient when they are told that it is safe to do so.

- Explain the nature of the procedures in simple terms. If resuscitation is unsuccessful, explain why the attempt has been stopped.

If the patient dies, advise the relatives that there may be a brief interval while equipment is removed, after which they can return to be together in private. Under some circumstances, the coroner may require certain equipment to be left in place. Offer the relatives time to think about what has happened and the opportunity for further questions.

Hospitals should develop policies to enable relatives to observe the attempted resuscitation of their loved one.

Caring for the recently bereaved

Caring for the bereaved compassionately will ease the grieving process. Adapt the following considerations to the individual family and their cultural needs:

- early contact with one person, usually a nurse;

- provision of a suitable area for the relatives to wait, e.g. relatives' room;

- breaking bad news sympathetically and supporting the grief response appropriately;

- arranging for relatives to view the body;

- religious and pastoral care requirements;

- legal and practical arrangements;

- follow up and team support.

Early contact with one person

Ideally this should be the person who has supported the relatives during the resuscitation attempt. If the resuscitation attempt was not observed allocate a member of the care team specifically to support the relatives. Communication between the emergency services and the receiving hospital should ensure that the arrival of relatives is anticipated for an out-of-hospital arrest. A warm, friendly and confident greeting will help to establish an open and honest relationship.

Provision of a suitable room

This should provide the appropriate ambience, space and privacy for relatives to ask questions and to express their emotions freely.

Breaking bad news and supporting the grief response

An uncomplicated and honest approach will help avoid mixed messages. The most appropriate person (not necessarily a doctor) should break the bad news to the relatives. It may be more appropriate for the nurse who has been accompanying the relatives to break the news,

although relatives may take comfort from talking to a doctor as well and this opportunity should always be offered. When preparing to talk to the relatives, consider the following:

- Prepare yourself mentally and physically. Check your clothing for blood, wash your hands and tidy your clothing.

- Confirm that you are talking with the correct relatives and establish their relationship to the deceased. Briefly establish what they know and use this as the basis for your communication with them.

- Use tone of voice and non-verbal behaviour to support what you are saying. Smiles, nods, eye contact, the use of touch, facial expression and gestures can help support verbal communication.

- Use simple words and avoid medical jargon and platitudes that will be meaningless to the relative.

- Sit or position yourself next to the relative so that you are on the same level.

- Do not enter into a long preamble or start to question the relative about issues such as premorbid health. They want to know immediately whether their loved one is alive or dead.

- Introduce the word "dead", "died" or "death" at the earliest moment and reinforce this on at least one further occasion, so that there is no ambiguity.

- After breaking the news, do not be afraid to allow a period of silence while the facts are absorbed.

- Anticipate the different types of reaction/emotional response you may experience after breaking the bad news.

Possible responses to grief include:

- Acute emotional distress/shock

- Anger

- Denial/disbelief

- Guilt

- Catatony.

These stages are not linear and individuals may move from one to another, returning to some repeatedly. An individual's gender, age and cultural background will influence the response to grief. Respect cultural requirements and, where possible, provide written guidelines for individual ethnic groups.

Arranging viewing of the body

Many newly bereaved relatives value the opportunity to view their loved ones. Their experience is likely to be affected by whether the deceased appears in a presentable condition. Advise relatives what to expect before viewing the body. People are less concerned about medical devices and equipment than is generally believed. If the deceased has mutilating injuries, warn the relatives. Being in the physical presence of their loved one will help them work through the grieving process. Ensure the opportunity to touch/hold the deceased is given. Staff should accompany relatives during the viewing process and they should remain near by to offer support or provide information as required.

Religious requirements, legal and practical arrangements

Variations in handling the body and expressions of grief are influenced by the patient's religious convictions. The resuscitation team should take into account the beliefs, values and rituals of the patient and the family. There is an increasing emphasis on the need for care practice to be culturally sensitive, as a way of valuing and respecting the cultural and religious needs of patients. Religious representatives from the patient's denomination or faith are usually available to attend in hospital. Hospital chaplains are a great source of strength and information to families and staff. Prayers, blessings, religious acts and procedure are all important in ensuring that relatives are not distressed further.

Legal and practical arrangements are equally important. These include:

- notification of the coroner or other appropriate authority;

- notification of the patient's family doctor;

- organ donation decisions;

- provision of information about what to do in the event of death;

- involvement of religious ministers;

- adhere to hospital procedure in the return of patients property and valuables;

- information concerning the social services that are available;

- information concerning post mortem examination where indicated;

- follow-up arrangements, which may involve long-term counselling;

- provision of a telephone contact number for relatives to use and a named staff member who they can call should they have any further questions.

Staff support and debriefing

When possible, make arrangements for staff to discuss with the team leader and the rest of the team issues that emerged from the resuscitation event. This is an extremely powerful educational tool.

Key learning points

- Many relatives want the opportunity to be present during the attempted resuscitation of their loved one. This may help the grieving process.

- Communication with bereaved relatives should be honest, simple, and supportive.

Further reading

Adams S, Whitlock M, Bloomfield P, Baskett PJF. Should relatives watch resuscitation? BMJ 1994;308:1687-9.

Axelsson A, Zettergren M, Axelsson C. Good and bad experiences of family presence during acute care and resuscitation. What makes the difference? Eur J Cardiovasc Nurs 2005;4:161-9.

Kent H, McDowell J. Sudden bereavement in acute care settings. Nursing Standard 2004;19:6.

McMahon-Parkes, K: Moule, P; Benger, J The views and preferences of resuscitated and non resuscitated patients towards family witnessed resuscitation : a qualitative study. International Journal Nursing Studies. 2009; 46 (2): 220-229.

Moons P European Nursing Organizations stand up for family presence during cardiopulmonary resuscitation: A joint position statement. International perspectives on cardiovascular nursing 2008:136 -139.

Resuscitation Council (UK). Should relatives witness resuscitation? London, Resuscitation Council (UK), 1996.

Royal College of Nursing. Witnessing Resuscitation: Guidance for Nursing Staff. Royal College of Nursing, London, April 2002.

Watts, J Death, Dying and Bereavement: Issues for practice. Dunedin 2010.

ALS

ALS

Appendix A Drugs Used in the Treatment of Cardiac Arrest

Drug	Shockable (VF/Pulseless VT)	Non-Shockable (PEA/Asystole)
Adrenaline	• Dose: 1 mg (10 ml 1:10,000 or 1 ml 1:1,000) IV • Given after the 3rd shock once compressions have been resumed • Repeated every 3 - 5 min (alternate loops) • Give without interrupting chest compressions	• Dose: 1 mg (10 ml 1:10,000 or 1 ml 1:1,000) IV • Given as soon as circulatory access is obtained • Repeated every 3 - 5 min (alternate loops) • Give without interrupting chest compressions
	Adrenaline has been the primary sympathomimetic drug for the management of cardiac arrest for 40 years. Its alpha-adrenergic effects cause systemic vasoconstriction, which increases coronary and cerebral perfusion pressures. The beta-adrenergic actions of adrenaline (inotropic, chronotropic) may increase coronary and cerebral blood flow, but concomitant increases in myocardial oxygen consumption and ectopic ventricular arrhythmias (particularly in the presence of acidaemia), transient hypoxaemia because of pulmonary arteriovenous shunting, impaired microcirculation, and increased post cardiac arrest myocardial dysfunction may offset these benefits. Although there is no evidence of long-term benefit from the use of adrenaline, the improved short-term survival documented in some studies warrants its continued use.	
Amiodarone	• Dose: 300 mg bolus IV • Given after the 3rd shock once compressions have been resumed • Further dose of 150 mg if VF/VT persists	• Not indicated for PEA or asystole
	Amiodarone is a membrane-stabilising anti-arrhythmic drug that increases the duration of the action potential and refractory period in atrial and ventricular myocardium. Atrioventricular conduction is slowed, and a similar effect is seen with accessory pathways. Amiodarone has a mild negative inotropic action and causes peripheral vasodilation through non-competitive alpha-blocking effects. The hypotension that occurs with intravenous amiodarone is related to the rate of delivery and is caused by the solvent, rather than the drug itself. Amiodarone should be flushed with 0.9% sodium chloride or 5% dextrose. When amiodarone is unavailable, consider an initial dose of 100 mg (1 - 1.5 mg kg^{-1}) of lidocaine for VF/VT refractory to three shocks. Give an additional bolus of 50 mg if necessary. The total dose should not exceed 3 mg kg^{-1} during the first hour.	
Magnesium	• Dose: 2 g given peripherally IV • May be repeated after 10 - 15 min • Indicated for VT, torsade de pointes, or digoxin toxicity associated with hypomagnesaemia	• Dose: 2 g given peripherally IV • May be repeated after 10 - 15 min • Indicated for supraventricular tachycardia or digoxin toxicity associated with hypomagnesaemia
	Magnesium facilitates neurochemical transmission: it decreases acetylcholine release and reduces the sensitivity of the motor endplate. Magnesium also improves the contractile response of the stunned myocardium, and may limit infarct size.	

Drug	Shockable (VF/Pulseless VT)	Non-Shockable (PEA/Asystole)
Calcium	• Dose: 10 ml 10% calcium chloride (6.8 mmol Ca^{2+}) IV • Indicated for PEA caused specifically by hyperkalaemia, hypocalcaemia or overdose of calcium channel blocking drugs	
	Calcium plays a vital role in the cellular mechanisms underlying myocardial contraction. High plasma concentrations achieved after injection may be harmful to the ischaemic myocardium and may impair cerebral recovery. Do not give calcium solutions and sodium bicarbonate simultaneously by the same route.	

Sodium Bicarbonate	• Dose: 50 mmol (50 ml of an 8.4% solution) IV
	
	• Routine use not recommended
	
	• Consider sodium bicarbonate in shockable and non-shockable rhythms for
	
	    ○ cardiac arrest associated with hyperkalaemia
	
	    ○ tricyclic overdose.
	
	Repeat the dose as necessary, but use acid-base analysis to guide therapy.	

	Cardiac arrest results in combined respiratory and metabolic acidosis as pulmonary gas exchange ceases and cellular metabolism becomes anaerobic. The best treatment of acidaemia in cardiac arrest is chest compression; some additional benefit is gained by ventilation. Bicarbonate causes generation of carbon dioxide, which diffuses rapidly into cells. This has the following effects: • it exacerbates intracellular acidosis; • it produces a negative inotropic effect on ischaemic myocardium; • it presents a large, osmotically-active sodium load to an already compromised circulation and brain; • it produces a shift to the left in the oxygen dissociation curve, further inhibiting release of oxygen to the tissues. Do not give calcium solutions and sodium bicarbonate simultaneously by the same route.	
Fluids	Infuse fluids rapidly if hypovolaemia is suspected. During resuscitation, there are no clear advantages in using colloid, so use 0.9% sodium chloride or Hartmann's solution. Avoid dextrose, which is redistributed away from the intravascular space rapidly and causes hyperglycaemia, which may worsen neurological outcome after cardiac arrest.	
Thrombolytics	• Tenecteplase 500 - 600 mcg kg^{-1} IV bolus • Alteplase (r-tPA) 50 mg IV bolus (British Thoracic Society guidelines for the management of suspected acute pulmonary embolism. Thorax 2003;58:470–484)	
	Fibrinolytic therapy should not be used routinely in cardiac arrest. Consider fibrinolytic therapy when cardiac arrest is caused by proven or suspected acute pulmonary embolus. If a fibrinolytic drug is given in these circumstances, consider performing CPR for at least 60 - 90 min before termination of resuscitation attempts. Ongoing CPR is not a contraindication to fibrinolysis.	

Appendix B Drugs Used in the Peri-arrest Period

Drug	Indication	Dose
Adenosine	• Paroxysmal SVT with re-entrant circuits that include the atrioventricular (AV) node (AVNRT and AVRT)	• 6 mg IV bolus • If unsuccessful, give up to two doses of 12 mg after 1 - 2 min intervals
	Adenosine is a naturally occurring purine nucleotide. It blocks transmission through the AV node but has little effect on other myocardial cells or conduction pathways. It has an extremely short half-life of 10 - 15 s and, therefore, is given as a rapid bolus into a fast running intravenous infusion or followed by a saline flush. Warn patients of transient unpleasant side effects; in particular, nausea, flushing, and chest discomfort. It is contraindicated in patients with asthma.	
Adrenaline	• Second-line treatment for cardiogenic shock • Bradycardia (alternative to external pacing) • Anaphylaxis	• 0.05 - 1 mcg kg^{-1} min^{-1} • 2 - 10 mcg min^{-1} • See Chapter 12
	An adrenaline infusion is indicated in the post-resuscitation period when less potent inotropic drugs (e.g. dobutamine) have failed to increase cardiac output adequately. It is indicated also for bradycardia associated with adverse signs and/or risk of asystole, which has not responded to atropine, if external pacing is unavailable or unsuccessful.	
Amiodarone	• Control of haemodynamically stable monomorphic VT, polymorphic VT and wide-complex tachycardia of uncertain origin • To control a rapid ventricular rate caused by accessory pathway conduction in pre-excited atrial arrhythmias (e.g. AF) and/or achieve chemical cardioversion • After unsuccessful electrical cardioversion, to achieve chemical cardioversion or to increase the likelihood of further electrical cardioversion succeeding	• 300 mg IV over 10 - 60 min (depending on haemodynamic stability of patient) • Followed by 900 mg over 24 h
	Intravenous amiodarone has effects on sodium, potassium and calcium channels as well as alpha- and beta-adrenergic blocking properties. In patients with severely impaired heart function, intravenous amiodarone is preferable to other anti-arrhythmic drugs for atrial and ventricular tachyarrhythmias. Major adverse effects (caused by the solvent, not the active drug) are hypotension and bradycardia, which can be minimised by slowing the rate of drug infusion. Whenever possible, intravenous amiodarone should be given via a central venous catheter; it causes thrombophlebitis when infused into a peripheral vein, but in an emergency it can be injected into a large peripheral vein.	

Drug	Indication	Dose
Aspirin	• Acute coronary syndromes	• 300 mg oral loading dose followed by 75 mg daily
	Aspirin improves the prognosis of patients with acute coronary syndromes, significantly reducing cardiovascular death. The efficacy of aspirin is achieved by anti-platelet activity and preventing early platelet thrombus formation.	
Atropine	• Sinus, atrial, or nodal bradycardia or AV block, when the haemodynamic condition of the patient is unstable because of the bradycardia.	• 500 mcg IV • Repeated doses to maximum of 3 mg
	Atropine antagonises the action of the parasympathetic neurotransmitter acetylcholine at muscarinic receptors. Therefore, it blocks the effect of the vagus nerve on both the sinoatrial (SA) node and the AV node, increasing sinus automaticity and facilitating AV node conduction. Side effects of atropine are dose-related (blurred vision, dry mouth and urinary retention). It can cause acute confusion, particularly in elderly patients. Asystole during cardiac arrest is usually caused by primary myocardial pathology rather than excessive vagal tone and there is no evidence that routine use of atropine is beneficial in the treatment of asystole or PEA.	
Beta-adrenoceptor blockers	• Narrow-complex regular tachycardias uncontrolled by vagal manoeuvres or adenosine in patients with preserved ventricular function • To control rate in atrial fibrillation (AF) and atrial flutter when ventricular function is preserved.	*Atenolol (beta$_1$)* • 5 mg IV over 5 min, repeated if necessary after 10 min *Metoprolol (beta$_1$)* • 2 - 5 mg IV at 5-min intervals to a total of 15 mg *Propranolol (beta$_1$ and beta$_2$ effects)* • 100 mcg kg^{-1} IV slowly in three equal doses at 2 - 3 min intervals *Esmolol* • short-acting (half-life of 2 - 9 min) beta$_1$-selective beta-blocker • IV loading dose of 500 mcg kg^{-1} over 1 min • followed by an infusion of 50 - 200 mcg kg^{-1} min^{-1}
	Beta blocking drugs reduce the effects of circulating catecholamines and decrease heart rate and blood pressure. They also have cardioprotective effects for patients with acute coronary syndromes. Side effects of beta blockade include bradycardia, AV conduction delay, hypotension and bronchospasm. Contraindications to the use of beta-adrenoceptor blocking drugs include second- or third-degree heart block, hypotension, severe congestive heart failure and lung disease associated with bronchospasm.	
Verapamil	• Stable regular narrow-complex tachycardias uncontrolled or unconverted by vagal manoeuvres or adenosine • To control ventricular rate in patients with AF or atrial flutter and preserved ventricular function	• 2.5 - 5 mg intravenously given over 2 min • In the absence of a therapeutic response or drug-induced adverse event, give repeated doses of 5 - 10 mg every 15 - 30 min to a maximum of 20 mg.
	Verapamil is a calcium channel blocking drug that slows conduction and increases refractoriness in the AV node. These actions may terminate re-entrant arrhythmias and control the ventricular response rate in patients with atrial tachycardias (including AF and atrial flutter). Intravenous verapamil should be given only to patients with narrow-complex paroxysmal SVT or arrhythmias known with certainty to be of supraventricular origin. Giving calcium channel blockers to a patient with ventricular tachycardia may cause cardiovascular collapse. Verapamil may decrease myocardial contractility and critically reduce cardiac output in patients with severe LV dysfunction.	

Drug	Indication	Dose
Digoxin	• Atrial fibrillation with fast ventricular response	• 500 mcg IV over 30 min
	Digoxin is a cardiac glycoside that slows ventricular rate by increasing vagal tone, decreasing sympathetic activity by suppression of baroreceptors, and prolonging AV node refractory period.	
Positive inotropic drugs	• Hypotension in the absence of hypovolaemia • Cardiogenic shock	*Dobutamine* 5 - 20 mcg kg^{-1} min^{-1} *Dopamine* 1 - 10 mcg kg^{-1} min^{-1} *Noradrenaline* 0.05 - 1 mcg kg^{-1} min^{-1}
	Dobutamine is often the positive inotropic drug of choice in the post-resuscitation period. Its beta agonist activity also causes vasodilation and an increase in heart rate. It is indicated when poor cardiac output and hypotension cause significantly reduced tissue perfusion. It is useful particularly when pulmonary oedema is present and hypotension prevents the use of other vasodilators. Dopamine is the precursor of the naturally occurring catecholamines adrenaline and noradrenaline. It has a dose dependent positive inotropic effect. Noradrenaline is a potent vasoconstrictor but also has a positive inotropic effect. It is indicated in the post resuscitation period when hypotension and poor cardiac output cause reduced tissue perfusion.	
Magnesium	• Polymorphic ventricular tachycardia (torsade de pointes) • Digoxin toxicity	• Dose: 2 g given peripherally (IV) over 10 min • May be repeated once if necessary
	Magnesium facilitates neurochemical transmission: it decreases acetylcholine release and reduces the sensitivity of the motor endplate.	
Nitrates	• Prophylaxis or relief of angina • Unstable angina pectoris • Myocardial infarction • Acute and chronic left ventricular failure	• GTN: Sublingual 300 - 600 mcg (spray or tablet); isosorbide mononitrate or dinitrate 30 - 120 mg oral per day (various preparations and dosing frequencies); transdermal 5 - 15 mg daily • GTN: Sublingual 300 - 600 mcg (spray or tablet); buccal tablets 2 - 5 mg; IV 10 - 200 mcg min^{-1}; isosorbide mononitrate or dinitrate 30 - 120 mg oral per day (various preparations and dosing frequencies) • GTN: Sublingual 300 - 600 mcg (spray or tablet); buccal 2 - 5 mg; IV 10 - 200 mcg min^{-1} • GTN: 10 - 200 mcg min^{-1} IV; isosorbide mononitrate or dinitrate 30 - 120 mg oral per day (various preparations and dosing frequencies); transdermal 5 - 15 mg daily
	After conversion to nitric oxide, nitrates cause vascular smooth muscle relaxation. The resultant dilation is more marked on the venous than the arterial side of the circulation, and it is this venodilatation, reducing left ventricular diastolic pressure, that is mainly responsible for relieving angina. Nitrates also dilate the coronary arteries and relieve spasm in coronary smooth muscle. Nitrates are contraindicated in hypotensive patients (systolic blood pressure < 90 mmHg)	

ALS

Appendix C Useful Websites

www.resus.org.uk	**Resuscitation Council UK**
www.erc.edu	**European Resuscitation Council**
www.ilcor.org	**International Liaison Committee on Resuscitation**
www.americanheart.org	**American Heart Association**
www.ics.ac.uk	**Intensive Care Society**
www.aagbi.org	**Association of Anaesthetists of Great Britain and Ireland**
www.bestbets.org	**Best evidence topics in emergency medicine**
www.bcs.com	**British Cardiac Society**
www.escardio.org	**European Society of Cardiology**
www.feel-uk.com	**Focused Echocardiography in Emergency Life Support**

NOTES

ALS

NOTES

NOTES

NOTES

NOTES

NOTES